LEON WEISBERG, M.D.

Department of Psychiatry and Neurology,
Tulane University School of Medicine,
New Orleans, Louisiana

CHARLES NICE, M.D.

Department of Radiology,
Tulane University School of Medicine,
New Orleans, Louisiana

MYRON KATZ, Ph.D.

University of New Orleans, Lakefront,
New Orleans, Louisiana

Cerebral Computed Tomography

A Text-Atlas

SECOND EDITION / W. B. SAUNDERS COMPANY / Philadelphia
London
Toronto
Mexico City
Rio de Janeiro
Sydney
Tokyo

1984

W. B. Saunders Company: West Washington Square
                           Philadelphia, PA   19105

                           1 St. Anne's Road
                           Eastbourne, East Sussex BN21 3UN, England

                           1 Goldthorne Avenue
                           Toronto, Ontario M8Z 5T9, Canada

                           Apartado 26370—Cedro 512
                           Mexico 4, D.F., Mexico

                           Rua Coronel Cabrita, 8
                           Sao Cristovao Caixa Postal 21176
                           Rio de Janeiro, Brazil

                           9 Waltham Street
                           Artarmon, N.S.W. 2064, Australia

                           Ichibancho, Central Bldg., 22-1 Ichibancho
                           Chiyoda-Ku, Tokyo 102, Japan

Library of Congress Cataloging in Publication Data

Weisberg, Leon A., 1941–
  Cerebral computed tomography, a text-atlas.

  Includes bibliographical references and index.
  1. Brain—Diseases—Diagnosis. 2. Brain—
Radiography. 3. Tomography. I. Nice, Charles M.
(Charles Monroe) II. Katz, Myron, 1948–
III. Title. [DNLM: 1. Brain—Radiography.
2. Tomography, X-Ray computed. WL 141 W426c]
RC386.6.T64W44   1984   616.8'097572   83–
7825
ISBN 0–7216–1077–3

Cerebral Computed Tomography   ISBN   0-7216-1077-3

Last digit is the print number: 9   8   7   6   5   4   3   2   1

*To my wife Laurie
and
our children—Stuart, Alec, Michael, and Melissa—
whose support and inspiration
made this book a worthwhile endeavor*

Preface

The introduction of computed tomography (CT) for the investigation of intracranial and orbital pathological conditions has revolutionized clinical management of patients with neurological disorders. Since the initial description of CT by Hounsfield and early clinical studies reported by Paxton and Ambrose, CT has been proven to be an extremely sensitive, accurate, and safe diagnostic procedure. Acceptance of CT by the medical community has occurred very rapidly. Within one decade there have been rapid technical advances, e.g., rapid scan time, finer matrix systems, thin tissue sections, and improved spatial and contrast resolution, multiplanar (coronal, sagittal) projections. These improvements have required continual upgrading of existing scanners to provide higher quality images; however, this has substantially increased cost. Because of the high cost of this rapidly expanding CT technology, it is necessary to understand its role in neurodiagnosis.

Initial clinical CT studies consisted of retrospective analyses in patients who had their diagnosis confirmed by other neurodiagnostic studies and by surgical or necropsy findings. These studies emphasized radiological and pathological correlation. They confirmed that image reconstruction computed tomography was a significant advance in neurodiagnosis. However, no attempt was made to study prospectively the value of CT in the evaluation of patients with specific neurological symptomatology or to establish the role of CT relative to other diagnostic studies. Many early studies provided conflicting clinical correlations with CT findings. This was the result of basing conclusions on limited numbers of patients as well as of the effects of sampling bias.

This text has been developed as an introduction to the utilization of CT in evaluating patients with intracranial and orbital disorders. It is oriented toward the neurologist, neurosurgeon, internist, pediatrician, radiologist, and other physicians who will be ordering this study in the course of their investigation of patients with neurological symptoms. It is the purpose of this book to familiarize the physician with a logical and systematic approach to the proper utilization of CT. This must be based upon knowledge of its sensitivity and accuracy as well as its limitations. It is important for the physician to be cognizant of the general principles of image reconstruction technology to be able to utilize CT in the most efficacious manner. The organization of this book emphasizes the role of CT in specific clinical problems as these initially present to the practicing physician. The role of CT is compared with that of other traditional diagnostic studies. With the information contained in this text, it is hoped that CT will be utilized in the most cost-effective manner, and that this will lead to improved patient care and cost containment.

LEON WEISBERG

CHARLES NICE

MYRON KATZ

Acknowledgments

There have been many changes in the technology and clinical practice of cranial and orbital computed tomography which have occurred since the first edition of this textbook. Therefore we believe that this revision will be helpful in providing the reader with the current state of the art of CT. Almost all the clinical cases and illustrations are different from those utilized in the first edition. The majority of the scans included in this edition were performed at the Tulane Medical Center; we utilized an updated EMI Mark 1 head scanner or a high resolution Picker Synerview body scanner. Some scans were also performed at the Charity Hospital of New Orleans utilizing a General Electric CT/T 8800 high resolution body scanner; others were generously referred to us by colleagues at other medical centers in the New Orleans region. Drs. Thomas Naidich, Earl Hutchins, and Jack Greenberg lent us several scans. The high quality of the scans in this book is due to the diligence and skill of our radiology technicians. We owe special thanks to Mary Villemartette, Lela Harris, Neil Lockett, and Monnie Mullens at the Tulane Medical Center and Lucien Fortier, Michael Hauck, and Alvin Collins at the Charity Hospital. Allen Davillier of the General Electric Company and John Barni of Picker International spent much time answering our multiple questions concerning technical aspects of CT. Many house officers in neurology, neurosurgery, and radiology at Tulane and Louisiana State Medical Centers provided help in collating clinical data. Several chapters were carefully reviewed by Dr. James Kenning and David Dunn and their incisive critiques strengthened the quality of the clinical information. Special thanks are given to all my colleagues in the Department of Neurology and Psychiatry for sharing their clinical experiences. We are grateful to Dr. Robert Ledley of the Computerized Radiology Society for permitting reprint of scans previously published by us in that journal and also to my colleagues in the American Society of Neuroimaging for their intellectual inspiration. My wife Laurie provided invaluable secretarial, editorial, and organizational assistance which permitted rapid and efficient completion of this revision. And lastly my thanks to Mr. Carroll Cann and Ms. Edna Dick of W. B. Saunders who were most helpful and supportive in seeing the revision to completion.

LEON A. WEISBERG

Contents

Part
I

*Overview of
General Principles,
Performance,
and
Normal Anatomy
of
Computed Tomography*

Chapter 1

INTRODUCTION

The impact of computed tomography (CT) upon evaluation of patients with neurological disorders is best appreciated by comparing sensitivity and accuracy of CT with other neurodiagnostic procedures. Within a short time interval, CT has obviated utilization of several procedures, e.g., echoencephalography, radionuclide scan and air study. CT has expanded our knowledge of evolution and resolution of certain neuropathological diseases. The relative safety and low radiation dosage has allowed observation of serial changes in certain normal neurological conditions such as aging and development. We have obtained much morphological information of gross brain changes; however, biochemical and physiological correlations are not clearly established. These correlations only can be inferred from CT findings. More precise delineation of these biochemical and physiological changes will probably require newer complementary imaging techniques such as positron emission tomography and nuclear magnetic resonance. In one early study performed at Massachusetts General Hospital, CT altered use of traditional diagnostic studies and modified treatment in 19 percent of patients.[1]

The clinical material presented in this book has been derived from diverse sources. These include (1) Charity Hospital of New Orleans, a large public (municipal and county) hospital, (2) Veterans Administration Hospital of New Orleans, and (3) Tulane Medical Center, a private university-based medical teaching facility. These facilities have active neurological and neurosurgical services. The data are based on an analysis of more than 25,000 patients who had head or orbit CT scans. The indications for referral to have a CT study are listed in Table 1–1. Of those scanned, two thirds were in-hospital patients and one third were outpatients. Thirty-eight percent of patients were ambulatory, 29 percent were in wheelchairs, and 33 percent were on stretchers. Of the initial 2750 patients, 20 percent had a postcontrast scan, whereas 53 percent of the 2750 patients tested subsequently had an enhanced scan. This compares with a range of 50 to 70 percent of contrast scans reported from other centers. During the last three years, two thirds of our patients had a postcontrast scan; in approximately 30 percent an enhanced scan was done without an initial noncontrast scan.

The increased use of contrast studies in CT results from two factors: (1) certain lesions are isodense on plain scan and seen only on postcontrast scan and (2) additional diagnostic information is sometimes obtained on a postcontrast scan, which causes certain lesions such as cerebral infarction, angiomata, metastases and abscesses (Table 1–2) to enhance. The intravenous administration was performed by rapid bolus injection or drip infusion.

An unexpected consequence of the high-dose intravenous infusion study was increased frequency of prominent enhancement patterns in certain conditions such as cerebral infarcts or hematomas. This initially resulted in a 20 percent increase in the number of angiograms performed during the first 36 months. Angiography was believed necessary to differentiate enhancing cerebral infarct or hematoma from other conditions such as neoplasm, angioma and abscess. This trend toward increased use of angiography has slowed as a result of gains in clinical experience with CT as our knowledge of temporal and spatial characteristics of enhancement patterns has expanded. Subsequently, there has been a marked decrease in the number of angiograms performed.

Following introduction of CT, the number of neurological and neurosurgical patients with

3

TABLE 1–1. Reason for CT Scan Referral in 20,000 Patients

Referral	Initial 2750 (percent)	Subsequent 2750 (percent)	Last 10,000 (percent)
Specific disorders	76	65	62
cerebrovascular disease	15	12	12
seizures	10	8	9
dementia	8	7	7
head trauma	7	9	9
suspected primary tumor	12	11	9
supratentorial	10.5	10	7
infratentorial	1.5	1	2
suspected metastases	6	5	5
visual or endocrine disorder and sella abnormality	1	1	1
disturbed consciousness	2	1	1
evaluation of previously documented lesion	2	1	1
post surgery or irradiation	6	4	2
orbital lesion	2	2	2
increased intracranial pressure			
pediatric	1	1	1
increasing head size	1	1	1
poor neurological development	1	1	1
hearing loss	1	1	1
Nonspecific disorders	24	35	38
headache	10	16	19
dizziness	8	10	10
syncope	2	4	4
vague psychiatric symptoms	1	2	2
weakness	3	3	3

intracranial disease admitted to Charity Hospital increased by 25 percent over the immediately preceding years. Because of certain carefully monitored economic restraints imposed upon physicians of Charity Hospital and Veterans Administration Hospital, all CT scan requests were initially triaged. These requests were reviewed and then approved by the attending physician who had formal training in neurodiagnostic techniques. The direct consequence of this policy was that not all patients with neurological symptoms or abnormal neurodiagnostic studies (EEG or skull radiogram) who had requests for CT were scanned. This policy was necessary because of limited scanning facilities; it was hoped that this would allow the most efficacious use of CT. When this system was utilized, more than 58 percent of CT scans were abnormal. This represented an incidence of positive results higher than those for other neurodiagnostic studies during this time period.

TABLE 1–2. Enhancement in Differential Diagnosis

	Frequency of Enhancement		
Pathological Condition	50 CC BOLUS (PERCENT)	100 CC BOLUS (PERCENT)	300 CC DRIP INFUSION (PERCENT)
cerebral infarction			
nonhemorrhagic	5	10	60
hemorrhagic	0	0	40
intracerebral hematoma	0	0	15
extradural hematoma	0	0	15
neoplasm			
meningioma	90	90	100
glioma	85	85	95
pituitary adenoma	100	100	100
craniopharyngioma	60	50	50
acoustic neurinoma	100	100	100
pinealoma	100	100	100
aneurysm	0	0	40
angioma	10	10	100
abscess	33	50	100

While this policy may be effective in defining a high percentage of abnormal studies, it is possible that this policy is restrictive and arbitrary. The system may deny CT to patients who actually require it.[2] As this triage system became more flexible, 44 percent of CT studies were shown to be abnormal. This decrease in abnormal studies may reflect two possible trends. Firstly, the most tenable conclusion is that less discrimination was employed in patient selection for CT. An alternative explanation is that CT was utilized as a screening procedure to eliminate the need for more invasive diagnostic studies or subsequent hospitalization. The lower incidence of abnormal studies is also believed to reflect an increase in the number of scanning facilities available with a decrease in the waiting time period. In addition, during this time period, physicians with no formal training in neurological disease began to order CT.

In the initial five-year scanning experience at these three medical centers, 90 percent of studies were referred by neurologists or neurosurgeons; 58 percent of these studies were abnormal. With increasing access to scanning facilities, the frequency of referrals from physicians who have had no formal training in neurological diagnosis has increased to 33 percent; only 39 percent of these CT studies were abnormal. By altering the triage system to allow all physicians to order CT without an initial neurological consultation, it did not seem that we had established a system that was cost-effective. CT was utilized by non-neurologically oriented physicians as an expensive triage procedure to replace a complete clinical neurological history and examination. This is reflected by an increase in the number of patients referred for CT because of vague and nonspecific neurological symptoms (see Table 1-1). At one of our referral hospitals, 34 percent of head scans are currently being performed without initial neurological consultation. Only 11 percent of these patients who had no initial neurological assessment showed an abnormal CT finding to adequately explain the neurological symptomatology that formed the basis for the referral; however, 38 percent of these were reported as having abnormal scan findings. These were diffuse abnormalities, e.g., cerebral infarction, unilateral calcification, subdural hematoma and cysts. In 10 percent of these cases, abnormal CT findings led to subsequent neurological consultation; however, in no case was clinical management or outcome altered by the initial CT abnormal findings. These results indicate that patients should have initial neurological consultation prior to CT. In addition, the finding of a significant number of CT abnormalities in which only a limited number were related to the initial neurological symptoms suggests that cost-efficient utilization value of CT should not be assessed simply by number of abnormal scans. It is important to determine the number of cases in which CT findings explained neurological symptoms and influenced management. We compared one hundred consecutive patients evaluated in the emergency department at Charity Hospital who were comatose. Because of severe impairment of consciousness, those patients had immediate CT scan. Those patients evaluated by a neurologist or neurosurgeon prior to CT showed lesions that were the probable etiological factor for coma in 86 percent, whereas those without prior neurological consultation showed causal lesions in only 36 percent, but abnormal CT patterns in 68 percent.

Following installation of a CT scanner at the Mayo Clinic, the number of neurological and neurosurgical patients increased by 15 to 20 percent. During this time, the number of electroencephalograms (EEG) also increased; however, utilization of isotope scan, echoencephalogram and air studies decreased markedly. Angiography remained at a constant level.[3] At the Mallinckrodt Institute[4] there was a marked reduction in air studies (66 percent), angiographies (34 percent) and isotope scans (24 percent). At the Dent Neurological Institute, the clinical work load represented by patient volume increased by 30 percent. The need for air studies and isotope scans was almost completely eliminated; angiography was decreased by 20 percent.[5]

Many concepts of neurological disease have been changed because of CT findings. Prior to CT, incidence of Grade I and II tumors in representative series of astrocytomas was only 5 to 7 percent; with CT these low-grade gliomas comprise 30 percent of all histologically proven cases. Despite earlier diagnosis, there has been no evidence of improved prognosis.[3] In the pre-CT era, incidental meningiomas—not associated with neurological symptomatology—were detected only by necropsy examination. In our experience, we have identified eight such meningiomas in neurologically asymptomatic patients and in patients in whom other diagnostic studies were negative.[6] Our experience has shown a marked increase in the early diagnosis of posterior fossa lesions. Diagnosis has been made before development of clinical findings of increased intracranial pressure. Clinically occult intracranial metastases from bronchogenic carcinoma are detected more frequently with CT than with isotope scans. No clinically symptomatic intracerebral hematoma has been missed by CT. Cerebellar hemorrhages are easily detected; this rapid diagnosis has led to an improved clinical outcome. In patients with suspected intracranial inflammatory disease, CT diagnosis has dramatically affected management and decreased mortality.

Wortzman and Holgate analyzed cost effectiveness of neurological evaluation utilizing CT scans. This was assessed specifically in regard to need for invasive contrast procedures and hospitalization. They evaluated the importance of CT in 203 patients in influencing the decision for angiography or air studies. In these patients angiography was not necessary in 61 and air study was avoided in 89; in 11 instances these studies were necessary. Of 241 patients, CT findings obviated hospitalization in 140, prompted admission in 28 and was not a crucial factor in 73 cases.[7] The most effective utilization of CT occurs in medical centers that have active neurological and neurosurgical services capable of implementing further diagnostic studies and therapy on the basis of CT findings. It seems reasonable that all such medical centers should have immediate access to a CT scanner.

REFERENCES

1. Fineberg HV, Bauman R, Sosman M: Computerized cranial tomography. Effect on diagnostic and therapeutic plans. JAMA 238:224–227, 1977
2. Brust JCM, Dickenson PCT, Healton EB: Failure of CT sharing in a large municipal hospital. N Engl J Med 304:1388, 1981
3. Baker HL: CT and neuroradiology: a fortunate primary union. Am J Roentgenol 127:101, 1976
4. Evens RG, Jost G: Economic analysis of computed tomography units. Am J Roentgenol 127:191, 1976
5. Oldendorf WH: The quest for an image of brain. Neurology 28:517–533, 1978
6. Weisberg LA: Incidental focal intracranial computed tomographic findings. J Neurol Neurosurg Psychiat 45:900, 1982
7. Wortzman G, Holgate RC, Morgan PP: Cranial computed tomography: an evaluation of cost effectiveness. Radiology 117:75, 1975

Chapter 2

PRINCIPLES AND TECHNIQUES OF IMAGE RECONSTRUCTION WITH CT

Myron Katz, Ph.D.

Neuroradiographic diagnostic procedures attempt to demonstrate normal and abnormal intracranial structures with the highest image quality while utilizing noninvasive modalities with low radiation dose. Image quality is measured by spatial and contrast resolution. These refer to the ability of the imaging system to discriminate objects of limiting size or proximity and differing density.

Skull Radiography

Conventional shadow radiography provides excellent spatial resolution perpendicular to the path of the x-ray beam (0.3 mm); however, its limited contrast demands that objects must differ in attenuation values by more than 2 per cent to be detected. Poor contrast is caused by these characteristics inherent in shadow radiography: (1) extensive x-ray scattering, (2) limited response of photographic film and (3) the additive nature of recorded attenuation. The major shortcomings of conventional radiography include limited contrast and superimposition of tissue. It is not always possible to localize a particular structure even if it is sufficiently different in density to be visually discriminated.

Conventional Tomography

To improve spatial resolution and overcome the problem of structure superimposition, conventional tomography was developed. This technique eliminates (by blurring out) unwanted information not in the plane of inter-

est, while tissue attenuation properties in the plane of interest remain in focus, free from any shadows or interference from overlying contiguous regions. In conventional (or geometric) tomography, an x-ray tube and a photographic plate are moved simultaneously in opposite directions within parallel planes. If the x-ray source is moved at the same speed as the film, a planar section of the patient half the distance from the film to the x-ray source will have a projection that moves with the photographic plate. The planar section remains "in focus" on the tomogram while the remainder of the intervening tissues are blurred out of focus. The region remaining in focus has a particular section thickness that diminishes as the magnitude of angular displacement (tomographic angle) increases. Consequently, contrast diminishes with increasing spatial resolution because of the blurring. It also causes spurious or phantom images. Because not all unwanted planes are adequately blurred out when a linear path is used, other planar paths (circular, elliptical, spiral or hypocycloidal) have been utilized. Despite these modifications, contrast has remained poor in geometric tomography, but because of good spatial resolution, this technique remains useful in assessing areas that are of high inherent contrast, such as sella turcica and petrous bone.[1, 2]

Contrast-Enhanced Neuroradiography

To improve contrast, it has been necessary to inject foreign materials (air into CSF spaces and iodinated contrast material into cerebral blood vessels) to create sufficiently large differences in x-ray attenuation values to permit imaging of ventricles, subarachnoid spaces and blood vessels. These techniques are invasive and traumatic—consequently, potentially dangerous. Air studies and angiography sometimes provide only indirect signs of intracranial lesions. For example, mass lesions are localized by the finding of displacements of ventricles or blood vessels. Despite these shortcomings, air studies and angiography remained our most sophisticated neurodiagnostic studies prior to introduction of CT.

Computed Tomography

Computed tomography represents an imaging technique in which a computer reconstructs the internal structure of a brain section (slice) on the basis of sets of x-ray measurements taken at a multitude of angles. The mathematical basis for reconstruction of the structure of an object from the infinite set of all of its projections was established in 1917 by Radon,[3] an Austrian mathematician. It was not realized until Smith et al.[4] in the early 1970's that despite Radon's theorem, reconstruction from projections depended, in a general sense, on an inherently discontinuous process. Perhaps because this was not known, a variety of scientists using approximative techniques developed reconstruction algorithms. In 1956, Bracewell, in an application to radioastronomy, led the way.[5] Oldendorf developed an apparatus that represents the first medical application of image reconstruction.[6] As a practicing neurologist with a biomedical engineering background he recognized the potential for this technique in the study of biological systems; however, he lacked the mathematical basis and computer technology to develop his idea into a practical clinical imaging system. At approximately the same time a physicist, A. M. Cormack, developed an extensive theory of image reconstruction from x-ray projections.[7] Soon after this De Rosier and Klug began work on an application to electron microscopy.[8] An alternative method to improve radiographic contrast was experimented with by D. E. Kuhl.[9] He used a computer to process data collected by a gamma detector at various axial (radial) angles after intravenous injection of radionuclides. The image produced was a reconstruction that represented a cross-sectional planar section containing the paths of detected gamma rays. Despite the fact that only passable contrast was obtained with this technique, it presented the breakthrough that all of the following approaches share: since no overlying structures were sampled by radiation, these structures could not blur the image. It remained for G. N. Hounsfield, an engineer and computer expert working for the Central Research Laboratories of EMI, Ltd., to develop the first practical model of a computerized reconstructive transmission tomographic scanner.[10] This era of experimentation could have ended a few years after the first scanners were in widespread use because at that time mathematical proof for a practicable design was published.[11] Despite this, there is little evidence that present CT devices conform to existing mathematically sound designs. In fact, as demonstrated in the section on image quality, there is evidence to the contrary.

Computed tomography is a diagnostic imaging system that utilizes a thinly collimated x-ray beam, detector system, computer and display system. For CT of the brain, multiple attenuation measurements are obtained at various angles through a planar brain section. These measurements are then stored and processed by the computer. Utilizing a suitable algorithm, the computer reconstructs an approximation to the structure of the brain section in the specific plane (axial, coronal, sagittal) as an array of numerical values that are to be compared to brain-tissue linear x-ray attenuation values. CT depends upon the mathematical effects of the computer algorithm to decompose the additive attenuation effects on each datum. Only the plane of interest affects the x-ray beam detected—far better than the radiographic techniques in conventional tomography. By virtually eliminating the influence of scattered radiation on the attenuation data (scattering also degrades contrast in conventional tomography), CT markedly improves contrast: tissue constituents of only slightly differing composition may be distinguished.

The CT system consists of two kinds of components: *hardware,* including x-ray tube, fixed and variable aluminum and copper filters, lead collimators, gantry or frame, detector system, computer, data storage system, and display system, and *software,* including various data preprocessing tools, reconstruction algorithms with interchangeable filters, and viewing aids such as multiformat display, capability for making attenuation measurements and histogram analyses, cursors for region of interest studies, and image reversal capability. CT scanning involves several basic processes, including x-ray generation and beam collimation, photon-tissue interaction, photon detection, scanner geometry, computer reconstruction and image quality.[12-15]

X-RAY GENERATION AND BEAM COLLIMATION

X-ray Source

Formerly, conventional x-ray tubes were used to generate photons for CT. The x-ray tube consisted of a fixed stationary anode with a large focal spot. This was energized to 120 kVp (penetrating power of the x-ray beam) and utilized a tube current of 30 mA (number of photons per second). Disadvantages of these tubes included high noise level accompanied by an insufficient photon sampling for each scan section and significant radiation exposure caused by the large focal spot, with attendant extensive collimation. Some newer scanners utilize a rotating anode. These may run continuously or may be pulsed to deliver bursts of photons; they operate at tube currents around 600 mA. Radiation exposure has decreased because their smaller focal spot requires less collimation—thus reducing x-ray scatter. With a pulsed beam that moves continuously around the patient, photons are delivered very rapidly; this makes subsecond scans possible. Problems associated with the pulsed beam include the need for heavy-duty x-ray tubes and more efficient tube cooling systems. This modification is important for body rather than head scans.

Filtration

The sensitivity of softer (lower energy) x-rays causes significant problems. Because they are more easily absorbed by human tissue, they greatly increase patient dose, particularly on the side closest to the x-ray source. This nonisotropic effect undermines the central assumption upon which data collection is interpreted and consequently the effectiveness of the computer's reconstruction algorithm. (See discussion on the spectral-shift artifact.) Therefore, when they are abundant, most need to be removed. An aluminum filter is utilized to absorb lower energy (softer) x-rays before collimation. In this way, the filter hardens the x-ray beam, that is, produces a beam with fewer, less penetrating photons. Bow tie–shaped filters, that is, filters that cause the effective path length of all x-ray beams to equalize, are employed to facilitate data collection and interpretation. (See discussion on detector system and on high contrast–related artifacts.)

Collimation

Once generated and filtered, the x-ray beam must be collimated into a thin pencil or fan-beam geometrical pattern. Lead materials define a rectangular aperture that controls the shape of the beam. These collimators may be placed at the x-ray tube and again in front of the detectors. The former determine section thickness by reducing radiation divergence, while the latter help isolate adjacent detectors to improve the statistical independence of their data. (See the last paragraph of the next section.) In early scanners, section thickness was 13 mm; however, newer scanners usually have a 10 mm section thickness for routine head scans. Other collimators, which may be as narrow as 2 mm, are available for petrous orbit and sella regions.

PHOTON-TISSUE INTERACTION

When a monochromatic x-ray beam of intensity I passes through an object, the attenuation, ΔI, causes fewer x-rays to pass through to the detector. The linear x-ray attenuation coefficient, μ, expresses the instantaneous ratio $\frac{\Delta I/I}{\Delta x}$ at any point along the path of the beam. For a homogeneous object, μ is constant and the penetrating intensity, I, can be related to the incident intensity, I_o, by $I = I_o e^{-\mu x}$ where x expresses the thickness of the transmitting object and e = 2.718. The result is that the intensity of the transmitted beam decreases exponentially as the thickness of the attenuator increases.

Attenuation is defined as the reduction in intensity of the x-ray beam as it passes through an object. Two processes significantly diminish the number of x-ray photons that penetrate the objects in computer tomography. More important at lower x-ray energies is the photoelectric effect. On the other hand, Compton scattering of x-rays by water is more than nine times as likely as the photoelectric effect if the energy of the incident photon exceeds 57 keV.

True absorption of x-rays is called the *photoelectric effect*. An impinging *photon* can be absorbed via excitation (increase in energy) of an electron of an atom—thereby causing that electron to jump to a higher energy level or even escape from the atom. The photoelectric effect is more probable with inner shell electrons since they can more easily accept incident energy at x-ray frequencies. The "potential well" is deeper (energy required for escape is greater) with larger atomic number (Z). The probability of photoelectric absorption per gram, that is, per unit mass, varies as Z^3. For example, since oxygen has Z = 8 and calcium has Z = 20, an electron of calcium is almost 16 times as likely to photoelectrically absorb an impinging photon as is an electron of oxygen.

Like the photoelectric effect, Compton scattering can occur as an interaction between photon and electron. This process is most probable when the photon interacts with outer loosely bound atomic electrons. Similarly, a transfer of energy occurs, but the over-riding concern is the change in direction of the altered photon. It is a question of density, or more precisely the number of electrons per cubic centimeter, that most accurately predicts the probability of Compton scattering. This may partially explain the significantly lower x-ray attenuation of fat than protein.

Attenuation of the x-ray beam is generally proportional to the number of electrons encountered, since electrons are responsible for both effects. However, the atomic number of atoms in tissue greatly affects the probability of photoelectric absorption. A scale of attenuation has been named after the inventor of CT, G. N. Hounsfield. One Hounsfield unit represents a 0.1 percent change in attenuation relative to water.

Another aspect of the passage of the x-ray beam through living tissue results in a change in the nature of the spectrum of the incident beam, since the x-ray source is not monochromatic. Lower energy photons are more likely to be absorbed, as photoelectric absorption varies inversely as the cube of the energy of the incident photons. This results in a change in the spectrum of the penetrating x-ray beam toward higher energies. Such high-energy photons are characteristically more penetrating, or harder. This beam-hardening alters the

probability of an average x-ray photon from the beam to undergo Compton scattering or photoelectric absorption and favors the former effect.[16]

The attenuation coefficient expresses the amount of scattering plus absorption per unit length of a particular kind of living tissue and a particular spectrum (i.e., distribution of wavelengths) of x-rays. It is generally assumed that the attenuation coefficient observed for any part of the body will be the same for each projection, but beam-hardening invalidates this assumption mildly. To minimize this error, 4 to 5 mm of aluminum is used to (filter) preharden the beam.

Another important aspect of attenuation results from the distribution of scattering angles accompanying the Compton effect. In an x-ray beam with an average energy of 73 keV (generated by an accelerating potential of 120 keV), more than half of the scattered photons are deflected through an angle of less than 45°. As the energy of the photon increases, the average deflection angle decreases. This means that the geometry of data collection and beam-hardening plays a major role in contrast and noise in the data. Some authors report that in conventional radiology over 90 percent of photons incident on the film are forwardly scattered (i.e., through an angle less than 90°).

DETECTOR SYSTEM

Detectors record the number of photons deposited by the x-ray beam after traversing the patient. There are two types of detectors: scintillation crystals (composed of sodium iodide, calcium fluoride, cesium iodide, or bismuth germinate) and high pressure xenon gas detectors.

Scintillation detectors produce a signal by allowing x-rays to excite electrons in the crystal. When an electron returns to an empty orbital of the lattice, flashes of light (scintillations) are produced. This signal is amplified via an optically coupled photomultiplier tube that produces an electronic impulse. Since the time required for the crystal to reach its unexcited state can be comparable to the time between consecutive data collections, this "afterglow" effect can produce distortions near transitions between bone and air. Scintillation detectors provide high amplification of input x-ray intensity and are very efficient. They are bulky and expensive, however. Because of afterglow, sodium iodide detectors can be used only in scanners that filter out high-speed intensity changes with devices such as the water bag (used in the original EMI head scanner) or the bow tie filter (commonly employed in modern scanners); this is why the other crystal compounds are used in newer scanners. Some new scanners have replaced the photomultiplier with solid-state electronics.

High-pressure xenon gas detectors act like Geiger counters. When a photon knocks out an orbital electron of xenon, the resulting ions carry an electrical current between wires that are kept at a constant potential. This current provides a weak electrical signal for data collection. The multiwire gas chambers are utilized when the design calls for a large number of detectors that must be packed closely together. They have no afterglow but are less effective at photon detection than the scintillation type.

An important advantage of these photon–electronic detector systems compared with photographic film is that the spectrum of response available more than matches variations in transmission intensities of the x-ray beam. It was necessary, however, to regularly recalibrate the detector system to ensure the accuracy of their response. When detectors malfunction, inaccuracies will result. Techniques for detector calibration differ for each individual scanner model. As expected, improvements in detector systems resulted in improved image quality and some of these were solid-state in design. The stability of detector systems has markedly improved in the last five years.

SCANNER GEOMETRY

The Meaning of a Projection

Imagine that an object is composed of various thicknesses of materials, each with its characteristic attenuation coefficient: μ_1, μ_2, μ_3, ... μ_n and particular thicknesses: x_1, x_2, x_3, ... x_n. The observed transmitted intensity I of the incident beam with intensity I_o would be given by:

$$I = I_o e^{-\mu_1 x_1} e^{-\mu_2 x_2} e^{-\mu_3 x_3} \ldots e^{-\mu_n x_n}$$
$$= I_o e^{-(\mu_1 x_1 + \mu_2 x_2 + \mu_3 x_3 + \ldots + \mu_n x_n)}$$

or equivalently

$$\ln (I_o/I) = \mu_1 x_1 + \mu_2 x_2 + \ldots + \mu_n x_n.$$

The idea of computed tomography is to treat the x_i's as known and try to determine the μ's. This is plausible if the problem is viewed as a linear system in which unknowns can be remotely sampled via a sufficient set of simultaneous equations. To get the required set of linear equations, an object can be assumed to have unknown but constant attenuation on uniform (usually square) subregions—each subregion having a known position and shape. Then the planar object can be represented by an array of attenuation coefficients:

$$\begin{matrix} \mu_{11} & \mu_{12} & \mu_{12} & \cdots & \mu_{1n} \\ \mu_{21} & \mu_{22} & \mu_{22} & \cdots & \mu_{2n} \\ \vdots & \vdots & \vdots & & \vdots \\ \mu_{n1} & \mu_{n2} & \mu_{n3} & & \mu_{nn} \end{matrix}$$

(Similarly, a three-dimensional object could be represented by a three-dimensional array of attenuation coefficients.) Simultaneous equations can be obtained by taking projections along the rows, giving n equations, along the columns, giving n more equations, upper left to lower right and upper right to lower left, giving 4 n − 2 more equations. Similarly, projections can be taken in other directions. Clearly, at least n^2 equations would be needed to determine the n^2 unknowns that specify a planar object—therefore the need for a large number of projections to get the required data. The decision to allow n^2 numbers to specify the distribution of the attenuation coefficients in an arbitrary object is part of choosing a reconstruction space. Having made this choice, the problem is to make measurements that will allow the determination of the best reconstruction of the x-ray attenuation distribution among the class of reconstructions that can be specified by such an array. (A three-dimensional object can be imaged by independently imaging each two-dimensional cross-section.) The engineer concerned with data collection will endeavor to provide, with a minimum of error, the required values of $\ln(I_o/I)$ for those equations.

Parallel and Fan Beam Systems

First-generation machines employed a parallel technique of data collection. This required both translational and rotational motions. Each projection was a series of data collections in which the beam passed through a single row of attenuation values. If we call the projection angle in the direction of the rows 0° then n data would be collected: I_1, I_2, I_3, . . . , I_n. These data would then be considered the projection data for the 0° direction. The ith datum, I_1, provides $\ln (I_o/I_i) = \mu_{i1}x_1 + \mu_{i2}x_2 + \ldots + \mu_{in}x_n$. Data are collected via the transmission of parallel beams. Motion of the x-ray source and detector was a translation perpendicular to the direction of the paths of the x-rays. After data for this direction had been collected, the gantry rotated to a new projection angle and collected another set of data, which became the projection data for this angle. After each pass the gantry was rotated one degree. Transmission data were collected at 180 different angles. Transmitted radiation was measured 160 times during each translational movement to provide 28,800 (160 × 180) readings. There was a single pencil beam and a single pair of sodium iodide crystal detectors. The head was surrounded by a water bag that provided a more uniformly hardened x-ray beam, but this restriction limited scanning to the axial plane. Scan time was four to five minutes per pair of scan sections. The mechanical characteristics of the translate-rotate movement limited scan speed. Each complete scan consisted of 4 pairs of scans; scan sequence required 20 minutes. Having collected the data, the reconstruction algorithm produced a two-dimensional image on an array of squares, or pixels. The size of the array of pixels was either 80 × 80 with each pixel being 3.0 × 3.0 mm or 160 × 160 with each pixel being 1.5 × 1.5 mm. As the number of pixels increases, potential image quality improves; the image quality of the 160 × 160 array was superior to that of the 80 × 80 system. Slice thickness was 13 mm. The x-ray tube was energized to 120 kVp with tube current of 30 mA. Slow scan time limited scanning to head and orbital regions since patient motion artifacts (stomach peristalsis and respiratory movements) frequently degraded image quality in other regions.

Second-generation CT employed multiple simultaneous pencils (fan-beam geometry) rather than a single pencil beam, and used an increased number of detectors. It retained translational and rotational motions of x-ray source and detector array. This form of data collection can be viewed as equivalent to parallel-beam geometry: the information that is collected by a particular detector collects only parallel beams of photons within a single translational pass. For example, if a linear array had five detectors, projection data that are collected would be virtually equivalent to information available in five repetitions of "translate then rotate" in first-generation scanners. This reduced scan speed because of the fan-beam geometry and multiple detector array. There were usually 10 to 30 scintillation crystal detectors. With reduction in scan time to approximately 20 to 30 seconds, degradation of image quality resulting from respiratory motion was overcome and body scanning became possible. Since the water bag was no longer necessary when afterglow was minimized, scanning in alternative planes (coronal, sagittal) became possible.

Third-generation scanners further reduced scanning time to approximately 1 to 10 seconds. This was accomplished utilizing a continuously rotating unit containing the x-ray source and detector array. This is true fan-beam geometry and data collection. The critical improvement was the complete removal of translational motions. To accomplish these higher scan speeds, wider fan beams and many more detectors were employed—necessitating faster photon delivery. Rotations to the full 360° were also employed. Xenon detectors were the rule, but some scanners used bismuth germinate crystals. The amount of data collected increased about 50-fold from early-generation scanners. This made possible apparently more accurate and higher spatial resolution reconstructions with resulting marked improvement in image quality. Impetus to find a better design included a problem with detector recalibration: with this system, each detector collects data for parts of the reconstruction outside of a specific circle; moreover, the smaller the circle the less redundant were other data collected. This meant that a faulty detector in the array (particularly if centrally located) would cause a circular artifact that could not be removed by ignoring the data from that detector or averaging data from nearby detectors. It was soon realized, however, that statistically predictable error averaging and the approximations upon which the reconstruction algorithm were based pointed to the expectation that even larger amounts of data would increase accuracy. The next design afforded this opportunity. The manufacturers of third-generation machines have now significantly improved the stability of the detector system so that the apparent need for the fourth-generation design has largely evaporated.

In fourth-generation scanners, the x-ray tube moves, but a full circle of detectors remain stationary. The x-ray tube rotates through an arc of 360 to 398° while it creates a wide fan beam. An extensive detector array (exceeding 600 in number) encircles the patient. Each detector views a rotating x-ray source like we would see the rising and setting sun. In this way data collections are spatially defined by the position of the x-ray source much more than the width of the detector—affording higher spatial resolution and the opportunity to collect much more data. Although much less critical to this design, recalibration of the detectors is facilitated and can be accomplished twice per rotation. However, with the improvement in detector stability, recalibration can be done weekly. Subsecond scans are possible with this design. Since many of the improvements on the fourth-generation scanners are more necessary for body than head or orbit scanning, these technical options will not be treated here since they depend upon the specific region being scanned. Besides the high cost of such an extensive detector array, this design has a greater difficulty with collimation of diverging radiation—causing a need for a greater patient radiation dose to get the same quality transmission data as a third-generation machine.

Resolution of the Data

Since data must be discrete to be measured, it is necessary to separate x-ray photons into compartments so that the intensity within each can be measured independently. In the fan-beam models this is accomplished spatially by use of an array of detectors. Separation of the compartments chronologically can be done by an internal clock within the computer or by pulsing the x-ray source as it is rotated. The physical positions of the x-ray source and detectors during photon collection determines the spatial resolution of the data. A glass and lead grid, called the *graticule*, provided the spatial and chronological separation of photons in the first-generation machines.

Although each system has a clearly defined spatial resolution of collected projection data, the utility of those data depends as well on contrast, statistical expected accuracy of measurements: If σ is the standard deviation of error in measurement of the intensity of the emerging x-ray beam when, for example, 150 photons originally entered the patient, then the expected standard deviation of the measurement when N times 150 photons enter the patient will be $\sigma/\sqrt{N}$. Therefore, if $N = 10^4$, then the standard deviation of error in the measurement will decrease by a factor of 10^2. This would suggest that if a finer graticule were used, say twice as fine, and everything else remained the same, then the spatial resolution of the data will improve by a factor of two but the contrast of the data will degrade by a factor of $\sqrt{2}$. The situation regarding the trade-off between the contrast and spatial resolution of the data of the fan-beam systems is important. Using the fixed ring of detectors, spatial resolution is easily refined (by increasing the number of measurements recorded per degree of rotation of the x-ray tube), but because of the effects of forward scattering, the standard deviation of error in the measurements is high and the statistical independence of these data is poor. Since time can be critical (in full body studies), higher photon fluxes (x-ray tube amperage) are required in order to compensate or improve the contrast.

Slice Thickness

When a three-dimensional object is considered to be a stacked array of two-dimensional planar arrays, rectangular parallelopipeds are usually specified as the uniformly shaped subvolumes. There are clear advantages to having the thickness of the slice or equivalently the height of each of these parallelopipeds as small as possible. This would provide good spatial resolution in the vertical direction and minimize the partial volume phenomenon (discussed later). Unfortunately, the available methods for collecting data for a thin region necessarily diminish the number of photons that reach the detectors: The x-ray beam is collimated before entering the patient so that only the particular slice is irradiated; in actual practice, a wedge-shaped region is sampled by the beam. Collimating the beam at the exit eliminates the counting of the only slightly scattered x-rays which, in turn, further decreases the number of photons reaching the detectors.

Another difficulty associated with the use of thinner slices is time. If thinner slices are used, more slices may have to be studied. To preserve accuracy, thinning the slice increases the amount of time needed to collect data for that slice. Therefore, thinning the slice dramatically increases the amount of time necessary for adequate examination.

COMPUTER RECONSTRUCTION

Reconstruction Algorithms

Although fundamentally different algorithmic processes have been explored, the basic idea behind the prominent methods for passing from radiological projection data to the reconstruction is described in the *back-projection*, or *summation*, *method*. This technique produces a reconstruction by overlaying a series of spread-out or back-projected images that can be obtained from the data in each projection: i.e., the value at each point in the reconstruction is the sum of the densities of each ray passing through that point. If the test object consists of a single disk in a homogeneous background and four projections are made, the reconstruction would be similar to an eight-pointed star (Fig. 2–1). The back-projection method is not accurate, since the original disk has been spread out in eight

directions. In the example of the disk reconstruction, the simple nature of the original object is reflected in the single star pattern created. However, if more general objects are imaged with this technique, spurious details may be hard to recognize. It is also obvious that the reconstruction does not have projection data that agree with the original data provided.[17, 18]

To improve the back-projection image, spurious details can be avoided by a process that removes star-shaped or point-spread effects; such an algorithm is named *Convolution*, or *filtered back-projection*. Alternatively, it is possible to concentrate on the production of a reconstruction whose projection data agree with the original data; the algebraic reconstruction technique (ART) is the best-known such algorithm. Both kinds of algorithms utilize the back-projection process, but only after they employ rules to alter the projection data. The key difference lies in the way data are

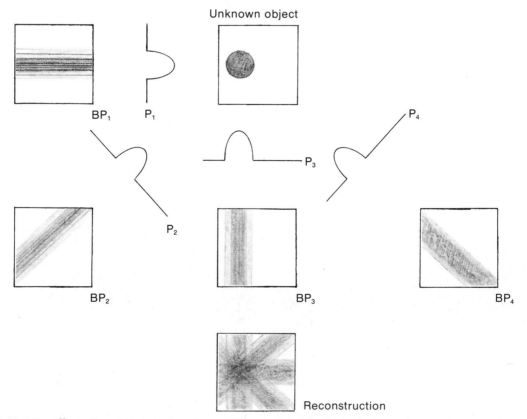

Figure 2–1. Illustration of the BACK-PROJECTION reconstruction algorithm. The unknown object is top central. Given information is the set of projection data: P_1, P_2, P_3, P_4. The back-projected images, BP_1, BP_2, BP_3, and BP_4, are the spread out values of the corresponding projections. The reconstruction is obtained by adding together or overlaying the back-projected images.

transformed. ART proceeds iteratively by altering data for each projection angle in a way that depends on the present guess for the reconstructed image. When these data are back-projected, the new image agrees with the original data at that projection direction. Convolution uses a single rule to change or filter each individual projection datum in a way that is both independent of its result on the reconstruction and all other projection data collected (or to be collected) from other directions.

The prototype EMI scanner programmed the computer to calculate the reconstruction using the ART algorithm because of the following: (1) When data are error-free, ART tends to pick the reconstruction (from the reconstruction space of 160 × 160 arrays of real numbers) that agrees with the projection data and is closest (in a least sum of the squared deviation sense) to the zero array, i.e., the 160 × 160 array of zeros. It is not in the nature of ART to introduce spurious images when perfect data are available. Nothing so clear-cut has been deduced about the Convolution algorithm; a reconstruction produced by Convolution may not even tend to agree with the provided projection data. (2) Compared to Convolution, ART is less affected by noisy data in its choice of reconstruction as long as the noise level in the data exceeds a modest figure. (3) ART's mathematical description is flexible enough to accept the introduction of additional information (called *constraints*); this flexibility has allowed creation of various other algorithms in the same family. (4) ART allows use of projection data that do not span a full semicircular arc; this was not realized for Convolution until late in the 1970's. (5) ART has a capability to depict more accurately large local fluctuations in attenuations without a concomitant amplification of the effects of noise in the data as compared with Convolution.

With demand for faster scanning, rise in confidence in data collection, increasing amounts of data collected and larger reconstruction arrays, EMI switched to Convolution; they may have considered the following reasons: (1) ART is a significantly more time-consuming algorithmic process than Convolution. Even in the first-generation scanners Convolution utilized only one third of the amount of computer time; this was not an issue when gantry motions required 4.5 minutes, but newer machines operated in one

third to one twentieth of these times. (2) Because of the iterative nature of ART—it proceeds by utilizing projection data at each angle in isolation and then continues to the next angle, continuing for a number of cycles—and the fact that real projection data will not match any feasible reconstruction (with probability 1.0), the current guess will tend to wander among virtually equivalent reconstructions after a few cycles of iterations. Convolution's two-step nature (first filter all of the data, then back-project) does not present this difficulty. (3) Since ART tends to wander, some criterion must be used to end its execution; this stopping criterion affects the accuracy of the reconstruction but has not been logically linked to that accuracy. Convolution requires no such arbitrary condition.

Other results further suggest implementation of Convolution. (1) Convolution has been shown to be equivalent to another technique called Fourier filtering under various ideal conditions; this near equivalence has lent more credence to the algorithm and provided insights into and guidelines for its implementation.[19] (2) Under conditions generally available in current practice, Convolution has been shown to be statistically reliable. In particular, with past limits on computer time, Convolution performed better than ART in the representation of small fluctuations of brain matter (when such matter is at least a small distance from the skull), when the projection data have low error content. (3) Currently, the filter function of Convolution can be varied at the beginning of each new scan sequence. This provides a flexibility to the user who knows how to take advantage of it. (See the last paragraph of this chapter.)

The current emphasis is on speed, since fan-beam geometries have greatly reduced scanning time. "Real time" computational speed refers to the amount of time required to complete the computation of a reconstruction on a computer when the speed of concurrent data acquisition is recognized as a limiting factor. It is difficult to surpass Convolution's time of execution because it is "real time constrained." Since the eventual effect of the projection data at any angle on the reconstruction is independent of the data collected at other angles, this effect can be calculated while the data are collected at the next projection angles. Some scanners utilize this fact in their display system. New algorithms will probably have to demonstrate improved reliability and scientific accuracy or require less data acquisition in order to replace Convolution; in particular, with computing power so cheap, the speed of execution of the algorithm is no longer a controlling issue.

CT Numbers

The array of CT or Hounsfield values produced by a computer is a discretized approximation of the linear attenuation coefficient (LAC) values of tissue constituents in a single section. As already explained, LAC values depend upon both the physical density and the atomic numbers of the constituents of the tissue components. Each discrete component of the reconstruction, or pixel, represents a rectangular parallelopiped of tissue whose size and position can be manipulated by the operator of the CT device. CT numbers are computed via the following definitions:

$$\text{CT number} = k \frac{\mu_p - \mu_w}{\mu_w}$$

where

$$k = \text{magnifying constant,}$$

μ_p = average linear attenuation coefficient of the pixel,

and

μ_w = linear attenuation coefficient of water.

Using a magnifying constant of 1000, attenuation lies in a 2000-unit range: dense bone has a value of +1000, water is 0, and air is −1000. The statistical accuracy is affected by the photon flux, the signal-to-noise ratio of the data, and the pixel size. Such measurements of "accuracy" are used despite their total inability to provide absolute bounds on the error in any particular reconstruction. Nevertheless, the published accuracy is given by 0.5 percent (5 CT units).

IMAGE QUALITY

Techniques of Display

Since CT numbers can be displayed as a digital printout as well as the more common gray scale image on a cathode ray tube, familiarity with the significance of those numerical values can provide important guides to diagnosis. As normal brain tissue (ventricles, subarachnoid spaces, blood vessels, gray and white matter) are represented by a 50-unit range (2.5 percent of the total scale), it is possible to examine this range more carefully by increasing the apparent contrast in a particular range by decreasing the "window width." The window width represents the range of the attenuation scale selected for study and the "window level" is the mean value of this range. The optimal settings will vary with different scanner models. For example, in a routine head scan, a window width of +76 and window level of +38 may be optimal; all values higher than +76 will appear white, those less than 0 will appear black, and all values between 0 and +76 will appear as shades of gray. This provides adequate visual contrast to recognize most normal and pathological structures. Be advised that such settings vary with each model of scanner. To study areas of low contrast (small differences in attenuation), a small window width should be used. Regions with high contrast such as orbits, petrous bone and sinus regions require a large window width. This ability to manipulate output data by altering apparent contrast differentiates CT from other radiographic techniques.

Representation of a Reconstruction

A reconstruction or CT image is a finite dimensional approximation of the x-ray attenuation distribution in a given section (axial, coronal or sagittal). Within this paragraph alone, "image quality" refers to how accurately the internal structure of the object is demonstrated. The problem of image quality in CT is *not* analogous to that which occurs in photography. When a photographic image is enlarged such that grain size is apparent, such a photograph still contains all information available in the negative. If one subsequently examines this image at a greater than normal distance, high-resolution spurious details are blurred out and only coarser but more accurate aspects remain. On the other hand, by remaking the choices that specify critical aspects of the CT system (including the "resolution of the data" and the "meaning of a projection"), which are analogous to choosing enlarging parameters, a reconstruction can be created to depict information at a finer (higher) spatial resolution. If the choice of that resolution is inappropriately fine, the reconstruction can be unpredictably inaccurate in its representation of details. The distinction be tween CT and photography lies in the fact that unlike photography, choosing to over-enlarge a reconstruction for CT cannot be redeemed by any method: These inaccuracies in the image cannot be subsequently removed by a more carefully designed reconstruction algorithm. Rigorous theories place a strict limit on the spatial resolution available from a particular data collection scheme; if an attempt is made to synthesize an image beyond this resolution, misleading image features may appear. These spurious features will not be removed by viewing the image subsequently at a lower resolution.[11] Figure 2–2 clarifies this point. This means that careful consideration must go into the choice of the (mathematically determined) spatial resolution of the reconstruction.

To further emphasize this point, it is beneficial to examine a feature available on some scanners. It is possible to have the computer display an "enlargement" of a user-selectable subregion of the original image after the data for the standard reconstruction have been collected and the resulting reconstruction displayed. This enlargement is done without collecting more projection data. The number of pixels in the new "enlargement" is identical to the number of pixels in the old standard image. One can repeat this request at will, until the region being imaged on the entire screen represents only 2 mm × 2 mm of the original, yet the reconstruction presented retains its array size. This feature runs in the face of the previous warning. There is, consequently, virtually no scientific basis for the accuracy of such "enlargements" obtained from the original data. This viewing technique is a wholesale abuse of the ignorance of the user.

Resolution

Spatial resolution is the ability of the imaging system to discriminate objects of limiting size or proximity. Factors that influence spatial resolution include (1) mathematical design of the CT imaging system, (2) pixel size, (3) aperture (size) of the detectors and (4) the reconstruction algorithm.

Contrast resolution is the ability of the imaging system to discriminate differences in optical density. Contrast may be most precisely described as the size of the *signal-to-noise ratio*, the quotient of the expected value of any pixel over the standard deviation of the

expected error in that value. The denominator is called the size of the noise while the signal strength is given by the numerator. In CT, statistical fluctuation within a picture element can be influenced by the number of photons and their energy levels, patient dose, detector system efficiency, section thickness and attenuating properties of the object scanned.

Detectability of a feature of an image is inextricably dually dependent on spatial and signal-to-noise ratio issues. For example, Barrett et al.[19] demonstrated that with a fixed signal-to-noise ratio, the same local contrast that will almost definitely occur by accident many times, independently and in random isolation on a single pixel within the same reconstruction, will accidently and simultaneously occur on four adjacent pixels only 1 in 10,000 times. Furthermore, the published characteristics of CT images state that it has a spatial resolution of 3 mm and can detect an attenuation difference of 0.5 percent of 5 CT units. It should *not* be expected that these qualities apply simultaneously. The spatial measurements may be made with a high-contrast object while the contrast measurement with a large object varying only slightly from its background.

Simultaneous application of these features requires a signal-to-noise ratio increase by a factor of four, which would demand a 16-fold increase in patient dose. However, in regions of high contrast, spatial resolution can reach 1.5 times pixel size.

In areas of high contrast, the partial-volume phenomenon, a problem caused by volume averaging, is most obscuring. In the pineal gland or choroid plexus, a small area of calcification easily overwhelms the imaging system because it can tilt the average attenuation of the pixel toward calcium—causing the entire pixel to appear white. Representing such a pixel white is not, however, indicative of a spurious or faulty reconstruction. As always, the attenuation value chosen for a single pixel causes a square to appear homogeneous and uniform; the inability of the reconstruction to demonstrate such highly localized variations in attenuation is not a reflection of deficient contrast response but instead the result of the design choice to utilize pixels that are too big to isolate the desired spatial features. This demonstrates that the size of pixels, which could ultimately limit spatial resolution, can, at times, affect the apparent contrast response of the system. In pixels that overlie the bound-

```
-50  -50  -50  -50  -50  -50  -50  -50  -50  -50  -50  -50

-50  -50  -50  -40   20   30   30   28   14  -50  -50  -50

-50  -50  -20   30   13    3    3   13   30   15  -50  -50

-50  -40   30    8    3    3    3    3    3   30  -40  -50

-50   15   15    3    3    3    3    3    3   18   15  -50

-50   30    3    3    3    3    3    3    3    5   30  -50

-50   30    3    3    3    3    3    3    3    3   30  -50

-50   15   13    3    3    3    3    3    3   13   20  -50

-50    5   30    6    3    3    3    3    6   30  -40  -50

-50  -50   10   30    6    3    3    7   30  -20  -50  -50

-50  -50  -50   10   30   30   30   30  -20  -50  -50  -50

-50  -50  -50  -50  -50  -50  -50  -50  -50  -50  -50  -50
```

```
-50  -50  -50  -50  -50  -50  -50  -50  -50  -50  -50  -50

-50  -50  -50  -40   20   31   29   28   14  -50  -50  -50

-50  -50  -20   29   13    3    3   13   31   15  -50  -50

-50  -40   31    8    3    4    2    3    3   29  -40  -50

-50   15   15    3    3    3    3    3    3   18   15  -50

-50   29    3    2    3    3    3    3    4    5   31  -50

-50   31    3    4    3    3    3    3    2    3   29  -50

-50   15   13    3    3    3    3    3    3   13   20  -50

-50    5   29    6    3    4    2    3    6   31  -40  -50

-50  -50   10   31    6    3    3    7   29  -20  -50  -50

-50  -50  -50   10   30   29   31   30  -20  -50  -50  -50

-50  -50  -50  -50  -50  -50  -50  -50  -50  -50  -50  -50
```

Figure 2–2 Although these two images are diagnostically different, they could not be distinguished from their projection data. This is an example of insufficient design. The two simulated reconstructions are displayed on a 12 by 12 array. (This represents an array of uniform squares, each over a centimeter on a side.) Each number is chosen to be approximately one tenth of the appropriate EMI number for slices taken through a patient's head. If projections of these two images are taken at exactly eight equally spaced projection angles, then the corresponding projection data will not disagree more than one part in one thousand at any datum. Notice that the lower image shows diagnostically significant fluctuations that are not present in the upper image; in particular, consider the 4's in the intracranial portion of the array.

aries between brain and skull, bone tissue may fall into pixels that also represent superficial brain parenchyma, artificially increasing the values assigned to such pixels. A bone correction subprogram contained in the reconstruction algorithm must degrade the accuracy of the image, but it could reduce the inconvenience caused by apparently overbrightened pixels near such boundaries.

In areas where adjacent tissue elements provide low contrast (differing in linear attenuation coefficient by about 1 percent), discrimination depends more critically upon photon flux, slice thickness and object size. Increasing photon flux can improve contrast. Decreasing slice thickness degrades contrast unless compensated for by an increase in photon flux. As a rule, it is not usually possible to image such objects if they are smaller than 6 mm; however, iodide enhancement can improve contrast and consequently spatial resolution, as explained earlier.

Artifacts

In order for physicians to draw accurate conclusions about data, it is essential to understand both the meaning and reliability of the data. Since even the best CT images are at least mildly inaccurate, physicians should be able to decipher information from misleading details in each reconstruction. This skill must be developed from experience, but a guide through the reasons for artifacts (inaccuracies) in a reconstruction should be helpful.

Mathematical Design–Related Artifacts

Despite the statistical unlikelihood of this occurrence, as demonstrated by phantom experiments, mathematical proof has established the existence of grossly inaccurate reconstructions that exactly match error-free projection data. Although manufacturers claim that attenuation coefficients exhibited in reconstructions are most often accurate to within about 2 to 5 CT units, it has been shown that by choosing to represent a reconstruction at a resolution that exceeds the information content of a particular class of projection data, both a healthy looking and a pathological image can have the same projection data. Mathematical justification of the resolution provided by existing scanning equipment should be available on demand. In particular, the collection of consistent and error-free x-ray projection data is not always sufficient to determine a reconstruction at any resolution (see Fig. 2–2).

Computer Algorithm–Related Artifacts

Projection data are not completely consistent or error-free, but the magnitude of such discrepancies is small. The Convolution algorithm performs well with data that are not error-free. It is important to understand that the Convolution algorithm represents inconsistencies in the error in a characteristic fashion. The reader should realize that the total error is a sum of consistent and inconsistent components. No reconstruction algorithm can distinguish the accurate data from the inaccurate consistent data; therefore it will present an image derived from their sum. However, the inconsistent part of the data is also exhibited in a reconstruction by the Convolution algorithm. When such inconsistent information is processed, back-projection patterns or streaked patterns that are generated are not damped out by compensating streaks from other directions. Since the Convolution algorithm imposes an oscillating character to projection data before back-projection occurs, uncompensated streak artifacts will tend to leave an oscillating or ringing effect. The presence of a ringing or an alternating anomaly in the reconstruction frequently results from inconsistencies in the data. If an object within a patient is involved with erroneous data collection, that object is usually near the presented ringing artifact in the reconstruction. Experience indicates that if a detail within a reconstruction is spatially removed from all suspiciously oscillating features, that detail is likely to be more reliably depicted. This applies to reconstructions that have not been post-processed to remove these oscillations. The consistent component of the error in projection data will produce artifacts that are not flagged by ringing features.

The filter function (the rule used to reorganize the projection data just before back-projection) employed by a particular Convolution algorithm represents a compromise between two goals. It would be desirable to be able to represent large local fluctuations in x-ray attenuation coefficients. On the other hand, it is also important that high-frequency error in the data not be amplified to a point that distorts the reconstruction. These goals are contradictory for the Convolution algorithm in that they make opposite demands on the filter function that, in any case, is not capable of only filtering out the inconsistent data. The effect is that a filter function is chosen that removes the worst part of the high-frequency error while living with the less common medium-frequency type. The filter function is chosen to best match the expected error and expected relief in the data. This means that either an unusually fast change in the x-ray attenuation in the patient or a significant increase in moderate frequency error will overwhelm the filter function, thereby causing a streaked, ringing artifact in the former case or a grainy image in the latter.

Data Collection–Related Artifacts

Artifacts associated with data collection can be presented starting from the obvious artifacts associated with the most inconsistent kinds of data to the least discernible artifacts that are associated with more consistent data. For reconstructions produced by the convolution algorithm, the more inconsistent the data, the more streaked and oscillating will be the reconstruction.

Grossly inconsistent data can be collected because of hardware malfunctions. Brief drops in the x-ray source output or faulty detector connections can produce extremely pronounced black and white bands. Herringbone patterns imposed on a reconstruction can be caused by inaccurate scanner rotation. Misalignment of the center of rotation of the scan literally shifts correct data to inappropriate equations and can effect gross inconsistencies. In third-generation scanners recalibration of each detector during scanning is not feasible; this means that drift in sensitivity cannot be easily compensated. When this happens, one or more concentric circles of artifacts are produced; this is called the "onion" artifact. However, very stable detectors have largely obviated this problem.

Patient Motion–Related Artifacts

The most common form of artifact is associated with patient motion. In most cases small degrees of patient motion do not cause significant inconsistencies; this is not the case, however, when a bone structure is greatly displaced. Motion artifacts are usually quite visible and distinctive. When an in-and-out motion, i.e., along the axis perpendicular to the scan, occurs, streaks are most visible in the reconstruction near areas in which there is the greatest change in attenuation. In basal sections slight in-and-out motion can reveal or hide the petrous pyramids. Side-to-side or rotary motions are frequently displayed by vertically oriented bands, often seen exterior to the skull. Similarly, up-and-down motions are indicated by horizontal streaks of oscillating gray levels. When a water bag is used, air trapped near the temporal hollow (or other places) can shift significantly, even with slight motions of the patient. This creates streaks that emanate from the offending region. Even motion of fluid within the body can cause serious artifacts; paranasal sinuses have been so implicated.

At least two remedies to patient motion problems have been employed. One provides the operator of the scanner with a "patient motion correction" option. This allows the collection of data at 225° instead of the normal 180°, and an auxiliary program discards up to 45 projections before Convolution is applied. Another device performs the Convolution reconstruction algorithm on the display console as data are collected. The operator can recognize a forming motion artifact and stop the scan sequence. In reconstructions marred by motion artifacts, the resolution will be degraded everywhere and not always in a homogeneous manner. With scanners that use a full circle of data collections, each beam direction is measured twice, naturally reducing the significance of erroneous data caused by patient motion.

Spectral-Shift Artifact

Probably the most pervasive and difficult-to-remedy defect in data collection is associated with the beam-hardening problem (the spectral-shift artifact). This error results from the polychromatic nature of the x-ray beam. As explained in the section on photon-tissue interaction, the probability of attenuation caused by photoelectric or Compton effects not only depends on the nature of the transmitting tissues but also on the energy of the photon. This means that as the beam passes through tissue the more probable photoelectric effect filters out the less energetic photons, which causes the transmitted beam to experience a different average attenuation than it would have had had it not just passed through that tissue. This causes some tissues such as bone to seem less dense if located nearer the exiting surface than the entering surface of the body. Judging from the nature of the artifact produced in a head scan, the erroneous part of the data seems to have a large consistent component; this means that the reconstruction algorithm per se would not be expected to remove the artifact. The characteristic spectral-shift artifact seems to make the skull thicker (2 to 5 mm). Errors in reconstructions caused by this type of artifact are typically associated with areas near to the skull, and are progressively more pronounced as the skull is approached. This artifact, which depends on the hardness of the penetrating beam, can be grossly described as a cusped discrepancy. Other bony regions present characteristic artifacts. The region between the petrous pyramids is frequently exhibited with depressed attenuation values; it is called the Hounsfield bar. The first procedure that is used to remove the spectral-shift artifact is extensive filtering of the beam before it enters the patient so that the spectrum of the beam is less sensitive to the tissue encountered. Another technique requires the computer to adjust collected data to a type that would result from more homogeneous attenuation phenomena. This type of preprocessing is quite successful in removing a large percentage of the artifact, but it necessarily creates one of its own since it must be based on a fixed percentage of brain matter to bone at each observed intensity level.

High Contrast–Related Artifacts

High-density regions or regions with a large local fluctuation in attenuation cause both data collection problems and difficulties for the convolution reconstruction algorithm. This effect is generated to some extent in every scan, since bone-to-air and bone-to-brain interfaces are universal. Previous diagnostic tests can leave residual matter that displays great local fluctuations in attenuation; residual Pantopaque or intraventricular gas left over from pneumoencephalography can detract from the clarity of a reconstruction. Metallic clips left by previous surgical procedures and metal casing of a valve or a tantalum plate can cause quite significant artifacts, the extent and severity of which vary with the size and proximity of the objects. An important error in data collection (apart from the effects of beam hardening) lies in the detector crystal that must accurately register intensity values, however abruptly these decrease during the scan. Because of afterglow in NaI, such a detector may not be able to provide the proper signal

to the computer memory. Afterglow in CaF_2 is shorter-lived, so it is used in some scanners. As previously mentioned, even slight motion can be a significant source of inconsistent data if large changes in attenuation result; therefore, high-density regions make data collection much more sensitive to movement. It was previously explained that too large a local fluctuation in attenuation values cannot be reconstructed with the convolution algorithm. Note that even when motion is not present, the reconstructions produced when high local fluctuations or extremes of attenuation are present are characterized by streaks (overshoots and undershoots) that pass through the unusual region. The most typical example of this kind of artifact appears as a thin line of relatively low attenuation values located about 5 mm from the skull. Such a streak does not result from inconsistent or even inaccurate data but from the choice of the filter function, which is inappropriate for this particular kind of error-free projection data.

REFERENCES

1. Gordon RR, Herman GT, Johnson S: Image reconstruction from projections. Sci Am 133:56, 1975
2. McCullough EC, Baker HL, Houser DW: Evaluation of the quantitative and radiation features of a scanning x-ray transverse axial tomograph: the EMI scanner. Radiology 111:709, 1974
3. Radon J: Uber die Bestimmung von Funktionen durch ihre Integralwerte langs gewisser manningfaltigkeiten. Ber Verh Sachs Akad 69:262, 1917
4. Smith KT, Solomon DC, Wagner SL: Practical and mathematical aspects of the problem of reconstructing objects from radiographs. Bull Am Math Soc 83(6):1227, 1977
5. Bracewell RN: Strip integration in radio astronomy. Austral J Phys 9:198, 1956
6. Oldendorf WH: Isolated flying spot detection of radiodensity discontinuities displaying the identical structural pattern of a complex object. IRE Trans Bio-Med Elect BME 8:68, 1961
7. Cormack AM: Representation of a function by its line integrals, with some radiological applications. J App Phys 34(9):2722, 1963
8. De Rosier DJ, Klug A: Reconstruction of three-dimensional structures from electron micrographs. Nature 217:130, 1968
9. Kuhl DE, Edwards RQ: Reorganizing data from the transverse section scans of the brain using digital processing. Radiology 91:975, 1968
10. Hounsfield GN: Computerized transverse axial scanning. Part I: Description of the system. Br J Radiol 46:1016, 1973
11. Katz MB: Questions of Uniqueness and Resolution in Reconstruction of Objects from their Projections. Lecture Notes in Biomathematics, Vol 26. Springer-Verlag, New York, 1979

12. Ter-Pogossian MM: Computerized cranial tomography: equipment and physics. Semin Roentgenol 12:13, 1977
13. Oldendorf WH: The quest for an image of brain. Neurology 28:517, 1978
14. Hounsfield GN: Computed medical imaging. J Comput Assist Tomogr 4:665, 1980
15. Seeram E: Computed Tomography Technology. W. B. Saunders Company, Philadelphia, 1982
16. Brooks RA, Di Chiro G: Beam hardening in x-ray reconstructive tomography. Physiol Med Biol 21:390, 1976
17. Edholm P: Image construction in transverse computer tomography. Acta Radiol (Suppl) 346:21, 1975
18. Herman GT, Rowland SW: Three methods for reconstructing objects from x-rays: a comparative study. Comp Graphics Image Proc 2:151, 1973
19. Barrett HH, Gordon SK, Hershel RS: Statistical limitations in transaxial tomography. Comput Biol Med 6:307 1976

Chapter 3

PERFORMANCE OF CT SCANNING

For routine head or orbit CT, patients should have no oral intake for three hours prior to scanning. This precaution is necessary because intravenous iodinated contrast medium administration may be necessary after the noncontrast scan. It is extremely helpful to explain certain features of CT examination to patients before they are positioned in the scanner. This explanation should include the following points: (1) type of equipment and potential irradiation, (2) length of the study, (3) movement of the machine, (4) importance of the subject remaining perfectly immobile, (5) noise of the machine and (6) possible need for contrast study. All metallic objects such as hair and wig pins, combs and earrings worn about the head should be removed because they may produce streak artifacts on CT. False teeth need be removed only for coronal studies. Some pediatric patients may have scalp intravenous apparatus. This equipment should be checked prior to CT scan to determine if there are any metallic parts. The needle is usually not large enough to cause significant artifact.

Patients are positioned supine on the x-ray table for routine axial CT scan. The head rests on a plastic holder built in the gantry aperture. The gantry has a directional light, which assists in centering the head. This may be a laser beam that may be potentially dangerous to the eyes; therefore, patients should be instructed to close their eyes.

The technician aligns the patient at the desired angulation. This may vary from parallel (zero angulation) to 25° relative to Reid's anatomical baseline (drawn from the superior orbital rim to the external auditory meatus). The desired angulation is achieved by tilting the head rest or the gantry. If the patient's head cannot be moved, the gantry may be tilted. The table top may be moved automatically through the gantry aperture via computer instructions or manually by the operator. The computer apprises the technician if the table measurements are accurate, as when the tissue section is 8 or 12 mm rather than 10 mm. The increments of table top movement are modified to determine slice section thickness. A computed radiographic image is obtained initially to delineate precise anatomical areas that are to be scanned (scoutview, topogram, pilot scan). This usually consists of a single lateral view but an anteriorposterior view is also possible. This is quite helpful in image localization (Fig. 3–1).

For routine brain scan, the sequence includes 10 to 13 sections, each slice being 10 mm in thickness. These extend from the skull base through the vertex region. The number of scan sections necessary for complete study will vary, depending on head shape and size; therefore, comparable anatomical landmarks are seen at varying scan sections in different patients. For example, in patients with dolichocephalic skulls several additional sections may be required to extend through the vertex region. It is important to obtain a complete study, as diagnostic errors may result from failure to include the high vertex region. Our routine axial scans are performed at approximately 20° angulation relative to the orbitomeatal line. The true axial plane (zero degree angulation) sometimes better visualizes the optic nerve and temporal horns of the lateral ventricles. For axial brain CT, we use a field size of 24 cm; however, a smaller field size of 15 cm provides better anatomical detail for axial orbital and sella studies and direct coronal views.

Following performance of complete noncontrast study, intravenous injection of iodinated

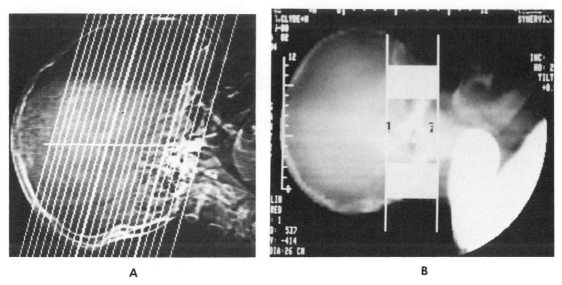

Figure 3–1. Scoutview (General Electric CT/T 8800) *(A)* and pilot scan (Picker Synerview) *(B)* showing scan sections.

contrast medium may be necessary. The specific type of contrast material used (Conray, Renograffin, Hypaque) does not seem to influence the quality of the enhanced scan. However, method of administration (bolus injection, drip infusion, bolus injection followed by drip infusion, drip infusion with bolus injection immediately before scan) is important because these may cause different plasma iodine concentrations. The technique therefore influences imaging of the intracranial anatomy. With bolus injection, the level of plasma iodine concentration rises rapidly within the initial 3 to 5 minutes followed by rapid decline, whereas with drip infusion, the rise of plasma iodine concentration is slower and does not achieve the peak seen with bolus injection. Other combinations have been utilized.

One technique is to administer bolus injection followed by drip infusion; however, the peak concentration is not higher than that achieved by bolus alone. This method increases iodine concentration but does not provide better enhanced images. With initial drip infusion followed by bolus injection performed immediately prior to scanning, highest peak concentrations are achieved with rapid fall-off. This technique is suited to scanners with rapid scanning times.[3] In adult patients, 40 grams of iodide is considered adequate; however, in some instances, larger (double) doses may be utilized.[1-4] Plasma concentration is determined by dose and rate of intravenous administration of contrast material. Renal function is an important variable because this determines

the rate of excretion of contrast. For pediatric patients, 1 to 2 ml per pound body weight of iodinated contrast (Renograffin–60, Hypaque–60) is used. If suspicious areas are identified on plain and enhanced study or if clinical findings direct attention to a specific region, e.g., pituitary fossa, posterior fossa, cerebellopontine angle or orbit, thinner sections or special scanning techniques such as coronal reconstructions provide important diagnostic information. Metrizamide or air cisternography CT are supplemental studies is selected cases when initial CT results are equivocal.

Patients must remain motionless during scanning because slight movement may significantly degrade image quality. This is a less common problem with rapid scan times. Motion-induced artifact still remains a significant problem in some patients, especially those with head trauma, and in small children. If sedation is utilized, cardiopulmonary complications are a potential risk. We utilize intravenous diazepam (Valium) initially in a dosage of 10 mg. This has been effective in 67 percent of adult patients; however, 30 percent require an additional dosage of 10 mg to complete the study. In 3 percent of patients, adequate sedation is not achieved with 20 mg; further increments significantly increase risk of oversedation and cardiopulmonary depression. Therefore, we usually terminate the study and reschedule the patient, utilizing an alternate method of sedation. Amobarbital (Amytal) is an effective short-acting sedative drug. This is administered intravenously at a rate of 50 mg per minute to a maximum dosage of 500 mg. Amytal should be utilized very carefully, especially if administered after diazepam, because these two drugs have potential synergistic cardiorespiratory toxicity. General anesthesia has been necessary only rarely in adults. Sedation is usually required in children younger than four years. Chloral hydrate is the safest and most efficacious drug. We utilize 50 to 75 mg per kilogram of this drug. This is administered orally 20 minutes prior to scanning. This dose may be repeated 40 minutes later if adequate sedation has not been achieved with the initial dose. In certain pediatric patients, a mixture consisting of meperidine (Demerol), chlorpromazine (Thorazine) and promethazine (Phenergan) is necessary to achieve sedation. General anesthesia has been necessary in less than 0.5 percent of children.

In positioning infants and young children in the scanner, it is imperative to avoid airway obstruction when flexing the head. Infants must be kept warm with blankets because the scanning room is usually quite cold (necessary for scanning machinery such as the computer) and these infants may have poor body temperature control.

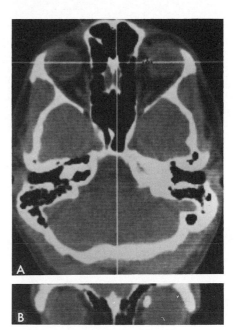

Figure 3–2. Axial scan shows a metallic object in the right medial orbital region with artifact (A). This is well delineated on reformated coronal sections (B).

SPECIAL SCANNING TECHNIQUES

Coronal Reconstructions

Large-aperture scanners make it possible to position patients for direct coronal (frontal, anterior-posterior) and sagittal (lateral) views. True coronal plane (90 degrees superior to orbitomeatal line) is achieved by hyperextending the head maximally with the patient in supine or prone position. The coronal plane may be modified with fewer degrees of head tilt. If the gantry is tilted, it may be possible to avoid streak artifact emanating from teeth or dense bone at the skull base and thereby compensate for patients who have limited neck mobility, as in cervical arthritis. However, movement of the gantry may alter the center of the scan field.

Computer-generated indirect coronal and sagittal reconstructions may be obtained by reformating projection profiles that have been obtained from thin (2 or 4 mm) axial sections. This technique is especially useful in scanning the pituitary and orbit regions (Fig. 3–2). This reformated technique avoids metallic artifact

emanating from teeth and eliminates the need to rescan the patient; however, it requires additional radiation to achieve thin section necessary for high-quality reformated images. Additional computer time may be necessary to process the reformated images.

Major indications for coronal CT include accurate intracranial localization in the following conditions: (1) infra- and supratentorial extension of lesions such as tentorial tumors and Dandy-Walker cysts, (2) intra- and extraventricular lesions such as tip of a shunt tube (3) intra- and extraaxial lesions, (4) juxta- and intrasellar position of lesions, (5) skull base lesions, (6) orbital lesions and (7) congenital anomalies to evaluate the relationship between malformed structures and normal anatomical landmarks.[5, 6]

Metrizamide Cisternography

Metrizamide is nonionic substituted amide. It is water-soluble iodide contrast material used for intrathecal enhancement. This material is rapidly reabsorbed and does not need to be removed by the examiner as is the case with Pantopaque. The isotonic solution contains 170 milligrams of iodine per milliliter; there is also hypertonic solution (190 mg per ml). In performing metrizamide cisternography, lumbar puncture is done under fluoroscopic control on a standard myelographic or CT table. Five milliliters of metrizamide are injected. After the subarachnoid position of the metrizamide is confirmed, the needle is removed and the patient is placed in supine position. The table is tilted downward and the patient is placed in Trendelenberg position on the CT table. Scan sections are usually 8 mm in thickness but may be thinner. We utilize a gray scale–window width setting of 150 and window level setting of 50. Metrizamide flows cranially to outline the CSF spaces. These CSF spaces that contain metrizamide are analyzed for displacement, distortion, effacement or enlargement.[7, 8] The filling patterns of ventricles (fourth, third, lateral) and cortical CSF spaces are analyzed (Fig. 3–3). This may be of help in differentiating normal pressure hydro-

cephalus from hydrocephalus ex vacuo (cerebral atrophy).

Metrizamide cisternography is indicated in these conditions if intravenous enhanced CT is nondiagnostic: (1) delineation of small isodense nonenhancing brain stem lesions; (2) verification of suspected acoustic tumors in the internal acoustic meatus or cerebellopontine angle region; (3) delineation of the precise location and communication of posterior fossa extraaxial cysts such as mega cisterna magna, Dandy-Walker cyst and subarachnoid cyst; (4) differentiation of intrasellar tumor from empty sella; (5) delineation of the presence or absence of communication of cysts with ventricles (Fig. 3–4); (6) differentiation of communicating hydrocephalus from hydrocephalus ex vacuo; (7) accurate localization of the site of CSF leak in patients with rhinorrhea.[9]

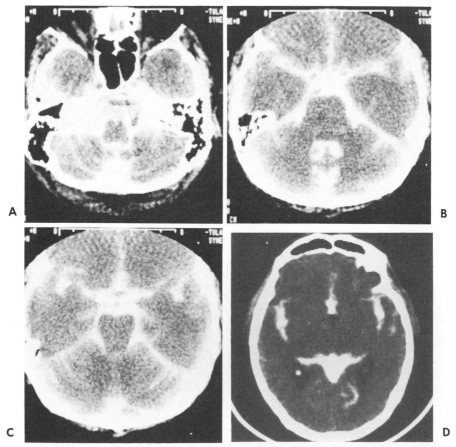

Figure 3–3. Metrizamide cisternogram outlines normal CSF-filled spaces. *A,* Lower brain stem with bilobed appearance of medullary pyramids; CPA cistern and vallecula are seen. *B,* Pontine level with flat surface of basis pontis and contrast in the floor of the fourth ventricle. Ambient, suprasellar and middle cerebral artery cisterns are seen. *C,* Midbrain level with heart-shaped appearance due to cerebral peduncles. Interpeduncular, perimesencephalic and suprasellar cisterns are seen. *D,* Pineal level outlining quadrigeminal and retrothalamic cisterns with contrast in the third ventricle and sylvian cistern.

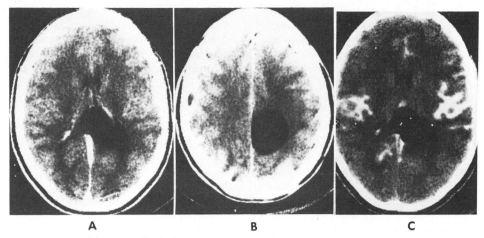

Figure 3–4. A 26-year-old woman had chronic seizure disorder controlled with phenytoin. EEG showed right parietal delta pattern. *CT findings:* hypodense sharply marginated lesion extending from the quadrigeminal plate region *(A)* to the parietal-occipital region *(B)*. With metrizamide cisternogram, no communication of the lesion with ventricles or subarachnoid spaces is seen *(C)*. *Operative findings:* subarachnoid cyst.

Gas (Air) Cisternography

This technique is utilized to detect small acoutic tumors located in the internal acoustic canal (intracanalicular) or cerebellopontine angle (CPA) that have not been detected with intravenous enhanced CT.[10] Patients are positioned in lateral decubitus position on the CT table with the side to be studied located superiorly. Lumbar puncture is performed; 5 ml of room air is injected intrathecally. The head of the CT table is tilted 10° to 20° upward. As air ascends to the CPA cistern, patients experience retroauricular pressure or pain. The patient is lowered to lateral decubitus position. The initial scan should be obtained at the level of the external acoustic meatus. Subsequent scans are obtained by moving patients to visualize the internal acoustic meatus and CPA cistern. Section thickness should be 2 to 5 mm. The gray scale viewing settings are different for analyzing bone detail (window width, 2000; window level, 475) and for demonstrating the presence of air in the CPA and internal acoustic canals (window width, 1500; window level, −200). Air provides more effective contrast than does metrizamide for detection of acoustic tumors. This is because air contrasts with dense petrous bone. It is not always possible to deliver air into the IAC or CPA cistern because of technical or anatomical factors such as adhesions and trabeculations; therefore, not all studies provide diagnostic information.

Intravenous-Enhanced CT

Indications for intravenous-enhanced CT remain controversial.[11] Some investigators recommend initial nonenhanced study supplemented by enhanced scan if indicated by clinical or radiographic findings. Others have questioned the need for initial nonenhanced scan in patients with certain conditions such as suspected CNS tumors; therefore, they recommend enhanced scan only.[12, 13] The performance of enhanced scan only reduces radiation exposure and shortens scan time for each patient. However, it leads to performance of an increasing number of contrast-enhanced studies and performance of intravenous study is time consuming.

We believe that nonenhanced scan should be performed initially in all cases for the following reasons:

1. Certain hypodense lesions may enhance sufficiently on enhanced scan to become isodense and therefore will not be detectable with only enhanced scan.

2. If enhanced scan shows a hyperdense lesion, it may not be possible to ascertain the components of this lesion (enhancement, calcification, hemorrhage) especially if all these components are present in same lesion, such as bleeding from angioma and hemorrhage into calcified neoplasm.

Indications for intravenous-enhanced scan reported in CT literature have included (1) lesion previously demonstrated by such other diagnostic studies as isotope scan, angiography, skull radiogram, biopsy; (2) suspicion of cerebral metastases; (3) posterior fossa or parasellar lesion; (4) vascular lesion such as aneurysm or angioma; (5) suspicion of recurrent intracranial tumor; (6) abnormal neurological findings such as memory loss, dementia, aphasia, hemiparesis and seizure history; (7) clinical findings of occlusive or hemorrhagic cerebrovascular disease; (8) head trauma; (9) evidence on nonenhanced scan of certain findings—shift of midline structures, asymmetry or effacement of ventricles, abnormal tissue density; (10) nonspecific symptoms such as headache, dizziness and seizures; (11) suspicion of an inflammatory disorder.[11]

Indications for enhanced scan have continued to broaden with increasing clinical experience. It has become almost routine to perform enhanced scan in many medical centers. The use of intravenous contrast radically changes the nature of CT from a noninvasive to an *invasive* procedure. Enhanced study requires patients to sign a consent form; and there is potential morbidity and mortality from administration of contrast agents. We believe that enhanced scan is indicated in the following situations:

1. Suspected parasellar lesion, as with endocrine symptoms of hypothalamic-pituitary dysfunction, visual symptoms of optic nerve or chiasmal involvement and radiographic evidence of sella turcica abnormalities. Five percent of parasellar lesions are detected only on enhanced scan.

2. Suspected cerebellopontine angle lesions as with sensorineural hearing loss, vertigo, gait unsteadiness, abnormal brain stem auditory evoked potentials and radiographic abnormalities of internal acoustic canal. Fifteen to 20 percent of these tumors are detected only on enhanced scan.

3. Suspicion of posterior fossa lesions such as neoplasm, angioma or inflammatory or vascular lesion. Two percent of these disorders show no abnormality on noncontrast scan.

4. Suspicion of recurrence of such intracranial pathological processes as neoplasm, abscess or aneurysm. In patients who have had prior surgery, radiotherapy or chemotherapy, it may be difficult to differentiate recurrence from tissue effects of these treatment modalities (radiation necrosis).

5. The finding of a positive isotope scan or angiogram.

6. If patients have systemic carcinoma and management will be modified by the finding of intracerebral metastases, enhanced scan should be performed even if patients are neurologically asymptomatic.[14]

7. If patients have intracranial hypertension without other neurological abnormalities and nonenhanced CT shows either ventricular dilatation or mass effect (distortion, effacement, midline shift), enhanced scan is necessary. In patients with intracranial hypertension if nonenhanced scan shows that ventricles are normal-sized without mass effect, it is possible that vascular malformation will be missed if enhanced scan and angiography are not performed. However, we have not seen examples of this occurrence and do not recommend enhanced scan in these patients.

8. Selected patients with suspected stroke syndromes. Ten to 25 percent of patients with cerebral ischemia or infarction show isodense enhancing lesion. All clinically symptomatic acute intracerebral hematomas are visualized on nonenhanced scan; however, ring enhancement may be seen at a later time.

9. In patients with suspected vascular malformations such as aneurysm or angioma. If plain scan or clinical findings suggest possible occurrence of aneurysm or angioma, enhanced CT may demonstrate characteristic findings due to the intravascular component of the vascular lesion.

10. In patients with acute head trauma, unenhanced scan provides complete diagnostic information. Because of impaired blood-brain barrier in these patients, enhanced scan may be potentially neurotoxic. In head-injured patients who are studied after the end of the first week, enhanced scan may be necessary to defined enhancement of isodense subdural hematoma or ring enhancement in hemorrhagic contusion.

11. In patients with suspected inflammatory disease, enhanced scan is necessary to delineate certain extra- and intracerebral lesions such as cerebritis, abscess formation and infarction due to vasculitis.

12. In patients with suspected demyelinating disorders, enhanced scan may define isodense enhancing periventricular lesions.

UNTOWARD REACTIONS DUE TO IODINATED CONTRAST AGENTS

Adverse reactions may develop following intravenous, intra-arterial or cisternal injection. Occurrence of these complications is variable; it depends upon route of administration and type of study performed—intravenous urography (5.6 percent), intravenous cholangiography (10 percent), cerebral angiography (2.3 percent). For intravenously enhanced brain and orbit CT scans, adverse reactions have ranged from 2.8 to 3.4 percent. It is surprising that the incidence of adverse reactions for CT is lower than for IVP because type, dosage and route of administration of contrast material are comparable. This difference in complication incidence may result from factors such as patient age, complicating medical illness and renal impairment.[15]

Adverse reactions to intravascular iodinated contrast medium have been graded as follows: (1) mild—no treatment needed, (2) moderate—treatment needed, (3) severe—hospitalization needed, (4) fatal. The incidence of severe reactions is 1 per 1000; fatal reactions occur in 1 of 10,000 cases. Type and incidence of adverse reactions are listed in Table 3–1.[15]

The incidence of adverse reactions to iodinated contrast material is similar in both sexes. If patients have a specific allergy to shellfish, chocolate, eggs, mild or a nonspecific allergy of any type, incidence of contrast reaction to iodine is 12 to 14 percent. If patients have had a prior specific reaction to contrast media, the incidence of subsequent reaction is 16 percent. Because iodinated contrast medium does not bind protein, specific antibody formation does not occur. Following initial con-

trast reaction, subsequent reactions are not inevitable and cannot be predicted. If a second reaction does occur, it will not necessarily be increasingly more severe than the initial reaction. Toxicity has been attributed to both cation and anion components of contrast material. Diatrizoate (Renografin, Hypaque), metrizoate (Isopaque), and iothalamate (Conray) are anions currently utilized. Their systemic toxicity is quite similar. The neurotoxicity of iothalamate is lower than that of diatrizoate salts. Recent studies have shown the importance of cation component; methylglucamine is considered less toxic than are the sodium salts.[16, 17]

In IVP studies, rapid bolus injection is associated with adverse reactions in 5.3 percent; drip infusion—in which the contrast is administered more slowly over 3 to 10 minutes—produces toxic reaction in 7.2 percent of cases. In contrast-enhanced brain and orbit CT studies, incidence of nausea and vomiting was 5 percent with bolus technique and 2 percent with drip infusion; however, incidences of other untoward reactions were comparable for both techniques. Nausea and vomiting occurred with equal frequency with half-dose, standard (40 grams of iodine) or double-dose studies; this suggests that these reactions are not dose related. It is speculated that nausea and vomiting are caused by the toxicity of the contrast agents on the area postrema of the medullary region.

The majority of adverse reactions occur at onset of injection. Delayed reactions may occur 30 to 60 minutes later. Neither acute nor delayed reactions are predictable or preventable. The most common adverse reactions are nausea and vomiting, which represent nonspecific reactions resulting from histamine release. Treatment should include removing the patient from the scanner to prevent aspiration and temporarily discontinuing contrast administration. The severity of this reaction may be diminished by having patients fast for three hours prior to the study. Because these reactions are precipitated by histamine release, treatment with diphenhydramine (50 mg intravenously) is usually initiated. Because of the sedative effect of antihistamines, outpatients should be cautioned about driving home alone. If nausea has been mild, it may be possible to resume infusion cautiously at a slower rate.

Specific untoward reactions to iodide contrast material are idiosyncratic and anaphylactoid. Mechanisms that have been postulated include iodide acting as antigen (which com-

TABLE 3–1. Type and Incidence of Adverse Reactions to Iodinated Contrast Agents*

Reaction	As a Percentage of Total Reactions
Vascular pain at site of injection	2.30
Flushing	12.47
Urticaria	15.58
Facial edema	2.61
Nausea	33.66
Vomiting	20.53
Drop in blood pressure	1.28
Ventricular fibrillation	.16
Cardiac arrest	.18
Circulatory collapse	.29
Difficulty breathing	3.19
Laryngeal edema	.41
Pulmonary edema	.08
Neurological findings	
convulsions	.15
paralysis	.09
coma	.03
Other	3.97

*From Shehadi WH: Adverse reactions to intravascularly administered contrast media. Am J Roentgenol 124:145, 1975.

bines with immunoglobulin E to cause liberation of histamine from mast cells), activation of alternative complement pathway and direct chemotoxic effect. Nausea and vomiting are not harbingers of anaphylactoid reaction. Hives and flushing are specific reactions usually caused by histamine release. These should *always* be treated because laryngeal spasm and edema may develop even if patients have no hoarseness or respiratory stridor. Treatment of this reaction includes diphenhydramine (50 mg intramuscularly or intravenously) or epinephrine in concentration of 1:1,000 (0.3 to 0.5 ml subcutaneously, which may be repeated 15 minutes later); this may require supplementation with hydrocortisone (200 mg intravenously). If bronchospasm is severe and persistent, aminophylline (400 mg administered at the rate of 25 mg per minute) may be necessary; however, this drug may worsen hypotension, precipitate cardiac arrhythmias or cause seizures.

There are two cardiovascular syndromes that may develop following use of iodinated contrast material. One includes an acute vagal reaction. This is characterized by a decrease in blood pressure and bradycardia. Treatment is atropine (0.6 mg intravenously every 2 minutes to a maximum dose of 3.0 mg). The other reaction is characterized by loss of effective intravascular volume and vasodilation. This results in hypotension, tachycardia and arrhythmias. Treatment of this iodine-induced shock syndrome is rapid fluid replacement (to produce volume expansion), epinephrine in concentration 1:1,000 (0.5 ml intravenously every 15 minutes for a maximum dose of 1.0 mg), hydrocortisone (500 mg intravenously) and diphenhydramine (50 mg intravenously).

If patients have had any type of previous adverse reaction, this increases the risk of a subsequent problem. These patients are usually quite anxious about repeat administration of contrast material. Recurrence of adverse reaction is not inevitable because reactions are not caused by specific antibody formation. Pretesting with a small amount of contrast medium is of no value because those reactions that occur after a full dose has been injected are minor and do not usually require treatment; more serious reactions occur immediately. Intradermal and subcutaneous pretesting is of no predictive value because false-positive response may occur because of nonspecific histamine release.

Pretreatment has been advocated in certain patients. This is premedication with prednisone (50 mg orally every 6 hours for 48 hours) or diphenhydramine (50 mg intramuscularly two hours before the scan). There is no clinical evidence that premedication with either drug is beneficial in decreasing incidence or severity of adverse reactions. If specific signs of adverse reaction develop in patients with a prior history of toxicity, the procedure should be terminated and treatment with epinephrine, cortisone and diphenhydramine should be immediately initiated.

Certain toxic reactions result from contrast extravasation into brain parenchyma through impaired blood-brain barrier due to increased capillary permeability. This direct toxicity may result in neurological disturbances—convulsions, paralysis, altered consciousness. Neurological symptoms usually develop immediately but may appear up to 24 hours later. The methylglucamine cation (salts) are believed to be less neurotoxic because their larger size causes less permeation of the blood-brain barrier. Renal toxicity may also develop.[18] This may be immediate or delayed. Risk factors for renal impairment include diabetes mellitus, multiple myeloma, azotemia (creatinine in excess of 4.5 mg percent) and dehydration. In patients who develop nephrotoxic reaction related to contrast media, renal biopsy shows necrosis of proximal and distal tubules. In patients with multiple myeloma, anuria with progressive renal failure resulting from precipitation of myeloma protein in renal tubules may develop. This is exacerbated if the patient is dehydrated. In patients with pheochromocytoma, iodide-containing contrast agents may precipitate hypertensive crisis. In patients with sickle cell disease, sickling episode may develop after these contrast studies.

Metrizamide (Amipaque). The isotonic solution contains 166 mg of iodine per ml.[19] It is supplied in bottles containing either 10 or 20 ml. In patients undergoing metrizamide myelography or cisternography, most common adverse effects are headache (43 percent), nausea (14 percent) and vomiting (12 percent). The occurrence of neurological toxicity correlates with the amount of contrast medium administered. Neurological symptomatology includes seizures, confusional states, cortical blindness, papillitis, central scotoma, aphasia and hemiparesis. These disorders may develop 2 to 36 hours after intrathecal administration. In a prospective study of patients undergoing metrizamide myelography, EEG abnormalities developed in 35 percent. These patterns include slowing, spike and sharp waves.[20] Because of increased cortical excitability caused by metrizamide, seizures may be precipiated. Phenothiazines have been reported to have synergistic toxicity with metrizamide. This combination of drugs may interact to induce seizures. These seizures may be prevented by prophylactic treatment with phenobarbital (initiated 8 hours before and continued for 24 hours after the study). In rare cases, encephalopathy characterized by tremor, myoclonus, seizures, focal neurological deficit and altered consciousness may develop. This disorder usually resolves within 24 to 96 hours.[21] Systemic toxicity due to venous reabsorption of cisternally injected contrast material may also rarely develop.

Radiation Exposure

The dosage delivered to the brain and orbit depends upon multiple factors.[22] Some of these variables are (1) x-ray tube characteristics of current (number of electrons flowing per second) and voltage (penetrating quality of irradiation), (2) collimation and filtration of x-ray beam (both before it enters the patients and at detectors), (3) exposure time, (4) section thickness, (5) scan angulation, (6) scanner geometry, (7) x-ray focal spot size and (8) type and number of detectors utilized.[23] Irradiation dose has been measured using thermoluminescent dosimeters (TLD) and plexiglass cylinder phantoms. For individual head scan consisting of 10 sections that are each 10 mm in thickness, irradiation exposure of the head has ranged from 1 to 20 rads. With modern microdose collimation systems available in third and fourth generation scanners, the dose is approximately 2 to 5 rads per study with a dosage of 1.0 to 2.5 rads to the central region of the head. This compares with doses for other radiological studies, with conventional skull radiogram consisting of four views (0.5 rads), angiogram consisting of 11 films in frontal and lateral plane (10 rads), air study with 18 films (3 rads) and isotope brain scan (0.2 rads). Organs that are located outside the scanned area received very low and probably negligible irradiation from two sources: scattered irradiation and secondary radiation due to slow leaks from the x-ray tube. For head and orbit CT, these may cause ovarian and gonadal exposure. This may be prevented by using lead apron shield. Radiation exposure to the lens of the eye is very low if the orbit is outside the area scanned. This is 10 to 20 percent of the dosage that is received by the skin within the scan field. Radiation dose may be more substantial in orbital CT since the lens is within the scan field, and it is highly susceptible to radiation-induced damage. Long-range effect of irradiation related to CT on the immature and developing brain of pediatric patients is not known.

REFERENCES

1. Norman D, Enzmann DR, Newton TH: Optimal contrast dosage in cranial computed tomography. Am J Roentgenol 131:687–689, 1978
2. Hayman LA, Evans RA, Hinck VC: Rapid dose contrast computed tomography of perisellar vessels. Radiology 131:121, 1979
3. Burman S, Rosenbaum AE: Rationale and techniques for intravenous enhancement in computed tomography. Radiol Clin North Am 20:15, 1982
4. Leppik LE, Thompson CJ, Ethier R: Diatrizoate in computed cranial tomography: a quantative study. Invest Radiol 12:21, 1977
5. Mass S, Norman D, Newton TH: Coronal computed tomography: indications and accuracy. Am J Roentgenol 131:875–879, 1978
6. Byrd SE, Harwood-Nash D, Fitz CR: Coronal computed tomography of the skull and brain in infants and children. Radiology 124:705–714, 1977
7. Drayer BP, Rosenbaum AE, Reigel DB: Metrizamide computed tomography cisternography: pediatric applications. Radiology 124:349–357, 1977
8. Drayer BP, Rosenbaum AE: Studies of the third circulation: Amipaque CT cisternography and ventriculography. J Neurosurg 48:946–958, 1978
9. Drayer BP, Wilkins RH, Boehnke M: Cerebrospinal fluid rhinorrhea demonstrated by metrizamide CT cisternography. Am J Roentgenol 129:149–151, 1977
10. Sortland D: Computed tomography combined with gas cisternography for the diagnosis of expanding lesions in the cerebellopontine angle. Neuroradiology 18:19–22, 1979
11. Kramer RA, Janetos GP, Perlstein G: An approach to contrast enhancement in computed tomography of the brain. Radiology 116:641–647, 1975
12. Latchaw RE, Gold LHA, Tourje EJ: A protocol for the use of contrast enhancement in cranial computed tomography. Radiology 126:681–687, 1978
13. Butler AR, Kricheff II: Noncontrast CT scanning: limited value in suspected brain tumor. Radiology 126:689–693, 1978
14. Davis JM, Davis KR, Newhouse J: Expanded high iodine dose in computed cranial tomography: a preliminary report. Radiology 131:373–380, 1979
15. Shehadi WH: Adverse reactions to intravascularly administered contrast media; a comprehensive study based on a prospective survey. Am J Roentgenol 124:145–154, 1975
16. Melartin E, Tuohimaa PJ, Dabb R: Neurotoxicity of iothalamates and diatrizoates. I. Significance of concentration and cation. Invest Radiol 5:13–21, 1970
17. Tuohimaa PJ, Melartin E: Neurotoxicity of iothalamates and diatrizoates II. Historadioautographic

study of rat brains with iodine tagged contrast media. Invest Radiol 5:22–29, 1970

18. Warren SE: Hazards of computerized tomography: renal failure following contrast injection. Surg Neurol 10:335–336, 1978

19. Granger RG, Kendall BE, Wylie IG: Lumbar myelography with metrizamide—a new nonionic contrast medium. Br J Radiol 49:996–1003, 1976

20. Ropper AH, Chiappa KH, Young RR: The effect of metrizamide on the electroencephalogram. Ann Neurol 6:222–226, 1979

21. Junck L, Marshall WH: Neurotoxicity of radiological contrast agents. Ann Neurol 13:469–484, 1983

22. McCullough EC, Payne JT: Patient dosage in computed tomography. Radiology 129:457–463, 1978

23. Seeram E: Computed Tomography Technology. W. B. Saunders Company, Philadelphia, 1982, pp. 139–151

Chapter 4

NORMAL CRANIAL AND ORBITAL CT SCANNING ANATOMY

Factors that determine anatomical image of the intracranial and orbital region visualized by axial CT include (1) scanning angulation; (2) slice thickness; (3) matrix size; (4) contrast resolution; (5) spatial resolution; (6) visual display mode of gray scale, e.g., window width and level; (7) enhanced study, e.g., dose and technique of contrast administration and (8) artifact. For routine brain scan, 10 to 12 tissue sections are necessary for a complete study. This represents infraventricular, low ventricular, high ventricular and supraventricular regions.[1, 2] It is important to be cognizant of normal anatomical landmarks, including those which are less constantly seen and may falsely simulate pathological conditions.

Infraventricular Anatomy (Fig. 4–1). Structures usually seen in the anterior region include orbital roof, sinuses (frontal, sphenoid), crista galli, sphenoid bone and anterior clinoids. Frontal lobes represented by gyrus recti are contiguous with the interhemispheric fissure; frontal gyri and sulci are seen laterally.

The superior frontal gyrus is anterior; the middle and inferior frontal gyri are located more posteriorly. The middle fossa is bounded anteriorly by the sphenoid bone, posteriorly by the petrous bone, medially by the cavernous sinus and pituitary fossa and laterally by the temporal bone. The superior and middle temporal gyri form the lateral boundary of the middle fossa; the medial temporal cortex (uncus) forms the suprasellar cistern lateral borders. The anterior tip of the temporal horn and the sylvian cistern are sometimes seen within the middle fossa. Dense bone at the skull base causes an artifact that degrades image quality; therefore, delineation of the normal frontal and temporal cortex is difficult to assess at this level, as are brain parenchymal density changes in the inferior brain regions.

The posterior fossa is bounded anteriorly by the petrous bone and posteriorly by the occipital bone. The occipital protuberance is located medially. The cerebellar tonsils appear as paired hyperdense nodules at the foramen

Figure 4–1. Infraventricular sections. *A,* Scan extends through the orbital roof, sphenoid bone, dorsum sella and petrous bone. The basilar artery is seen in the prepontine cistern. The midline triangular-shaped fourth ventricle is seen in the posterior fossa. *B,* Slightly higher post-contrast section shows a normal circle of Willis. Tips of temporal horns are seen in the middle fossa.

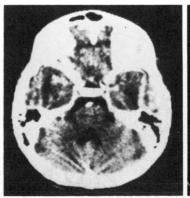
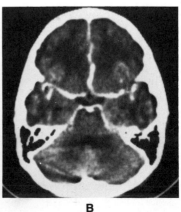

A

B

magnum. The cisterna magna is the most posterior and inferior cisternal space. It is usually a small midline hypodense triangular or ovoid-shaped structure appearing contiguous with the occipital bone. In some cases it may appear asymmetrical. It has variable width and may extend above the tentorium. The vallecula extends from the cisterna magna to the fourth ventricle. An enlarged (mega) cisterna magna may simulate a posterior cyst, but delineation of this normal variant is usually possible even without metrizamide cisternogram (Fig. 4–2). Mega cisterna magna does not distort the fourth ventricle or basal cisterns, and this structure does not cause hydrocephalus.[3]

The fourth ventricle is a triangular-shaped hypodense structure located in the midline of the posterior fossa. Because of the triangular shape of this ventricle and the tangential scanning plane through it, its size and appearance may vary. Lateral recesses of the fourth ventricle (foramina of Luschka) are identified as posterior extensions from the base of the triangularly shaped ventricle. Hypodense fanlike structures extending anterolaterally from the fourth ventricle represent cerebellar white matter. The fourth ventricular floor is covered by choroid plexus and is indented by the cerebellar nodulus and inferior vermis. These cerebellar structures appear hyperdense on plain scan; they may enhance (see contrast pseudotumors) following contrast administration. The inferior cerebellar cistern may appear as a hypodense midline structure, which may be misinterpreted as the fourth ventricle. The brain stem appears as a round mottled hyperdense structure anterior to the fourth ventricle and posterior to the dorsum sella and the pontine or interpeduncular cistern. The pontomedullary region is separated from the cerebellum by ambient cisterns that extend laterally into the cerebellopontine angle (CPA) cistern. At the pontine level, the anterior brain stem border is formed by the prepontine cistern. This cistern may be located directly behind the dorsum sella.

CPA cisterns are hypodense thin linear bands directly underneath the petrous pyramids. They may be indented by hyperdense nodules that represent cerebellar flocculus.[4] This structure may simulate acoustic tumor. Symmetrical jugular tubercles appear as calcified masses contiguous with petrous bones. If bone settings are utilized, internal acoustic canals may be assessed. Lateral cerebellar hemispheres have a homogeneous mottled hyperdense appearance relative to lateral cistern

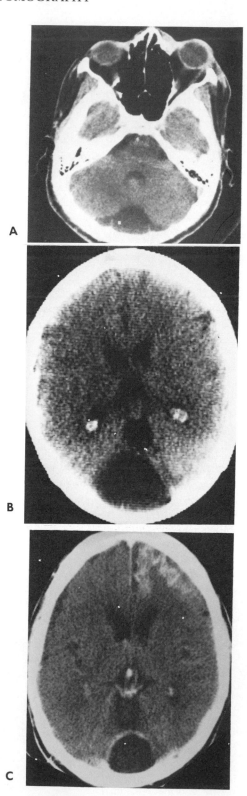

Figure 4–2. Mega cisterna magna. *A*, Triangular-shaped hypodense midline structure with normal-sized fourth ventricle. *B*, Round hypodense structure with supratentorial extension and *C*, there is enhancement in the surrounding dura. There is gyral enhancement in distribution of anterior cerebral artery.

and medial white matter. If there is cerebellar atrophy, horizontal fissures separating cerebellar folia appear as parallel horizontal bands extending across the posterior fossa. A linear horizontal hypodense band may extend across the brain stem region; this represents a well-recognized and constant artifact (Hounsfield bar).

The pituitary fossa (Fig. 4–3) and the suprasellar cistern (Fig. 4–4) are well visualized in axial sections; however, coronal and sagittal sections provide important supplemental data, including delineation of the pituitary gland. Paired hyperdense (calcified) round structures in the anterior portion of the pituitary fossa represent anterior clinoids, and sometimes planum sphenoidale is seen medial to the clinoids; a posterior horizontal hyperdense band represents the dorsum sella. These structures should not be confused with pathological juxtasellar calcifications. The pituitary gland is visualized poorly in axial section but is well visualized in coronal sections (Fig. 4–5). The pituitary fossa usually appears hypodense. This may reflect contributions from three types of structures: intrasellar CSF spaces, sphenoid sinus air cells and suprasellar cisterns. The pituitary gland appears isodense or hyperdense; its normal height is 2.6 to 6.7 mm. Its superior surface is outlined by CSF and appears flat; its inferior surface consists of sphenoid sinus roof. The pituitary fossa merges laterally with the caverous sinus, anterior clinoids and carotid artery.[7] The pituitary infundibulum is seen best on enhanced scan due to the hyperdense enhancing vascular plexus. This structure appears on axial sections as a round mass within the pituitary fossa or as a linear vertical band extending to the infundibular recess of the third ventricle on coronal sections.[8] The cavernous sinus is visualized on enhanced scan as symmetrical vertically oriented bands lateral to the pituitary fossa. Three round hypodense regions may sometimes be seen within the cavernous sinus. These represent cranial nerves (abducens, oculomotor, trochlear).[9]

The suprasellar (optic chiasmal) cistern is located directly above the pituitary fossa.[5] It is pentagonal or hexagonal in shape. The anterior border is formed by frontal lobes; this indentation creates a bilobed appearance. The cistern of lamina terminalis originates from the anterior interhemispheric fissure. An anterior-lateral extension of the suprasellar cistern is formed by the middle cerebral artery cistern

extending to the sylvian cistern. The lateral perimeter of the suprasellar cistern is formed by the temporal lobe (uncus). If the interpeduncular cistern forms the posterior border of

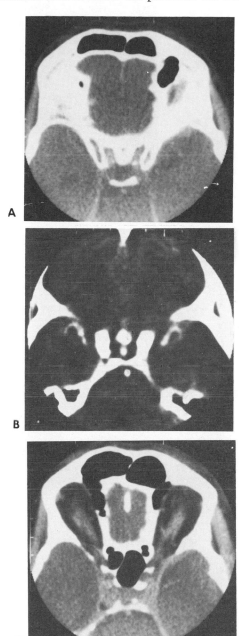

Figure 4–3. Pituitary fossa. *A,* Clinoid processes are dense structures lateral to the pituitary fossa. The dorsum sella is a dense horizontal band; the planum sphenoidale is a midline anterior structure. *B,* The pituitary gland is homogeneous round enhancing intrasellar structure. The basilar artery is seen behind the dorsum sella. *C,* Cavernous sinus appears as dense homogeneous enhancing linear bands lateral to the pituitary fossa.

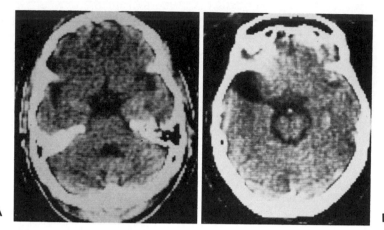

Figure 4–4. Suprasellar cistern. *A,* Pentagonal shape intersecting the pons. *B,* Hexagonal shape intersecting the midbrain.

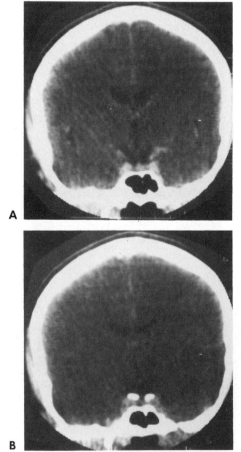

Figure 4–5. Coronal sections of the pituitary fossa. *A,* The pituitary gland has a dense linear horizontal band that merges laterally with the cavernous sinus. The carotid arteries are superior, and the middle cerebral arteries extend laterally. *B,* More anteriorly, the sella floor is seen with the sphenoid sinus inferiorly. Anterior clinoids are seen laterally.

the supresellar cistern, this perimeter appears bilobed because of the shape of the cerebral peduncles of midbrain; therefore, the suprasellar cistern appears hexagonal. The posterior edge is flat if the scan section intersects the pons; the suprasellar cistern therefore appears pentagonal. Paired optic nerves are visualized as hyperdense symmetrical paramedian round structures within the anterior suprasellar cistern. Optic chiasm appears V-shaped and hyperdense behind the optic nerves.

The perimeter of suprasellar cistern is well-outlined on enhanced scan by major vascular channels. The internal carotid arteries are located at anterolateral points. They may appear symmetrical or asymmetrical. The significance of slight asymmetries may be difficult to assess. The middle cerebral arteries extend laterally into the sylvian cistern; the anterior cerebral arteries outline the anterior suprasellar region. The infundibular vascular plexus appears as a round enhancing structure in the anterior midline suprasellar region. The basilar artery is located posterior to the suprasellar cistern behind the dorsum sella within the prepontine or interpeduncular cistern; however, with certain degrees of angulation, the basilar artery may appear to be located within the posterior portion of the suprasellar cistern. The posterior cerebral arteries originate from the basilar artery. They extend posterolaterally around the brain stem.

The brain stem appears as a round midline structure. It has a mottled (salt and pepper), hyperdense appearance. The pons is located between the fourth ventricle and the prepon-

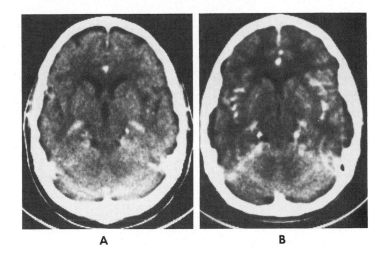

Figure 4–6. Low ventricular section. *A,* This includes frontal horns, third ventricle (anterior and midportion) and quadrigeminal cistern. The anterior cerebral artery is seen in the midline frontal region. *B,* Similar section showing insular branches of the middle cerebral artery in the sylvian cistern.

A   **B**

tine cistern. It is separated from the cerebellum by ambient cistern. The pons appears homogeneous, whereas the midbrain is more heterogeneous with a central hypodense region believed to represent cerebellar decussation.[10]

Low Ventricular Anatomy (Fig. 4–6). These sections include infra- and supratentorial structures. Infratentorial structures are medial and supratentorial structures are lateral to the tentorial leaves (Fig. 4–7). The inferior temporal gyrus is situated directly lateral to the tentorium; the middle and superior temporal gyri are more anteriorly located. The inferior frontal gyrus is located anterior to the superior temporal gyrus. At this level the sylvian fissure has a comma or Y-shaped configuration. The frontal lobes are separated by a midline linear hypodense band representing interhemis-

pheric fissure. The frontal horns and the anterior portions of the bodies of the lateral ventricles appear as symmetrical right-angled triangular structures. These portions of lateral ventricles are separated by a thin band representing the septum pellucidum. Cavities (cava) may occur within the septum pellucidum in several locations. Those cava located anterior to the fornices are cava septi pellucidi; those that are posterior, cava vergae (Fig. 4–8). These cava are normal anatomical variants without clinical significance and no associated ventricular enlargement; however, cysts may also develop in these locations.

Corpus callosal fibers are anterior to the frontal horns, but they are not directly visualized by CT. The caudate indents the lateral wall of the ventricular body. This surface is concave. The anterior limb of the internal

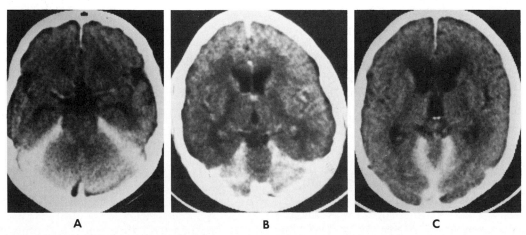

A   **B**   **C**

Figure 4–7. Tentorial anatomy. *A,* Section below the tentorium showing diverging enhancing bands. *B,* Level at the tentorium showing M-shaped configuration. *C,* Level above the tentorium showing Y-shaped configuration.

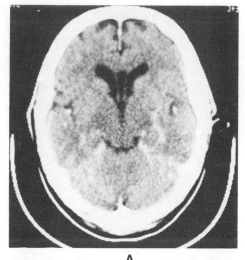

A

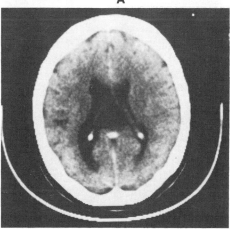

B

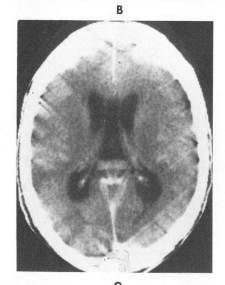

C

Figure 4–8. Ventricular cavum. *A*, Well-delineated cavum septum pellucidum separating the lateral ventricles. *B*, Cavum vergae involving the posterior third located posterior to the fornix. *C*, Intraventricular blood in the cavum vergae and occipital horns.

capsule separates the head of caudate from the lenticular nucleus (putamen, globus pallidus). The third ventricle appears as an elongated tubular structure (3 to 8 mm in width). It is wider in the posterior than in the anterior region. The upper brain stem appears directly posterior to the third ventricle. The superior colliculi create a bilobed indentation into the quadrigeminal cistern. Ambient cistern wings extend laterally from the quadrigeminal cistern. The temporal horns are seen as slit-like or comma-shaped hypodense structures pointing medially in the middle fossa. They are not always visualized in normal persons; however, with zero degree angulation they are more frequently seen. The choroid plexus is seen inferior to the temporal horn on enhanced scan. The junction of the temporal horn with the trigone atrium is seen on higher sections.

The next higher ventricular section shows the pineal body (Fig. 4–9). This structure is located within the quadrigeminal cistern. The pineal is usually visualized as a hyperdense structure even if it is not calcified. The superior vermis and midbrain are medial to the tentorial leaves and posterior to the quadrigeminal cistern. The lateral occipital gyrus is located lateral to the tentorium. The inferior, middle and superior temporal gyri extend anteriorly to the sylvian fissure; the frontal lobes are seen anteriorly. The frontal horn and bodies of the lateral ventricles have a similar appearance to that visualized on lower sections. The intraventricular foramina are visualized at this level. The anterior limb of the internal capsule separates the caudate and lenticular nucleus; the genu and posterior limb separate the lenticular nucleus and thalamus.

A more superior section demonstrates the junction of the posterior third ventricle and the quadrigeminal cistern.[11] The third ventricle becomes bulbous and diamond-shaped as it merges with the quadrigeminal cistern. The lateral borders of the third ventricle are formed by thalami. The massa intermedia is a commissural gray-matter bundle between two halves of thalamus. This appears as a hyperdense mass separating the anterior and posterior third ventricle. The walls of the third ventricle diverge posteriorly to form a triangle. At this level the quadrigeminal cistern is triangular; therefore, the junction of the third ventricle and the quadrigeminal cistern appears diamond-shaped. The telea choroidea may be seen as a thin band separating the third ventricle from the quadrigeminal cistern. The retrothalamic cistern extends laterally

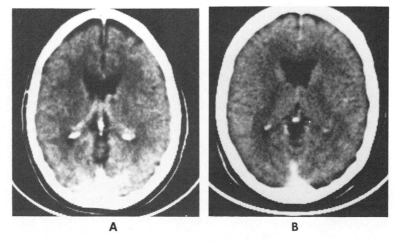

Figure 4–9. Third ventricle. *A,* This structure appears as a linear band as it originates from the anterior third ventricle and widens posteriorly. *B,* Diamond-shaped confluence with quadrigeminal cistern. This contains hyperdense pineal body. The superior cerebellar cistern is posterior. *C,* Choroid plexus of the third ventricle densely enhances. *D,* Paired internal cerebral veins are seen at the intraventricular foramen, and basal veins of Rosenthal are seen at the lateral border of the quadrigeminal cistern.

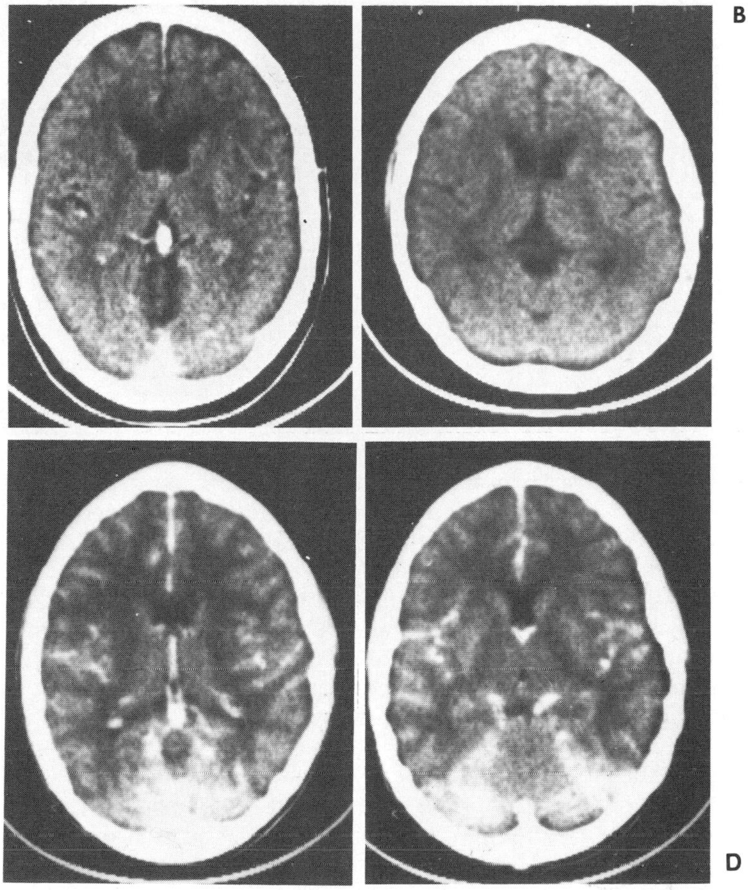

from the quadrigeminal cistern, and the superior cerebellar cistern is posterior to the quadrigeminal cistern. The cavum velum interpositum represents rostral (anterior) extension of the quadrigeminal cistern.

The lateral ventricle may appear as two separate regions at this level (Fig. 4–10). The frontal horns and body are anterior; the trigone and occipital horns are posterior. Glomeruli of the choroid plexus are dense regions seen within the lateral ventricle, the left portion being located posterior to the right. The internal capsule is most completely visualized at this level.[12] It includes anterior limb, lying

Figure 4–10. Midventricular level. *A,* Frontal horns are seen anteriorly and atrium-occipital horns are seen posteriorly. Choroid plexus is seen in the occipital horn. *B,* The internal capsule is seen as a hypodense region (anterior and posterior limb, genu).

A   B

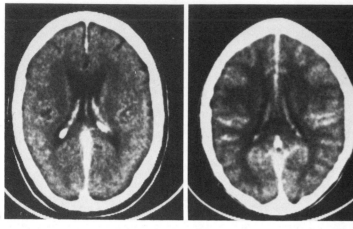

Figure 4–11. High ventricular level. *A*, Section shows body and occipital horns of the lateral ventricle. *B*, Posteriorly, vein of Galen and straight sinus drain into the confluence of the sinus. Choroid plexus densely enhances.

between the caudate and lenticular nucleus; the genu and posterior limb, lying between the lenticular nucleus and thalamus; and the retrolenticular portion, extending posterior to the lenticular nucleus and around the trigone. The posterior limb is less dense than other portions of the internal capsule; therefore, care must be exercised because not all posterior capsular hypodensities represent lacunae. The superior capsular portion passes lateral to the roof of the lateral ventricle at the junction with the corona radiata. Inferiorly, the internal capsule and cerebral peduncle junction is not seen. The insular cortex is lateral to the internal capsule; the sylvian cistern is lateral to the insula and is separated by the external capsule.[13]

High Ventricular Anatomy (Fig. 4–11). At this level the bodies of the lateral ventricles are continuous posteriorly with the occipital horns. The body of the caudate appears as a thin hyperdense band at the lateral edge of the ventricular bodies. Scalloped-edged irregularly marginated hypodensities of the corona radiata are seen lateral to the ventricles. The ventricular bodies are separated by the corpus callosum. Anterior to the corpus callosum is the interhemispheric fissure, which separates the frontal lobes. The posterior corpus callosum causes divergence of the lateral ventricles.[14]

The posterior interhemispheric fissure is located behind the corpus callosum; this structure separates the occipital lobes. The occipital horns may vary from small tent-like structures, which project from the trigone posteriorly, to well-developed finger-like projections extending to within 1 to 2 cm of the occipital bone. The occipital tips are rounded, bulbous, flared or tapered in shape. The calcar avis may

appear as hyperdense masses projecting into the medial wall of the occipital horn.

The central and sylvian fissures are constant landmarks. The frontal lobe comprises the region from the central sulcus to the interhemispheric fissure. This includes the precentral gyrus and the superior and middle frontal gyri. The parietal lobe (somesthetic cortex and anterior angular gyrus) is located between the central and sylvian fissures. The lateral hemispheric border includes the angular gyrus, parietal-occipital cortex and lateral occipital gyrus; the medial hemisphere consists of the calcarine cortex.

Superaventricular Anatomy (Fig. 4–12). The central region is represented by hypodense subcortical white matter and is surrounded by cortical gray matter. The interhemispheric fissure extends continuously from the anterior to the posterior region. A hyper-

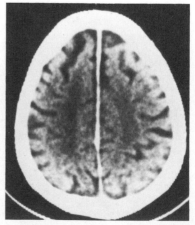

Figure 4–12. Supraventricular level. Section shows dense linear band representing falx and hypodense white matter. Sulcal spaces are well-visualized.

dense vertical band within the interhemispheric fissure represents falx. It is seen on both noncontrast and enhanced scans.[15] The lateral cerebral convexity is divided by the central sulcus. At this level the frontal lobe represents a small portion, with the major surface being parietal lobe. Vertex sections are angulated such that the parietal region projects quite far forward to comprise approximately three quarters of cortex scan at this level.

Postcontrast Anatomy[16]

ARTERIES. Normal arterial structures are rarely seen on nonenhanced scan; however, ectatic (vertebral-basilar, carotid) or calcified arteries may be visualized. On enhanced scan, major arteries are visualized.

Internal carotid arteries appear as round enhancing structures in the anterolateral suprasellar cistern. Middle cerebral arteries extend laterally to terminate in the sylvian cistern. Insular branches of the middle cerebral artery appear as round or curvilinear vertically oriented hyperdensities within the sylvian cisterns. The horizontal portion of the anterior cerebral arteries extends medially along the anterior suprasellar cistern. They take a 90° turn in the lamina terminalis cistern, and at this level the junction of the anterior cerebral and the anterior communicating arteries may be visualized. As these latter vessels curve around the corpus callosum, they are perpendicular to the scanning plane. They appear as round enhancing structures in the interhemispheric fissure. The basilar artery appears as a round enhancing mass within the interpeduncular or prepontine cistern. Paired posterior cerebral arteries extend posterolaterally around the midbrain. Vertebral arteries are paired at the foramen magnum; they diverge laterally into the cerebellopontine angle cisterns. The posterior inferior cerebellar arteries may be seen in the fourth ventricular floor.

VEINS. The thalamostriate veins appear as linear hyperdensities located anterolateral to the lateral ventricular choroid plexus. They curve medially through the intraventricular foramina to merge with the internal cerebral vein in the third ventricular roof. Paired internal cerebral veins appear as hyperdense round structures located at the intraventricular foramina. They course posteriorly through the third ventricular roof to join the vein of Galen. Caudate veins are lateral to the thalamostriate vein. The posterior portion of the basal veins of Rosenthal appear as linear hyperdensities passing posteromedially toward the third ventricular–quadrigeminal cistern to join the vein of Galen located in the superior quadrigeminal cistern. This vein appears as a round hyperdensity within the quadrigeminal cistern or tentorial apex. The vein of Galen drains into the straight sinus. The transverse (lateral) sinuses and the straight sinus drain into the confluence of sinus (torcular). This appears as a triangular hyperdensity with its base at the occipital protuberance.

DURA. Dural folds of the falx and tentorium may be visualized on plain scan and are better visualized on enhanced study. The falx appears as a vertically oriented linear band. The posterior segment of falx extends from the calvarium to the splenium of the corpus callosum; the intervening interhemispheric fissure is quite small. The anterior falx is thin, and the interhemispheric fissure is wider. The supracallosal portion (above the free edge of the falx) is seen as a continuous linear band. The tentorium delineates the supra- and infratentorial compartments on axial and coronal sections.[17] At the level below the torcular, tentorial bands diverge laterally toward attachment at the transverse sinuses. On a section obtained above the torcular, the tentorial leaves converge superiorly and medially toward the straight sinus to create a Y-shaped configuration of tentorium. If a section is obtained at the level of the torcular, the tentorial leaves have M-shaped configuration on it. Lateral uprights appear as diverging bands; the medial portion is V-shaped. In scans obtained at zero degree angulation, full extent of the tentorium is seen, extending from the anterior clinoids to the anterior portion of the straight sinus at the incisural apex. The midbrain and superior vermis are medial to the tentorial leaves. The inferior temporal cortex is lateral to the diverging tentorial leaves; the occipital cortex is lateral and posterior to the V-shaped tentorium.

CHOROID PLEXUS. The choroid of the lateral ventricular body extends from the intraventricular foramina to the glomus behind the thalamus. This choroid densely enhances. It is contiguous with deep veins that appear thinner and more sharply marginated. The choroid plexus glomeruli are located in the trigone and are usually calcified. The choroid of the temporal horn appears as crescent-shaped hyperdensities. The third ventricular choroid is located in the roof and appears as a vertical hyperdense band. The fourth ventricular choroid appears as a horizontal band in the posterior-inferior region.

CONTRAST PSEUDOTUMORS (Fig. 4–13). Nodular enhancement directly posterior and inferior to the fourth ventricle may originate from vermis, tonsils, or choroid plexus.[18] Enhancement within the CPA cistern may represent flocculus. Absense of mass effect effectively excludes posterior fossa mass. Hyperdensities and enhancement characteristics of the choroid plexus of the lateral and third ventricles may simulate intraventricular tumor, e.g., colloid cyst. Enhancement of the tentorium and the temporal horn choroid may be contiguous to create a ring blush. This blush may be unilateral if the patient has been asymmetrically positioned. An M-shaped tentorial enhancement may simulate that seen in inflammatory or neoplastic disorders. Cavernous sinus enhancement may be asymmetrical to simulate a parasellar pathological process. Subependymal venous enhancement may simulate periventricular neoplastic or inflammatory disorders. Subcortical gray matter structures (caudate, lenticular nucleus, thalamus) are hyperdense compared with contiguous CSF spaces and the internal capsule. They show a slight normal attenuation increase on enhanced scan.[19]

Orbital Anatomy (see Chapter 14). Orbital detail may be well delineated if thin sections and coronal reconstructions are utilized. The following structures should be analyzed; (1) paranasal sinuses, (2) face and orbital bone, (3) globe, (4) optic nerve, (5) extraocular muscles, (6) retro-orbital fat, (7) lacrimal gland, (8) superior ophthalmic vein, (9) middle fossa, (10) frontal lobe and (11) parasellar region. In most cases, noncontrast scan provides accurate diagnostic information; however, if parasellar extension of the lesion is suspected, enhanced scan is necessary.

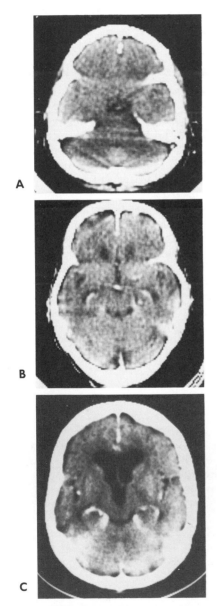

Figure 4–13. Contrast pseudotumors. *A*, Vermian enhancement. *B*, Temporal horn enhancement. *C*, Pseudoring due to choroid plexus of the temporal horn and tentorium.

REFERENCES

1. Huckman MS, Grainer LS, Clasen RC: The normal computed tomogram. Semin Roentgenol 12:27, 1977
2. Gado M, Hanaway J, Frank R: Functional anatomy of the cerebral cortex by computed tomography. Comput Assist Tomogr 3:1–19, 1979
3. Adam R, Greenberg JD: The mega cisterna magna. J Neurosurg 48:190–192, 1978
4. Daniels DL, Houghton VM, Williams AL: The flocculus in computed tomography. Am J Neuroradiol 2:227–229, 1981
5. Kuuliala I: The normal suprasellar space in computed tomography. Clin Radiol 31:155–159, 1980
6. Earnest F, McCullough E, Frank DA: Fact or artifact: an analysis of artifact in high resolution computed tomographic scanning of the sella. Radiology 140:109–113, 1981
7. Syvertsen A, Haughton VM, Williams AL: The computed tomographic appearance of the normal pituitary gland and pituitary microadenomas. Radiology 133:385–391, 1979
8. Hayman LA, Evans RA, Hinck VC: Rapid high dose (RHD) contrast computed tomography of perisellar vessels. Radiology 131:121–123, 1979

9. Kline LB, Acker JD, Post JDM: The cavernous sinus: a computed tomographic study. Am J Neuroradiol 2:299–305, 1981
10. Berns TF, Daniels DL, Williams AL: Mesencephalic anatomy: demonstration by computed tomography. Am J Neuroradiol 2:65–67, 1981
11. Messina AV, Potts DG, Sigel RM: Computed tomography evaluation of the posterior third ventricle. Radiology 119:581, 1976
12. Manelfe C, Clanet M, Gigaud M: Internal capsule; normal anatomy and ischemic changes demonstrated by CT. J Neuroradiol 2:149–155, 1981
13. Bierney JP, Komar NN: The sylvian cistern on computed tomography scanning. Comput Assist Tomogr 1:227–230, 1977
14. Wing SD, Osborn AG: Normal and pathologic anatomy of the corpus callosum by CT. Comput Axial Tomogr 1:183–192, 1977
15. Zimmerman RD, Yurberg E, Russell EJ: Falx and interhemispheric fissure on axial CT: 1. Normal anatomy. Am J Neuroradiol 3:175–180, 1982
16. Naidich TP, Pudlowski RM, Leeds NE: The normal contrast-enhanced computed axial tomogram of the brain. J Comput Assist Tomogr 1:16–29, 1977
17. Naidich TP, Leeds NE, Kricheff II et al: The tentorium in axial section. 1. Normal CT appearance and non-neoplastic pathology. Radiology 123:631, 1977
18. Kramer RA: Vermian pseudotumor: a potential pitfall of CT brain scanning with contrast enhancement. Neuroradiology 13:229, 1977
19. Osborn AG, Saville T: The basal ganglia on cranial computed tomography: normal anatomy and pathology. Comput Axial Tomogr 1:245–255, 1977

Part II

Evaluation of Specific Neurological Symptoms and Signs

Chapter 5

PROGRESSIVE NEUROLOGICAL DEFICIT

Localization of Lesions

FRONTAL

These lesions cause distinctive symptoms: (1) lateral convexity lesions present with focal motor or sensory seizures; (2) parasagittal lesions present with seizures and contralateral leg monoparesis; (3) basal-inferior lesions present with behavioral and personality disturbances, dementia, olfactory disturbances and papilledema; (4) bifrontal and corpus callosal lesions present with seizures, dementia, gait disorder and urinary incontinence. The combined findings of dementia and prominent primitive (release) reflexes such as suck, snout, grasp, and palmomental are most likely caused by frontal lesions. Middle and superior frontal gyral lesions are frequently associated with apathy, lethargy and confusional states; basal frontal lesions may cause excitement, psychosis and hallucinosis. If a frontal lesion causes gait and balance dysfunction, this may falsely suggest cerebellar disorder.[1]

Superficial frontal lesions may cause unilateral continuous high-voltage slow wave EEG pattern; whereas deep infiltrating tumors may cause bilateral polymorphic or monorhythmic slow wave pattern or cause no EEG abnormalities. Frontal masses show characteristic angiographic findings: proximal shift of the anterior cerebral artery, slight shift of the internal cerebral vein, posterior displacement of the anterior sylvian triangle vessels, posterior displacement and closing of the venous angle and a frontal mass that may be avascular (because of displacement and compression of normal vessels) or highly vascular (because of neovascularity). It is usually possible to differentiate between extra- and intra-axial lesions and to demonstrate the presence of abnormal vascularity. With CT, it is possible to obtain complementary information regarding the location.

Infarction

Anterior or middle cerebral artery occlusion may cause ischemia or infarction in the frontal region. CT shows a sharply marginated hypodense lesion. This lesion is rectangular- or triangular-shaped and conforms to specific vascular territories. There is usually minimal mass effect. Enhancement may occur in a superficial gray matter gyral pattern.

Intra-axial Lesions

Malignant Neoplasms. Most common lesions include metastases and gliomas. These lesions show frond-like hypodense projections extending into the deep white matter representing edema; however, gray-white interface is not inwardly (medially) deviated. Anterior frontal horns may be effaced and displaced (contralaterally and posteriorly), and there may be subfalcine herniation. The density pattern of these lesions is usually mixed and heterogeneous, reflecting pathological features of malignant neoplasms. These lesions usually enhance more densely with thicker rim on a ventricular than on a cortical surface (Fig. 5–1). The characteristic finding of intra-axial lesions is that enhancement thickens and widens anterior frontal horns, septi pellucidi and corpus callosum. Ruptured anterior cerebral–anterior communicating artery aneurysms may result in caval and septal hematoma that widens septi pellucidi and separates frontal horns; however, septal thickening and wid-

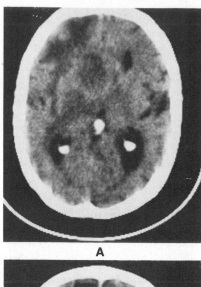

A

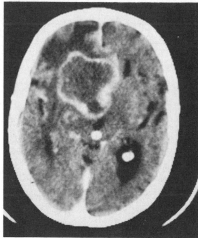

B

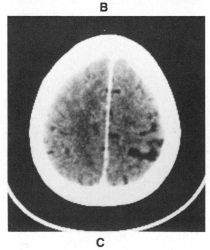

C

Figure 5–1. An 80-year-old man developed personality change. Findings were organic dementia and right pronator drift. *CT findings:* left frontal heterogeneous mixed-density lesion (A) with variable thickness ring enhancement extending across the corpus callosum (B). Left cortical spaces are effaced (C). *Operative finding:* glioblastoma multiforme.

ening of malignant neoplasms is specific only if present on enhanced study.[2]

Cerebritis and Abscess. These inflammatory lesions appear hypodense and round on plain scan; there is a thin, faintly hyperdense rim that enhances on postcontrast scan. Enhancement is usually thin and regular; it appears thicker on the peripheral cortical surface than on the white matter–ventricular surface (Fig. 5–2). There may be contiguous satellite nodular enhancing lesions; this is consistent with daughter abscesses. Subependymal enhancement caused by ependymitis and ventriculitis may simulate paraventricular tumor extension.

Intracerebral Hematoma. These appear as hyperdense noncalcified lesions. These are round or triangular in configuration with sharp margination. They may extend deeply into white matter and appear to point toward the ventricular surface. Frontal hematomas, which result from ruptured aneurysms, may show blood in the bifrontal, interhemispheric and caval-septal regions.

Extra-axial Lesions

Neoplasms. Meningiomas are commonly located in the subfrontal or falx region. They may be contiguous with bone or falx. Thickening of falx adjacent to the tumor is consistent with extra-axial lesion; however, falx thickening is sometimes also seen in gliomas and metastases. Meningiomas cause falx to be buckled posteriorly; and frontal horns, the septi pellicudi and callosal region are posteriorly displaced. Meningiomas are sharply marginated, regular in shape and usually homogeneous in density on plain scan and enhancement pattern. There is a usually thin hypodense surrounding rim (Fig. 5–3).

Extracerebral Hematoma and Empyema

These lesions are subdural or epidural in location. Epidural lesions extend across the midline and cause posterior falx bowing. They are usually well-circumscribed and lenticular-shaped. Subdural lesion extension is limited by dural membrane; therefore, these lesions do not cross the midline. These lesions are semilunar or lenticular-shaped and appear contiguous with bone. Dural membrane is sometimes seen on plain scan but is best delineated on enhanced scan.

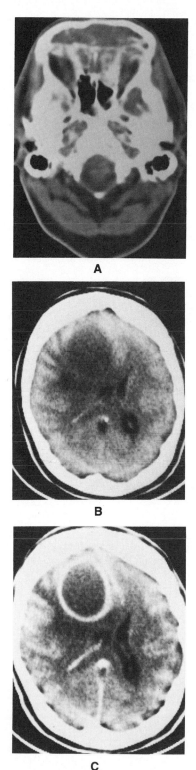

Figure 5–2. A 48-year-old acromegalic with chronic frontal sinusitis developed headache and left-sided weakness. *CT findings:* frontal sinus opacification (A) and left frontal hypodense sharply marginated lesion (B) with homogeneous peripheral rim enhancement (C). *Operative finding:* brain abscess.

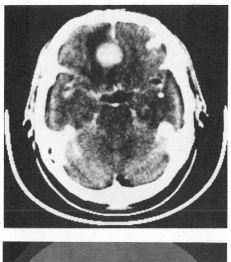

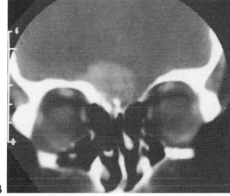

Figure 5–3. A 52-year-old woman who had a surgically excised melanoma developed anosmia. *CT findings:* subfrontal and sphenoid noncalcified enhancing lesion (A). The lesion is well delineated on coronal projection (B).

PARIETAL LESIONS

Superficial lesions may cause focal motor or sensory seizures. Characteristic symptoms include numbness or electrical-like or pins-and-needles sensation. Deep parietal lesions may cause painful sensations, including hyperpathia. Dominant hemispheric parietal lesions may cause aphasic disturbances or Gerstmann syndrome (right-left confusion, finger agnosia, agraphia, acalculia). Nondominant parietal lesions cause disorders of body schema perception, denial of illness and contructional apraxia. Visual field defect consisting of inferior homonymous quadrantanopsia is characteristic of parietal lesions.[3] Angiographic findings in parietal masses include: (1) distal shift of the pericallosal artery, (2) shift of the internal cerebral vein, (3) downward displacement of the sylvian triangle, (4) stretching of parietal arteries, (5) opening of the venous angle and (6) hypo- or hypervascular mass. With CT, it is usually possible to differentiate ischemic infarction from neoplasms and angiomas without angiography.

Vascular Ischemia and Infarction

With middle cerebral artery infarction, CT shows a sharply marginated wedge-shaped hypodense parietal lesion. Enhancement may occur in gray matter (superficial gyral or deep nuclear) regions with relative sparing of white matter. In infarcted areas, enhancement is most intense when mass effect is minimal, whereas in neoplasms, enhancement is present when mass effect is quite prominent. Isodense enhancing ischemic lesions may simulate some vascular malformations because both these lesions may cause minimal mass effect; however, follow-up CT shows decreased enhancement in ischemic lesions.

Intra-axial Lesions

Neoplasms. Malignant neoplams (glioma, metastases) consist of mixed density pattern and show heterogeneous enhancement. There are frond-like hypodense projections extending into white matter. The mass causes contralateral displacement of the lateral ventricle and may cause subfalcine herniation. Gray–white matter interface is not medically displaced; however, sulcal spaces may be effaced.

Non-neoplastic Lesions. Intracerebral hematomas are uncommon in this location; and their occurrence suggests underlying neoplasm or angioma. These hematomas do not usually extend into the ventricles. The CT findings of cerebritis and abscess cannot always be differentiated from malignant intra-axial lesions.

Extra-axial Lesions

These lesions cause medial (inward) displacement of gray–white matter border. Parietal and convexity meningiomas appear as sharply marginated isodense or hyperdense lesions. They are round or lenticular-shaped and contiguous with bone. They enhance in a dense homogeneous pattern. They may cause bone erosion. Because of their peripheral location and tendency to cause underlying cerebral atrophy, they produce less mass effect than intra-axial lesions. Meningiomas may simulate thrombosed angiomas or aneurysms. Subdural or epidural lesions are semilunar or lenticular-shaped. The gray–white matter interface is inwardly displaced by these lesions.

TEMPORAL LESIONS

Temporal lesions may be intra-axial (hematoma, abscess, glioma, metastases) or extra-axial (middle fossa or sphenoid wing meningioma, subtemporal subdural hematoma, epidermoid cyst [Fig. 5–4], subarachnoid cyst [Fig. 5–5], laterally extending juxtasellar lesion or supratentorial extension of incisural tumor). Symptoms of temporal lobe lesions

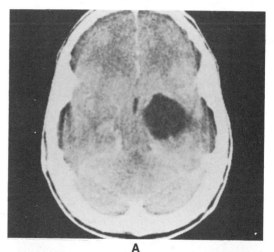

A

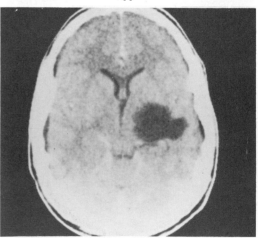

B

Figure 5–4. A 21-year-old man had one seizure. EEG showed right temporal spike focus; angiogram showed a temporal avascular mass. *CT findings:* irregularly marginated hypodense (A) nonenhancing medial temporal mass with elevation of the third ventricle (B). *Operative finding:* epidermoid cyst.

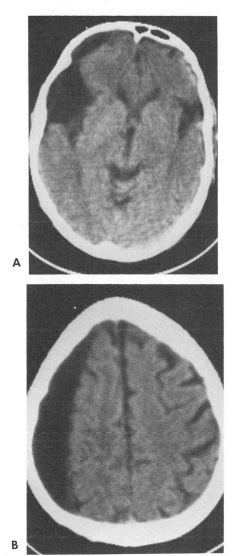

Figure 5–5. A 30-year-old man developed headache. Findings were right pronator drift and Babinski sign. EEG showed left temporal delta activity. Angiogram showed a temporal intracerebral mass. *CT findings*: temporal subarachnoid cyst (A) and convexity subdural hematoma with effacement of cortical sulcal spaces (B).

are psychomotor seizures, aphasia, and superior homonymous quadrantanopsia. Visual field defect is characteristic of intra-axial temporal lesions; trigeminal sensory disturbances suggest an extra-axial middle fossa lesion. The finding of unilateral or bilateral temporal EEG slowing or spike discharges may sometimes reflect the presence of a lesion located remote to the temporal region. Isotope scan uptake cause by temporal fossa lesions may be obscured by overlying temporalis muscle. Extra-axial temporal angiographic findings include

elevation and medial displacement of the middle cerebral artery, medial displacement of the anterior choriodal artery, and midline shift of both the anterior cerebral artery and internal cerebral vein. Intra-axial temporal angiographic abnormalities include superior displacement of the sylvian triangle, lateral displacement of the middle cerebral vessels, midline shift of the internal cerebral vein and elevation, stretching and draping of superficial vessels around the mass.

The limitations of angiography in this situation are that the location of the mass relative to the temporal horn is not defined, and that the paucity of inferior temporal superficial vessels makes it difficult to differentiate between extra- and intra-axial locations.

With CT, intra-axial temporal lesions show these features: (1) ovoid or round shape, (2) no evidence of bone erosion, (3) frond-like projections representing edema and (4) effacement of temporal horn and sylvian cistern. There may be distortion and effacement of the lateral suprasellar cistern surface that represents transtentorial herniation. Hematomas and abscesses may extend into the temporal horn. Extra-axial temporal lesions may cause the enlargement of the middle fossa, middle fossa bone erosion and displacement of the sylvian fissure and temporal horn. Coronal sections may be necessary to differentiate between extra- and intra-axial temporal lesions.

OCCIPITAL LESIONS

Homonymous hemianopsia is characteristic of occipital lesions; however, visual fields may be normal with lateral occipital surface lesions. Focal visual seizures are common symptoms. Intra-axial occipital lesions include gliomas and metastases; less common lesions include angiomas, abscesses, porencephalic cysts and hematomas. Meningiomas are common extra-axial lesions. Vascular occlusion in posterior cerebral artery distribution may cause occipital lobe ischemia or infarction. With occipital lesions, EEG shows suppression of normal alpha rhythm or polymorphic delta pattern. Angiographic findings of occipital lesions include normal position of the anterior cerebral artery, significant shift of the internal cerebral vein, anterior displacement of the sylvian triangle, opening of the venous angle and avascular or neovascular mass.[4]

With CT, extra-axial lesions may show these

features: (1) posterior falx thickening, (2) forward bowing of posterior portion of falx, (3) occipital bone erosion, (4) anterior displacement of occipital horn, (5) anterior displacement of gray–white matter interface and (6) regular-shaped and sharp margination. Intra-axial lesions may show these CT abnormalities: (1) extension into the splenium of the corpus callosum as manifested by enhancement of this structure (Fig. 5–6), (2) subependymal occipital horn enhancement, (3) effacement without displacement of gray–white matter interface, (4) jagged-edged margination, irregular shape and heterogeneous enhancement. In vascular infarction the hypodense region is sharply marginated; however, the gray matter gyral enhancement pattern may be serpentine and tortuous. This may extend into the thalamic and the inferior and posterior temporal regions.

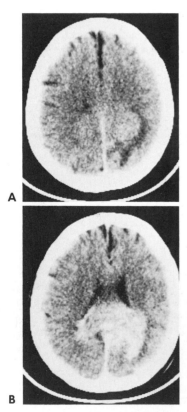

Figure 5–6. This 50-year-old man developed confusional episodes and memory loss. *CT findings:* mixed-density right occipital lesion (*A*) with heterogeneous enhancement extending across the splenium of the corpus callosum (*B*). *Operative finding:* Grade III glioma.

CORPUS CALLOSUM LESIONS

Lesions include gliomas, metastases and lipomas. Gliomas primarily originate from or secondarily invade the corpus callosum. The majority arise from the anterior callosal region. They may grow into the cingulate gyrus and thicken the septi pellucidi; they may grow unilaterally into the cerebral hemispheres. Posterior callosal gliomas spread into the splenium and occipital region. Lipomas originate in the anterior callosal region; they frequently are associated with callosal agenesis. Clinical symptoms of callosal neoplasms include increased intracranial pressure, personality and behavioral changes, seizures, alexia due to involvement of splenium, apraxia of the left hand because of anterior callosal lesions, and gait ataxia. Callosal tumors may be clinically silent for many years. Skull radiogram may show supratentorial midline calcification in lipomas, oligodendrogliomas, vascular malformations and epidermoid cysts. Lipomas show characteristic peripheral calcified rim, which surrounds central radiolucent regions. Air study findings characteristic of callosal tumors include lateral separation of frontal horns, effacement of the posterosuperior portion of the third ventricle, lateral ventricular enlargement and thickening of the corpus callosum and septum pellucidum. Angiography is utilized to demonstrate tumor stain of malignant neoplasms or vascular malformations.

With axial and coronal CT, callosal lesions are well-delineated. CT findings of callosal gliomas include: (1) abnormal midline callosal soft-tissue density, (2) lateral separation of frontal horns (Fig. 5–7), (3) thickening of septi pellucidi or splenium as manifested by dense contrast enhancement of these structures (Fig. 5–8), (4) ependymal enhancement consistent with periventricular tumor and (5) extension of tumor into cerebral hemispheres. Coronal sections demonstrate the location of the mass relative to ventricles, e.g., intra- or paraventricular. Septal hematomas caused by ruptured aneurysms appear as hyperdense nonenhancing hyperdense lesions separating the frontal horns. Lipomas have a hypodense central core and peripheral calcified portion (Fig. 5–9). In corpus callosal agenesis, frontal horns are widely separated, with superior extension of third ventricle. The third ventricular roof may appear dilated and extend to the inter-

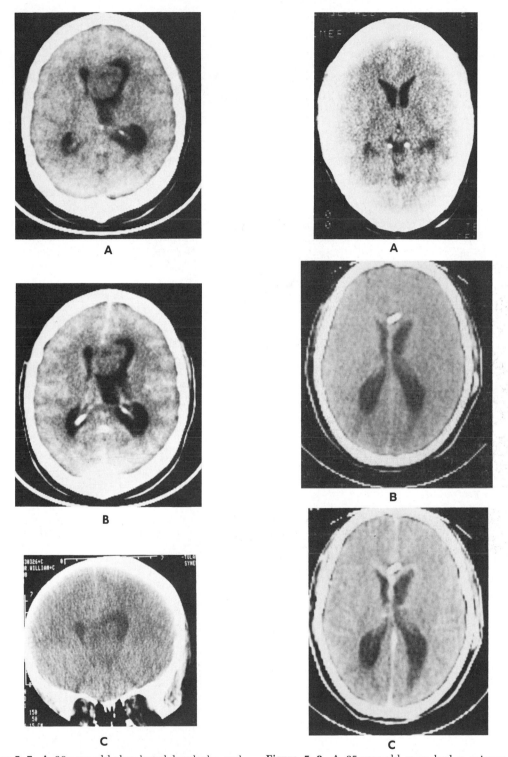

Figure 5–7. A 30-year-old developed headache and vomiting. Findings were papilledema and right lateral rectus paresis. *CT findings*: round hyperdense non-enhancing collosal lesion (A). The right lateral ventricle is dilated (B). Reformated coronal projections show the mass extending from the callosal region and intraventricular foramina into the third ventricle (C). *Operative findings*: callosal and intraventricular glioma.

Figure 5–8. A 25-year-old man had a seizure and subsequently developed neurological and behavioral symptoms. EEG showed left temporal delta activity; angiogram was negative. *CT findings*: plain and enhanced scans were negative (A). Three months later, he was markedly demented. Repeat CT shows marked thickening of the septi pellucidi (B) with dense septal and callosal enhancement (C). *Necropsy findings*: corpus callosal glioma.

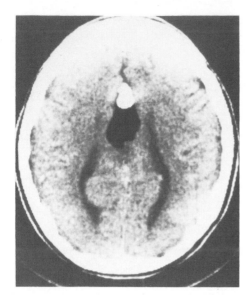

Figure 5–9. An 18-year-old woman had generalized seizure. This condition was well-controlled on anticonvulsant medication. *CT findings*: calcified anterior callosal mass with hypodense region (consistent with fat). *Diagnosis*: lipoma of corpus callosum.

hemispheric fissure; the associated cyst may be seen separating the frontal horns.[5]

LATERAL VENTRICULAR LESIONS

The most common tumors include choroid plexus papillomas, ependymomas, gliomas, meningiomas, dermoids and epidermoids. Meningiomas and choroid plexus papillomas are attached to the ventricular wall by a pedicle; gliomas do not have a distinct pedicle and infiltrate through the ventricular surface to the cerebral hemispheres. These tumors usually cause obstructive hydrocephalus, sometimes with localized dilation of the lateral ventricle contiguous with tumor. Focal neurological deficit results from localized dilatation of an obstructed loculated portion of the ventricle or infiltration of tumor into the cerebral hemispheres. In certain infiltrating intraventricular neoplasms, EEG and isotope scan findings may simulate deep hemispheric lesion. Diagnosis of intraventricular tumor is established by combined pneumography and ventriculography; this demonstrates hydrocephalus and may outline air-tumor interface. Angiographic displacement of choroidal arteries and veins delineates intraventricular location of tumor.[6]

CT has become the primary study to diag-

nose intraventricular tumors. It shows ventricular dilatation with a hyperdense enhancing intraventricular mass. If the mass is seen with surrounding localized ventricular dilatation, intraventricular location is established; however, localization by CT is not always possible without complementary ventriculography or angiography. Choroid plexus papilloma (Fig. 5–10) and meningioma (Fig. 5–11) appear as speckled hyperdense multilobulated calcified and enhancing lesions. Tumor pedicle that attaches to the ventricular wall may be visualized by coronal projections. Epidermoid and dermoid tumors are multilobulated and sharply marginated hypodense lesions with peripheral calcification. If the intraventricular mass is hypodense and nonenhancing, it may not be detected by CT because it has similar density to CSF. In these cases, ventriculogram may be required. Gliomas are heterogeneous irregularly marginated lesions with dense complex enhancement.[7] They usually extend

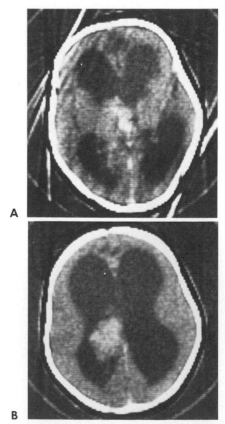

Figure 5–10. An 8-month-old child had progressive increase in head size. *CT findings*: left lateral ventricular hyperdense lesion (*A*) with calcified portion (*B*) with symmetrical lateral ventricular enlargement. *Operative diagnosis*: choroid plexus papilloma.

The putamen is separated from the insula by the external capsule. The globus pallidus is more medial and separated from the caudate nucleus by the anterior limb of the internal capsule and from the thalamus by the posterior capsular limb. The head of the caudate is lens-shaped and hyperdense relative to the contiguous frontal horn and internal capsule.[8] Pathological processes involving basal ganglia include: (1) calcification, (2) intracerebral hemorrhage, (3) inflammatory conditions such as abscess and granuloma, (4) neoplasms such as

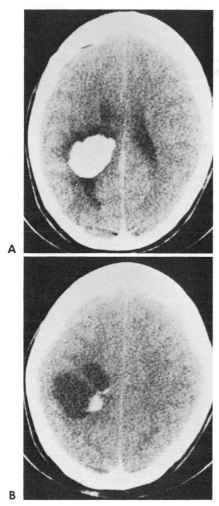

Figure 5–11. This 43-year-old woman developed right focal sensory seizures. EEG showed left parietal spike focus; isotope scan and skull radiogram were negative. *CT findings*: left atrial-occipital hyperdense calcified lesion (*A*) with enlargement of contiguous lateral ventricle (*B*). *Operative finding*: intraventricular meningioma.

into cerebral hemispheres. Intraventricular hemorrhages appear hyperdense; they conform to the shape of the ventricles. The presence of enhancement that has a serpentine pattern and surrounds the intraventricular hematoma has been seen with intraventricular angiomas (Fig. 5–12).

LESIONS OF THE BASAL GANGLIA

Basal ganglia consist of gray matter nuclear structures that are located medial to insula.

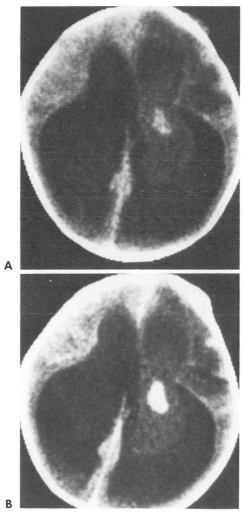

Figure 5–12. A neonate had enlarged head circumference but was neurologically normal. *CT findings*: marked lateral ventricular enlargement with right hyperdense (*A*) intraventricular enhancing lesion. (*B*) Angiogram showed parietal blush. *Operative findings*: hematoma due to intraventricular vascular malformation.

gliomas and metastases, (5) infarction, (6) vascular malformations such as angioma and aneurysm, (7) hypoxic-ischemic processes such as hypoglycemia and poisoning by carbon monoxide, cyanide and methanol, (8) degenerative conditions such as Huntington's disease and Wilson's disease.

Patients with basal ganglia tumors usually present with progressively worsening motor and sensory disturbances. There are clinical findings of corticospinal tract and sensory impairment caused by internal capsule involvement. Parkinsonism is a rare manifestation of basal ganglia tumors. If the tumor causes parkinsonism, the findings consist of unilateral resting tremor and rigidity; however, rarely these findings are bilateral. Hemiparesis replaces parkinsonian features when tumor extends into the internal capsule. Of five patients with CT evidence of basal ganglia tumors who presented with parkinsonism, all had unilateral findings.[9] EEG is usually normal or shows bilateral abnormalities; isotope scan rarely delineates abnormal uptake. Angiographic findings of basal ganglia lesions include lateral displacement of the lenticulostriate vessels, round shift of the anterior cerebral artery and opening of the venous angle.

With CT, diagnosis of basal ganglia lesions is readily accomplished. If a hyperdense ganglionic lesion is present, it is important to make precise attenuation measurements to differentiate calcification from hematoma. Calcification may be located in the globus pallidus but may be more extensive to involve the putamen; however, it does not extend across the internal capsule. Acute hematomas are usually unilateral and extend into the internal capsule. At a later stage hematomas may be less clearly hyperdense and show ring enhancement such that differentiation of hematomas from neoplasms is possible only with serial scans. Ring enhancement of basal ganglia hematomas may be quite dense and irregular; this is different from the smooth thin and regular enhancement of superficial supratentorial ring-enhancing hematomas. Middle cerebral and internal cartoid artery aneurysms may project into the basal ganglia. CT appearance depends upon pathological features of these aneurysms, that is, whether they are patent or thrombosed. Angiomas may be partially thrombosed. They may show calcification and abnormal enhancing vessels with CT; however, angiography is required to define these vascular lesions.

LESIONS OF THE THALAMUS

Patients with thalamic lesions have symptoms dependent upon the major vector of expansion. Lateral extension into the internal capsule causes hemiparesis and hemisensory deficit. Posterior extension into the midbrain and geniculate body causes impaired vertical eye movements, pupillary abnormalities and homonymous hemianopsia. Inferior extension into the subthalamus may cause hemiballism. If the tumor initially obstructs the third ventricle, intracranial hypertension and obstructive hydrocephalus result. EEG is normal in one half of patients; isotope scan is positive in only 30 to 40 percent of thalamic gliomas.[10] Angiographic findings of thalamic lesions in-

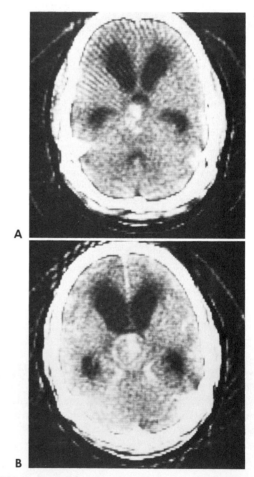

Figure 5–13. This 26-year-old man developed headache and right-sided weakness. Findings were papilledema and right pronator drift. *CT findings*: left medial thalamic hyperdense lesion is distorting and reversing shape of third ventricle (*A*). The rim and central portion enhance slightly (*B*). Lateral ventricles are enlarged. *Operative finding*: thalamic glioma.

and contralateral displacement of the third ventricle, (2) poor visualization of the third ventricle (Fig. 5–13), (3) distortion and displacement of the ipsilateral lateral ventricle, (4) lateral deviation of the ipsilateral temporal horn, (5) asymmetry of the quadrigeminal cistern, (6) posterior and lateral displacement of the atrial choroid plexus. Dense heterogeneous ring enhancement is usually seen; this may extend into the basal ganglia, corpus callosum, temporal region, ventricles (Fig. 5–14) or midbrain.

Thalamic metastases and lymphoma may show findings identical to those in gliomas;

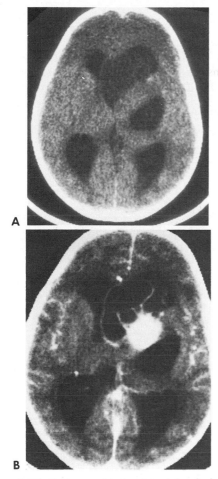

Figure 5–14. A 4-year-old developed headache and vomiting. Findings were papilledema and left hemiparesis. EEG showed monorhythmic frontal delta activity; isotope scan was negative. *CT findings:* right thalamic hypodense lesion that shows dense nodular (*A*) and subependymal enhancement (*B*). The third ventricle is effaced and the atrial region is displaced posteriorly. *Operative findings:* Grade II thalamic glioma with intraventricular extension.

clude (1) elevation of the middle cerebral artery; (2) lateral displacement of the middle cerebral artery to widen the arc between this vessel and the pericallosal artery; (3) stretching, elongation and enlargement of the anterior choroidal artery; (4) widening of the arc of the lateral posterior choroidal arteries and (5) elevation and shift of the internal cerebral and thalamostriate veins.[11]

The majority of thalamic tumors are gliomas. These usually appear as heterogeneous mixed-density lesions; less commonly they are hypodense or isodense. Mass effect is manifested by these findings: (1) elevation

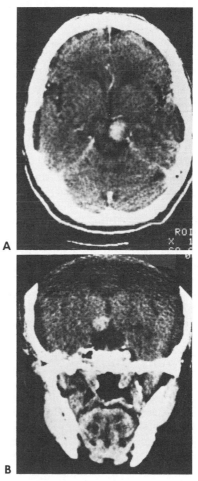

Figure 5–15. This 52-year-old woman had had an episode of headache followed by generalized seizure and left hemiparesis 13 years ago. She clinically improved with minimal residual motor weakness; however, she developed left-sided unilateral parkinsonism following phenothiazine mediation. *CT findings:* right subthalamic (*A*) hyperdense lesion with slight diffuse enhancement seen on coronal scan (*B*). Angiogram showed no abnormality. *Necropsy findings:* thrombosed subthalamic angioma.

however, these lesions are frequently multiple. Other lesions that simulate thalamic glioma include (1) ring-enhancing hematoma when mass effect and enhancement of these lesions spontaneously resolve within several weeks; (2) abscess with nodular or ring enhancement when the ring is thin and smooth; (3) infarcts that appear as sharply marginated hypodense or isodense enhancing lesions with minimal mass effect; (4) gliotic reaction in which lesions are hypodense or isodense and show enhancement and minimal mass effect; (5) thrombosed angiomas appearing as mixed-density lesions with calcified regions and tubular or serpiginous enhancing` structures (Fig. 5–15). Angiogram should be complementary to CT. Definitive diagnosis of thalamic glioma is established only by tissue biopsy. This should always be carried out prior to initiation of irradiation.[12]

ANTERIOR THIRD VENTRICULAR LESIONS

Colloid cysts originate in the anterosuperior third ventricle directly posterior to the intraventricular foramina. They are attached to the third ventricular roof. They may be small and do not cause ventricular dilatation. Larger lesions may obstruct the intraventricular foramina and result in lateral ventricular dilatation. Colloid cysts are round or oval-shaped. Cyst contents are thick because of high protein content.

Clinical findings are related to cyst size and ventricular obstruction. Small colloid cysts have been found as incidental necropsy findings. The most common clinical manifestation is headache, which is exacerbated by factors that increase intracranial pressure—change in head position, coughing and sneezing. Papilledema may be the only abnormal neurological finding. In other cases, clinical findings of dementia, gait ataxia and urinary incontinence may simulate normal pressure hydrocephalus. Prior to CT, ventriculography was the most reliable procedure to diagnose colloid cysts. Air studies demonstrate lateral ventricular dilatation and outline contour of cysts; however, small colloid cysts show ventricular dilatation without evidence of the mass. Angiography usually shows evidence of hydrocephalus only; however, utilizing magnification angiotomography, hypertrophied choroidal vessels supplying the cyst may also be seen.

We have defined both clinically symptomatic and asymptomatic cysts with CT. Colloid cysts appear hyperdense (70 percent) or isodense (30 percent). They are round or oval sharply marginated lesions located at the intraventricular foramina; they may project into the posteroinferior portion of the frontal horns (Fig. 5–16). Lateral ventricles are usually dilated and the third ventricle is not visualized. Coronal sections may demonstrate supplemental findings, as widening of the septi pellucidi and indentation and separation of the

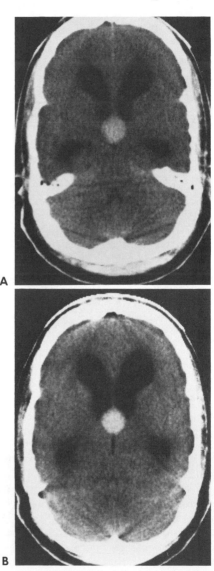

Figure 5–16. A 29-year-old man had headache and vomiting. Findings were bilateral papilledema. CT findings: sharply marginated hyperdense (A) enhancing (B) anterior third ventricular mass causing obstructive hydrocephalus. Operative finding: colloid cyst.

rarely intraventricular in location. They are calcified lesions that contain hypodense components with complex heterogeneous enhancement.[14]

POSTERIOR THIRD VENTRICULAR LESIONS

These tumors are classified as follows: (1) tumors of pineal parenchyma such as pinealoma, (2) teratomas including typical and atypical forms (germinoma) and (3) tumors of other types such as glioma, metastases, medulloblastoma and meningioma. Other lesions include vein of Galen aneurysm, quadrigeminal plate cyst (Fig. 5–18), thalamic hematoma and

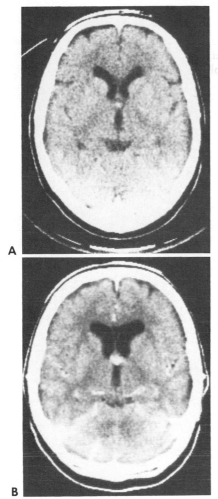

Figure 5–17. A 52-year-old woman developed visual blurring. Left homonymous hemianopsia was noted. *CT findings:* hyperdense (A) enhancing anterior third ventricular lesion (B).

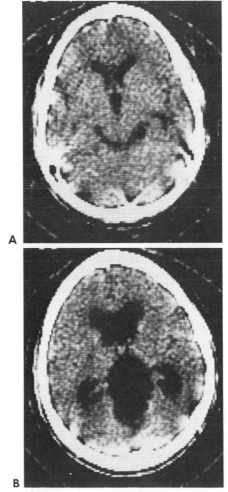

Figure 5–18. This 18-year-old developed vertical diplopia. Findings were isolated right superior oblique muscle paresis. *CT findings:* oval-shaped sharply marginated hypodense nonenhancing lesion (A). There is slight widening of the quadrigeminal cistern (B). Air study showed a quadrigeminal plate cyst.

inferior portion of the frontal horns. Contrast enhancement is varied. The hyperdense lesions show slight homogeneous enhancement (Fig. 5–17), and isodense lesions show homogeneous dense enhancement.[13]

Other anterior third ventricular lesions may simulate colloid cysts. These include basilar artery aneurysms, gliomas, craniopharyngiomas and meningiomas. The tips of basilar aneurysms project anteriorly and superiorly into the third ventricle; they do not extend to the intraventricular foramina. Meningiomas appear as hyperdense calcified densely enhancing masses. Intraventricular gliomas are sometimes calcified, eccentric in location, multilobulated in shape and show heterogeneous enhancement. Craniopharyngiomas are

primary thalamic and posterior fossa neoplasms. Patients with pineal tumors present
with symptoms of intracranial hypertension
caused by obstructive hydrocephalus. If the
quadrigeminal plate is compressed, symptoms
include upward gaze paresis and poorly reactive and dilated pupils. Characteristic endocrine symptoms of pineal tumors include precocious or delayed puberty. These tumors are
much more common in boys than in girls.

Diagnosis of pineal tumor is suggested by
the radiographic finding of pineal calcification
occurring in a child less than 10 years old. In
patients with teratomas, pineal calcification is
not usually detected, whereas germinomas
show prominent pineal calcification (Fig. 5–
19). Germinomas involving the anterior third

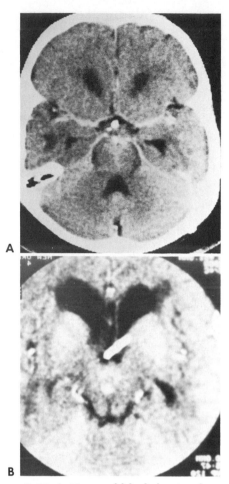

Figure 5–20. A 10-year-old had shunt and was irradiated for pinealoma 4 years previously. He developed
recurrent headache and vomiting. *CT findings:* shunt
tube is visualized in enlarged lateral ventricles (*A*).
There is an isodense enhancing (*B*) midbrain mass
representing pinealoma.

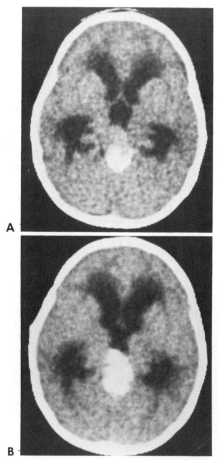

Figure 5–19. A 5-year-old became lethargic and had
episodic vomiting. Findings were papilledema, nonreactive dilated pupils and impaired upward gaze. *CT
findings:* hyperdense calcified (*A*) posterior third ventricular mass that densely enhanced (*B*). Lateral and
third ventricles are dilated with reversal of the convex
shape of the posterior third ventricle.

ventricle may show abnormal sella without
pineal calcification. The diagnosis of posterior
third ventricular tumor is usually established
by ventriculography. This shows hydrocephalus and a filling defect in the posterior third
ventricle. Angiographic findings include elevation of the internal cerebral vein and the
vein of Galen, with abnormal vessels supplying the tumor being derived from posterior
choroidal arteries.

Diagnosis of pineal tumors is well-established by CT; however, delineation of histopathological features is less reliably established. These tumors distort and displace the
posterior third ventricle. If there is anterior
concavity of the dilated posterior third ventricle, this suggests mass effect. Pineal tumors
frequently extend into the quadrigeminal, am-

bient and superior cerebellar cistern (Fig. 5–20). Pineal tumors are round and multilobulated. They may vary in size from several millimeters to three centimeters. Pinealomas

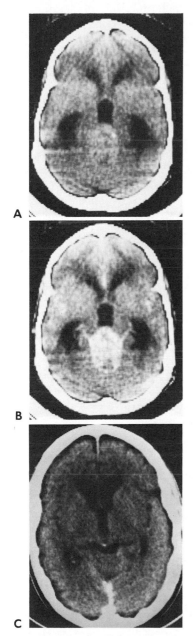

Figure 5–21. This 22-year-old developed headache, diplopia and gait instability. Findings were right-sided limb ataxia, dilated nonreactive pupillary response, bilateral Babinski signs. *CT findings*: sharply marginated hyperdense posterior third ventricular mass (A) with several interspersed calcified portions. There is dense enhancement (B). Two years following shunt placement and irradiation of a germinoma, ventricles are normal-sized (C) and there is no residual neoplasm.

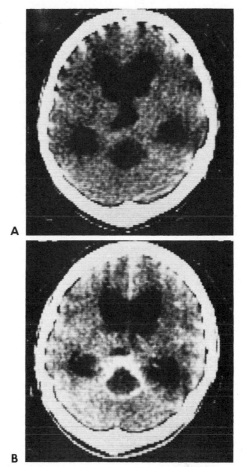

Figure 5–22. A 15-year-old developed headache and vomiting. Findings were papilledema, upward gaze paresis, nonreactive dilated pupils. *CT findings*: sharply marginated ovoid hypodense posterior third ventricular mass (A) with variable-thickness enhancing rim (B). *Operative finding*: cystic astrocytoma.

and teratomas show regions of interspersed calcification; glial tumors and metastases do not calcify.[15] Teratomas have a heterogeneous density pattern; the hypodense component is frequently caused by the cystic component and calcification is not prominent. Germinomas appear as multilobulated hyperdense lesions with interspersed calcification and dense enhancement (Fig. 5–21). Gliomas and metastases may be isodense; these tumors show dense enhancement. Pinealomas and teratomas may densely and homogeneously enhance and they are sharply marginated; gliomas show dense complex and irregular enhancement (Fig. 5–22). Subependymal and cisternal enhancement is consistent with paraventricular extension of pineal neoplasms.[16, 17]

TENTORIAL LESIONS

Meningiomas are the most common tentorial lesions. These may originate from supratentorial or infratentorial location. Patients present with clinical features dependent upon vector of expansion. These include trigeminal sensory disturbances, gait instability and intracranial hypertension. Skull radiogram and isotope scan are frequently negative with tentorial meningiomas.[18] Angiographic findings of tentorial meningioma include (1) anterior displacement of the basilar artery, (2) anterior displacement of the precentral cerebellar vein, (3) elevation of the superior cerebellar arteries and veins, (4) elevation of the posterior cerebral arteries, (5) prominent enlargement of the tentorial artery that originates from the internal carotid artery at the level of the cavernous sinus. The finding of persistent and homogeneous angiographic stain is characteristic of meningioma.

With CT, diagnosis of tentorial meningioma can be established at an earlier stage than with air studies or angiography. In the pre-CT era, the average duration of symptoms prior to diagnosis was 2.5 years; however, with CT, patients were symptomatic less than seven months prior to detection. Tentorial meningiomas are usually located contiguous with the petrous bone. They extend medially and superiorly to elevate the posterior third ventricle. They are sharply marginated hyperdense and homogeneously enhancing lesions. They are comma-shaped and extend to the incisural region. CT findings of transincisural extension include (1) effacement, distortion or elevation of the quadrigeminal cistern; (2) compression of the posterolateral portion of suprasellar-interpeduncular cistern; (3) elevation and lateral displacement of the posterior third ventricle; (4) anterolateral displacement of the dilated ipsilateral temporal horn. On axial sections, infratentorial components are located medially to the tentorial leaves (Fig. 5–23). Coronal sections are supplemental to delineate supratentorial and infratentorial components of these lesions.[19]

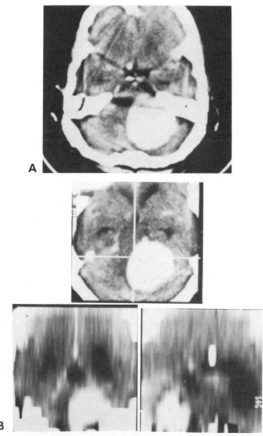

Figure 5–23. A 19-year-old developed headache, vomiting, gait instability. Findings were gait ataxia and papilledema. *CT findings:* right posterior fossa hyperdense enhancing mass extending to the tentorium (*A*). This is seen on reformatted coronal and sagittal projections (*B*). The contiguous cistern is enlarged, consistent with extra-axial tentorial meningioma.

POSTERIOR FOSSA LESIONS

Extra-axial

Those lesions that originate from meninges, nerve sheath and calvarium are extra-axial. In the posterior fossa, the most common extra-axial lesions are neurinomas (acoustic, trigeminal), meningioma (of cerebellopontine angle, tentorium, clivus, foramen magnum), extradural hematoma, chordoma, cholesteatoma, cyst (dermoid, subarachnoid), vascular malformations (angioma, aneurysm). CT findings of extra-axial lesions include (1) displacement of normal brain parenchyma (brain stem, cerebellum) away from bone with widening of contiguous subarachnoid cisterns or subdural spaces, (2) evidence of bone erosion, (3) sharp margination of lesion and (4) contiguity with the tentorium or foramen magnum.[20]

Intra-axial

These include lesions located within the posterior fossa structures (cerebellum, brain stem, fourth ventricle). Lesions involving the fourth ventricle may be intra- or extra-axial.

The most frequently occurring intra-axial lesions are cerebellar astrocytomas, medulloblastomas, ependymomas, cerebellar hemangioblastomas and brain stem gliomas. CT findings consistent with intra-axial lesions include (1) narrowing or effacement of basal cisterns as the mass displaces the brain outward toward the inner table; (2) no evidence of bone erosion; (3) indistinct and irregular margination of the lesion in some, e.g., brain stem gliomas, but not all cases, e.g., cerebellar astrocytomas. It is usually possible to differentiate CT findings of lesions in the brain stem, the cerebellum and the fourth ventricle. Intra-axial fourth ventricular masses are central in location and expand rather than displace the fourth ventricle as manifested by a surrounding hypodense rim, which represents expanded fourth ventricle.

BRAIN STEM LESIONS

Brain stem gliomas are most frequent in childhood; metastases and gliomas occur with equal frequency in adults.[21] Vascular malformations such as telangiectasia may simulate brain stem gliomas; however, onset of symptomatology is usually apoplectic rather than progressive.[22] Initial symptoms of brain stem gliomas include those resulting from facial and abducens nerve paresis or cerebellar dysfunction. One half of patients have initial symptoms of vomiting and headache to suggest possible occurrence of intracranial hypertension; however, brain stem gliomas usually present before there is obstruction of the aqueduct or fourth ventricle. Nausea and vomiting are usually caused by direct vagal nuclei medullary compression, and frontal headache may be caused by traction on the ophthalmic branch of the trigeminal nerve. Cranial nerve findings are present in 93 percent of patients, pyramidal tract and cerebellar signs in 75 percent; however, papilledema is uncommon and is present in less than 33 percent.

Air study has been the most reliable technique to demonstrate brain stem lesions. Characteristic findings are symmetrical enlargement of the brain stem and obliteration of mesencephalic, pontine and medullary cisterns. Tumor expansion may be eccentric; this may be exophytic and lateral into the cerebellopontine angle or medial into the fourth ven-

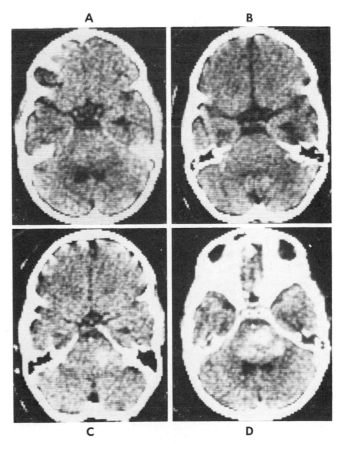

A   B

C   D

Figure 5–24. A 7-year-old girl developed gait instability and diplopia. Findings were bilateral abducens, facial paresis and gait ataxia. *CT findings:* widened brain stem as manifested by anterior displacement and straightening of the interpeduncular cistern and fourth ventricle flattened by an isodense nonenhancing mass (A). Following irradiation of presumed brain stem glioma, CT shows an isodense lesion (B) that now enhances. (C). Nine months later, she could not walk or swallow. *CT findings:* hyperdense brain stem mass with dense enhancement (D). *Necropsy finding:* brain stem glioma.

tricle. Vertebral angiography is supplemental; it may demonstrate tumor stain or vascular lesions that may simulate brain stem neoplasm. With air study and angiography the presence of brain stem mass is delineated; however, other etiologies for enlarged brain stem include focal encephalitis, demyelinated lesions, angiomas, intrapontine cysts, abscesses and granulomas.

With noncontrast and intravenously enhanced CT, we have detected 96 percent of brain stem neoplasms. The findings include (1) widening of the brain stem (symmetrical, 55 percent; asymmetrical, 45 percent); (2) flattening and posterior displacement of the fourth ventricle (100 percent); (3) anterior displacement and distortion of the interpeduncular cistern (80 percent); (4) distortion of the quadrigeminal cistern (25 percent); (5) anterior displacement of the basilar artery (10 percent) and (6) lateral displacement of the posterior cerebral arteries (10 percent). One sign of intrinsic brain stem enlargement is that the anterior part of the fourth ventricle is flat or anteriorly concave. A second sign is present when sagittal measurement of the pons (measured from the dorsum sella to the anterior fourth ventricle) is greater than the distance behind the fourth ventricle (Fig. 5–24). Hydrocephalus is present in 35 percent of cases; this is manifested by lateral and third ventricular enlargement with an abnormal fourth ventricle. These tumors may infiltrate into the thalamic–third ventricular or cerebellar peduncular region. Density pattern includes the following: (1) hypodense irregularly margined and nonenhancing (40 percent); (2) hypodense irregularly margined with nodular or heterogeneous enhancement (20 percent); (3) isodense enhancing (10 percent); (4) isodense nonenhancing (10 percent) and (5) heterogeneous mixed-density enhancing (20 percent). Evidence for brain stem infiltration is effacement of surrounding CSF-filled spaces and abnormal density in the brain stem. Brain stem gliomas are usually solid tumors; calcification, hemorrhage or cyst is rarely present. The presence of a sharply marginated hypodense lesion indicates cyst formation, and this finding suggests that surgical drainage may be of value. Contrast enhancement is seen in approximately one half of these neoplasms; this is usually slight and may occur in one portion of the tumor (Fig. 5–25). Dense, complex and extensive enhancement indicates glioblastomatous transformation.[23, 24] We have

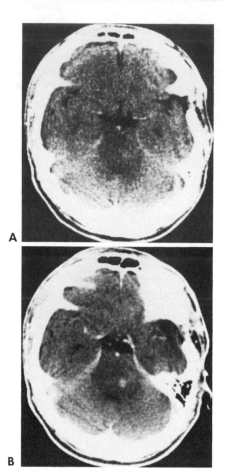

Figure 5–25. An 8-year-old developed vertigo. Findings included right abducens and facial paresis with gait ataxia. *CT findings*: hypodense brain stem lesion anteriorly distorting the interpeduncular cistern. It is also displacing posteriorly and flattening the fourth ventricle (*A*). There is a small nodular enhancing region (*B*). *Surgical finding*: brain stem glioma.

seen gliomas change with time in the following characteristic manner—no enhancement, small area of nodular enhancement and extensive complex and heterogeneous ring enhancement. Cisternal enhancement is not commonly seen with brain stem gliomas.

Anterior exophytic tumor extension is manifested by abnormal tissue densities located anterior to the basilar artery (which may be displaced); these densities project into the prepontine cistern. Posterior exophytic extension is manifested by enhancing tumor projecting posterior to the fourth ventricle (Fig. 5–26).

CT has been highly sensitive in demonstrating brain stem lesions. Metrizamide cisternography may be necessary in three situations: first, detection of small tumors, second, definition of those that originate in the medulla and extend posteriorly and third, detection of the presence of exophytic extension. Isodense enhancing brain stem lesions without evidence of brain stem widening suggest a non-neoplastic etiology such as demyelinated lesion or vascular ischemia; *spontaneous* disappearance of enhancement excludes neoplasm. Brain stem metastases may appear as isodense brain stem–enhancing lesions sometimes with minimal edema. Abscesses and granulomas may appear identical to metastases. The presence

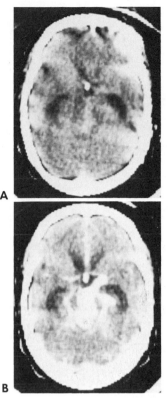

Figure 5–27. This 24-year-old woman developed sudden onset of headache, dizziness and gait unsteadiness. CSF was bloody. Ventriculogram showed brain stem mass and hydrocephalus. Angiogram showed brain stem angioma. She had diversionary shunt. *CT findings:* hyperdense brain stem lesion (A) with evidence of tortuous enhancement surrounding the brain stem and extending toward the posterior third ventricle (B).

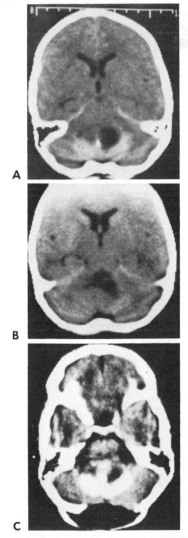

Figure 5–26. A 2-year-old developed facial weakness and difficulty swallowing. *CT findings:* hypodense round mass with enhancement posterior to the fourth ventricle (A). The fourth ventricle is tilted (B). Following operative biopsy of a brain stem glioma with exophytic extension, CT shows an isodense lesion, which densely enhances posterior to the fourth ventricle (C).

of intrapontine hematoma that occurs in normotensive patients is suggestive of angioma; in these cases angiography should be performed (Fig. 5–27).

CEREBELLAR LESIONS

These tumors arise in either the vermal or the hemispheric region. Midline vermal tumors cause gait and truncal instability with early evidence of intracranial hypertension due to fourth ventricular obstruction. Some patients present with intracranial hypertension without clear-cut cerebellar signs. If tumor is located in the cerebellar hemispheres, unilateral limb ataxia is usually the initial clinical disturbance.[25] Diagnosis of cerebellar tumor has been established by air study. Vertebral angiography is sometimes necessary to

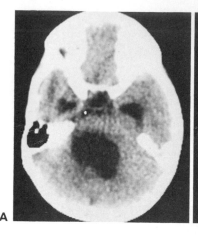

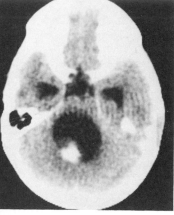

A

B

Figure 5–28. A 3-year-old girl fell frequently. Findings were gait ataxia and papilledema. *CT findings:* hypodense paramedian posterior fossa mass (*A*) with eccentric nodular enhancement (*B*). The fourth ventricle is not visualized and there is biventricular enlargement. *Surgical findings:* cystic astrocytoma with mural nodule.

exclude tumor nodule characteristic of hemangioblastoma. Angiographic findings of cerebellar tumors include forward displacement of the basilar artery, downward displacement of the posterior-inferior cerebellar artery and elevation of the superior cerebellar artery.

CT has been entirely reliable in diagnosis of cerebellar lesions. Hemispheric lesions are eccentric in location and cause contralateral fourth ventricular displacement. Vermal lesions are paramedian but eccentric; these cause displacement or effacement of the fourth ventricle. On the basis of attenuation characteristics and enhancement pattern, specific pathological features of certain cerebellar lesions may be delineated preoperatively. Cerebellar astrocytomas appear as round or oval sharply marginated hypodense lesions with an eccentric small hyperdense component that enhances densely. This pattern is characteristic of cystic cerebellar astrocytoma with mural nodule (Fig. 5–28). Other cystic cerebellar astrocytomas appear hypodense without enhancing mural nodule (Fig. 5–29). Because of the high protein content of neoplastic cysts, the attenuation value of cysts may be higher than CSF. Without evidence of mural nodular enhancement, hypodense cerebellar cysts of neoplastic origin cannot be differentiated from those of non-neoplastic origin. Solid cerebellar astrocytomas appear as heterogeneous mixed-density lesions with dense nodular or complex ring enhancement (Fig. 5–30). Other astrocytomas appear as dense globular and multilobuated calcified lesions without cystic or enhancing component. Obstructive hydrocephalus and fourth ventricular mass effect are invariably present in cerebellar astrocytomas.[26, 27]

Cerebellar hemangioblastoma is usually located in cerebellar hemispheres—less frequently, in vermal or intraventricular hemispheres. They may be solid or cystic, sometimes with central necrosis. Cystic tumors appear as round or oval sharply marginated hypodense lesions. The presence of a mural nodule is manifested by a dense nodular eccentric peripheral enhancing portion. Necrotic tumors appear as heterogeneous density lesions with variable-thickness ring enhancement. Solid hemangioblastomas appear as isodense densely enhancing lesions that are irregular in shape and multilobulated (Fig. 5–31). In hemangioblastomas, calcified or hemorrhagic portions are not seen.[28, 29] Angiography shows evidence of small dense tumor stain.

Less common cerebellar lesions are metastases, abscess, hematoma, infarction, vascular malformations, desmoplastic medulloblastomas (cerebellar sarcoma), entrapped fourth

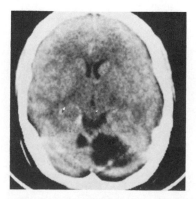

Figure 5–29. A 29-year-old developed episodic vertigo. Findings were right-limb ataxia and horizontal nystagmus. *CT findings:* hypodense nonenhancing lesion with contralateral deviation of the fourth ventricle. *Operative findings:* noncystic cerebellar astrocytoma.

ventricle,[30] cysts (subarachnoid, dermoid) and non-neoplastic gliotic cyst.[31] The presence of a thin, regularly shaped peripheral enhancing rim is characteristic of abscess; this rim is not usually seen with cerebellar astrocytomas. The peripheral enhancing rim of metastases is heterogeneous in shape and of variable thickness. Non-neoplastic gliotic cerebellar cysts appear as hypodense sharply marginated lesions. They usually do not enhance because there is no tumor nodule. It has been suggested that the finding of gliotic cerebellar cyst by CT and surgical findings do not exclude astrocytoma because a tumor nodule may be located in the white matter at some distance from the cyst rather than within the lumen of the cyst. An ntrapped fourth ventricle results from fourth ventricular outlet obstruction. CT shows a midline large triangular-shaped hypodense non-enhancing structure; this represents dilated

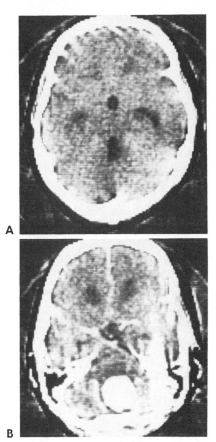

Figure 5–31. This 40-year-old women developed swallowing difficulty and slurred speech. *CT findings:* plain scan shows a tilted and anteriorly displaced fourth ventricle (A). There is dense homogeneous enhancement (B). *Operative finding:* solid hemangioblastoma.

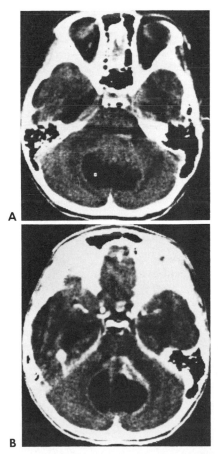

Figure 5–30. A 7-year-old developed staggering gait. Findings were gait ataxia and papilledema. *CT findings:* mixed-density (A) lesion with ring and heterogeneous (B) enhancement. *Operative finding:* noncystic cerebellar astrocytoma.

fourth ventricle. Lateral and third ventricle may or may not be enlarged; however, if lateral ventricles are enlarged, shunting does not result in decreased size of the fourth ventricle. Reduction of fourth ventricular size is accomplished by direct shunting of this encysted ventricle.

FOURTH VENTRICULAR LESIONS

Clinical findings of intracranial hypertension are early manifestations of intraventricular tumors. Medulloblastomas and ependymomas are the most common tumors. CT findings of fourth ventricular intra-axial lesions include (1) abnormal soft-tissue density midline mass, (2) surrounding hypodense rim, (3) fourth ventricle not identified as separate structure and (4) presence of a round midline hypodense

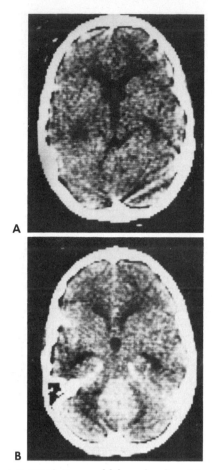

Figure 5–32. A 7-year-old boy developed headache and vomiting. He had papilledema and lateral rectus paresis. *CT findings*: isodense (*A*) enhancing midline posterior fossa mass with surrounding lucent rim (*B*) consistent with an expanded fourth ventricle. *Operative finding*: medulloblastoma.

cular rim may be located anterior to the tumor margin (if tumor is attached to fourth ventricular roof) or posterior to it (if it is attached to the floor of the fourth ventricle). As tumor invades the vermis and extends exophytically into the vallecula and cisterna magna, the posterior portion of the hypodense rim is effaced. Posterior pointing of the halo indicates exophytic extension. If tumor extends upward through the tentorium, the hypodense anterior rim that is convex posteriorly represents the quadrigeminal cistern.

Medulloblastomas originate from cells of the external granular layer of the inferior medullary velum representing the fourth ventricular roof. They grow anteriorly to fill the lumen of the fourth ventricle and posteriorly into the vermis and cisterna magna. Medulloblastomas are highly cellular vascular tumors that frequently seed into cisternal spaces. Degenerative change such as hemorrhage, calcification and cyst are uncommon. CT shows an isodense or hyperdense (noncalcified) homogeneous lesion that densely enhances.

A crescent-shaped hypodense rim located anterior to the mass represents the fourth ventricle and not the cystic component (Fig. 5–32). Exophytic extension that is reflected by cisternal enhancement (cisterna magna, cerebellopontine angle) is commonly demonstrated. The fourth ventricle usually appears dilated and filled with rounded tumor and there is biventricular enlargement. Desmoplastic medulloblastomas (cerebellar sarcomas) are usually located laterally in the cerebellar hemispheres (Fig. 5–33). They may cause intraventricular and exophytic cisternal extension. These tumors appear as heterogeneous mixed-density lesions that displace the fourth ventricle laterally. There is dense complex variable-thickness ring or nodular enhancement.[32, 33] These may simulate solid cerebellar astrocytomas or necrotic hemangioblastomas.

region that represents CSF space located between central tumor and expanded fourth ventricle. Hypodense rim may completely encircle the tumor; however, it may appear as a crescent-shaped hypodense rim. This semicir-

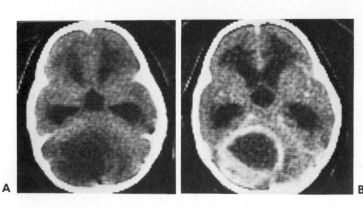

Figure 5–33. A 10-year-old boy developed clumsiness using his left hand. Findings were left-sided intention tremor, dysmetria and papilledema. *CT findings*: left cerebellar hypodense lesion (*A*) with irregular ring enhancement (*B*). The fourth ventricle is nonvisualized and there is biventricular enlargement. *Operative finding*: cerebellar sarcoma (medulloblastoma).

Ependymomas arise from the floor of the fourth ventricle. They may extend exophytically through the lateral recesses of the fourth ventricle into the cerebellopontine angle cisterns, vallecula, cisterna magna or cervical subarachnoid spaces; they may also extend into the cerebellum or brain stem. Ependymomas are multilobulated and highly vascular tumors that are not sharply marginated from surrounding parenchyma. They may contain cystic components and frequently have calcified (Fig. 5–34) or hemorrhagic components. CT findings reflect their pathological features. Most frequently, they appear as round or oval midline heterogeneous mixed-density irregularly marginated lesions. They contain multi-

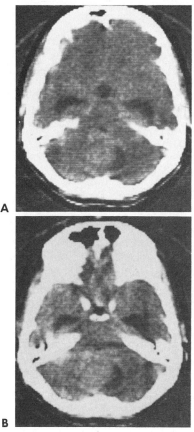

Figure 5–35. A 16-year-old had headache and vomiting. Findings were papilledema and vertical nystagmus. *CT findings:* isodense nonenhancing midline posterior fossa lesion (A) with surrounding cystic semilunar hypodense component (B) and this is seen on coronal view(s). *Operative finding:* ependymoma.

ple punctate calcified regions and hypodense portions that represent cyst (Fig. 5–35). Isodense and hyperdense regions show variable enhancement pattern, including dense homogeneous, variable thickness ring, and complex and heterogeneous. Surrounding hypodense halo is better visualized on enhanced than on noncontrast scan. The fourth ventricle is enlarged and is represented by central hypodense rim. There is lateral and third ventricular dilatation.[34] Differentiation of ependymomas from medulloblastoma or solid vermal astrocytomas may not always be possible.

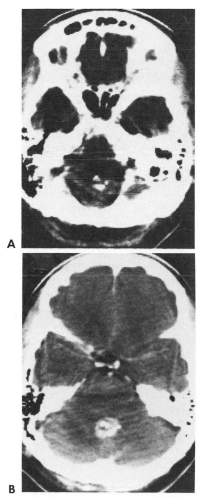

Figure 5–34. A 17-year-old developed dizziness. Examination and skull and cervical spine radiograms were negative. *CT findings:* calcified (A) and enhancing midline mass located posterior to the fourth ventricle (B). *Operative finding:* ependymoma.

REFERENCES

1. Botez MI: Frontal lobe tumors. *In* Handbook of Clinical Neurology, Vol 17. PJ Vinken, GW Bruyn (eds). North American Publishing Co., Amsterdam, 1974, pp. 234–280

2. Russell EJ, Naidich TP: The enhancing septal alveal wedge: a septal sign of intraaxial mass. Neuroradiology 23:33–40, 1982
3. Suchenwirth RMA: Parietal lobe tumors. In Handbook of Clinical Neurology, Vol 17. PJ Vinken, GW Bruyn (eds). North Holland Publishing Co., Amsterdam, 1974, pp. 290–307
4. Gassel MM: Occipital lobe tumors. In Handbook of Clinical Neurology, Vol 17. PJ Vinkin, GW Bruyn (eds). North Holland Publishing Co., Amsterdam, 1974, pp. 310–349
5. Wing SD, Osborn AG: Normal and pathologic anatomy of the corpus callosum by computed tomography. Comput Axial Tomogr 1:183–192, 1977
6. Boudreau RP: Primary intraventricular tumors. Radiology 75:867, 1960
7. Veiga-Pires JA, Dossetor RS: CT scanning for papilloma of choroid plexus. Neuroradiology 17:13–16, 1978
8. Osborn AG, Saville T: The basal ganglia on cranial computed tomography: normal anatomy and pathology. Comput Axial Tomogr 1:245–255, 1977
9. Sciarra D, Sprofkin BE: Symptoms and signs referable to the basal ganglia in brain tumor. Arch Neurol Psychiatr 69:450, 1953
10. Cheek WR, Taveras JM: Thalamic tumors. J Neurosurg 24:505, 1966
11. Lawrie BW: Radiology of thalamic tumors. Clin Radiol 21:10, 1970
12. Weisberg LA: Thalamic gliomas: clinical and computed tomographic correlations. Neuroradiology 7:210, 1938.
13. Zilkha A: Computed tomography of colloid cysts of the third ventricle. Clin Radiol 32:397–401, 1981
14. Ganti SR, Antunes JL, Louis KM: Computed tomography in the diagnosis of colloid cysts of the third ventricle. Radiology 138:385, 1981
15. Messina AV, Potts G, Sigel RM: Computed tomography evaluation of the posterior third ventricle. Radiology 119:581, 1976
16. Chang CG, Kageyama N, Kobayashi T: Pineal tumors: clinical diagnosis, with special emphasis on the significance of pineal calcification. Neurosurgery 8:656, 1981
17. Neuwelt EA, Glasberg M, Frenkel E: Malignant pineal region tumors. J Neurosurg 51:597, 1979
18. Barrows HS, Harter DH: Tentorial meningiomas. J Neurol Neurosurg Psychiatr 25:40, 1962
19. Naidich TP, Leeds NE, Kricheff II: The tentorium in axial section. II, Lesion localization. Radiology 123:639, 1977
20. Naidich TP, Lin JP, Leeds NE: CT in the diagnosis of extraaxial posterior fossa masses. Radiology 120:333, 1976
21. Panitch HS, Berg BO: Brain stem tumors of childhood and adolescence. Am J Dis Child 119:465, 1970
22. Zeller RS, Chutorian AM: Vascular malformations of the pons in children. Neurology 25:776, 1975
23. Bilaniuk LT, Zimmerman RA, Littman P: Computed tomography of brain stem gliomas in children. Radiology 134:89, 1980
24. Weisberg LA: Computed tomography in the diagnosis of brain stem gliomas. Comput Tomogr 3:145, 1979
25. Weisberg LA: Computed tomographic findings in cerebellar astrocytoma. Comput Radiol 6:137, 1982
26. Naidich TP, Lin JP, Leeds NE: Primary tumors and other masses of the cerebellum and fourth ventricle. Neuroradiology 14:153–174, 1977
27. Gado M, Huete I, Mikhael M: Computerized tomography of infratentorial tumors. Semin Roentgenol 12:297, 1977
28. Cornell SH, Hibri NS, Menezes AH: The complementary nature of computed tomography and angiography in the diagnosis of cerebellar hemangioblastoma. Neuroradiology 17:201, 1979
29. Jeffreys R: Clinical and surgical aspects of posterior fossa hemangioblastoma. J Neurol Neurosurg Psychiatr 38:105, 1975
30. Zimmerman RA, Bilaniuk LT, Gallo E: Computed tomography of the trapped fourth ventricle. Am J Roentgenol 130:503, 1978
31. Weisberg LA: Nonneoplastic gliotic cerebellar cysts: clinical and computed tomographic correlations. Neuroradiology 23:3, 1982
32. Zimmerman RA, Bilaniuk LT, Pahlajani H: Spectrum of medulloblastomas demonstrated by computed tomography. Radiology 126:137, 1978
33. Weisberg LA: Computed tomographic findings in medulloblastomas. Comput Tomogr 6:83, 1982
34. Swartz JD, Zimmerman RA, Bilaniuk LT: Computed tomography of intracranial ependymomas. Radiology 143:97, 1982
35. Segall HD, Zee CS, Naidich TP: Computed tomography in neoplasms of the posterior fossa in children. Med Clin North Am 20:237, 1982

Meningioma

Meningiomas constitute 14 to 20 percent of intracranial neoplasms.[1] They commonly occur in middle age with peak incidence at age 45. There is a female predominance, with 60 percent of cases occurring in women. Sites of predilection directly correlate with abundant arachnoid granulations: parasagittal and falx (26 percent), convexity (18 percent), sphenoid ridge (18 percent), olfactory groove (12 percent), parasellar (12 percent), posterior fossa (10 percent), intraventricular (2 percent), intraorbital (1 percent). Meningiomas are usually slow growing, extracerebral in location, have benign histological features and do not recur after surgical removal. They are classified as benign tumors because their total removal usually results in cure; however, they may grow to large size. Meningiomas may extend into surgically inaccessible locations such as venous sinuses, demonstrate local invasiveness and recur after surgery. Other meningiomas remain small and may be incidental necropsy findings (Fig. 5–36).

The presence of meningioma may be suspected clinically; however, diagnosis depends upon radiographic studies. Plain skull radiograms detect abnormalities in 30 to 60 percent of cases. These are hyperostosis, thinning of bone because of pressure erosion, speckled or globular calcification, and prominent vascular channels.[2] Isotope scan detects 85 to 90 percent of meningiomas; false-negative studies occur most commonly in parasellar, temporal, intraventricular or posterior fossa tumors and in those that are less than 15 mm in size.[3, 4] Angiography demonstrates the presence of symptomatic meningiomas in 95 percent of cases; false-negative results may occur with small parasagittal or lateral sphenoid (en plaque) meningiomas. Specific angiographic features may permit accurate preoperative diagnosis of meningioma in 70 percent of cases.

Meningiomas usually derive their blood supply from meningeal vessels; therefore, common carotid injection is necessary to demonstrate abnormal tumor circulation. Some falx meningiomas are supplied by terminal branches of pericallosal or middle cerebral arterial segments. Vascular blush is usually homogeneous sharply marginated opacification (sunburst pattern); it begins in the midarterial and persists into the venous phase. Tumor vessels are regularly aligned and have similar-sized caliber. This vascular pattern is consistent with the noninfiltrating and benign histological nature of the majority of meningiomas. In some cases meningiomas appear as avascular masses. Some angioblastic meningiomas show nonhomogeneous opacification with irregularly aligned vessels and early draining veins suggestive of malignant neoplasm. In rare cases superficial cortical gliomas or metastases infiltrate dura and derive part of their blood supply from dural vessels to simulate meningioma.

Angiography is necessary in patients with suspected meningioma to estimate size and mass effect, define the presence and type of tumor circulation, and demonstrate the source of the abnormal vascular supply and the relationship of tumor to contiguous arteries, veins and venous sinuses. This information is important to know preoperatively because invasion of the venous sinus by meningioma makes total removal quite difficult and invasion or encasement of major arterial structures is associated with higher morbidity and mortality.

Initial CT studies in patients with suspected meningiomas demonstrated 95 to 100 percent accuracy in detecting tumor with 85 percent specificity for meningiomas.[5-7] CT has detected meningiomas in neurologically asymptomatic patients who had negative skull radiogram and isotope scan. The smallest intracranial meningioma detected was 7 mm. On noncontrast scan, 62 percent of meningiomas appear as homogeneous speckled sharply marginated high-density lesions with regular contours (round, ovoid). The lesion appears separate from normal surrounding parenchyma. This is consistent with its encapsulated extracerebral nature. The hyperdense portion represents four possible pathological features: widespread psammomatous calcifications, high cellular tu-

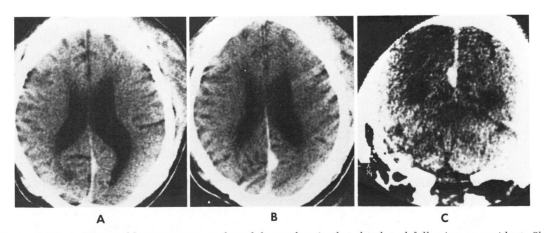

A   **B**   **C**

Figure 5–36. A 63-year-old woman was evaluated for neck pain that developed following an accident. She showed mild recent memory impairment only. *CT findings:* noncontrast scan shows localized dural thickening (A). Postcontrast scan shows dense homogeneous enhancement contiguous to the falx (B) and this is seen on coronal view (C). She died one year later and necropsy showed falx meningioma.

mor density, dense globular calcification and intratumoral hemorrhage. If meningiomas show attenuation coefficients of 200 to 500 units, this reflects dense globular calcification; however, dispersed psammomatous calcification may be found to have attenuation values below that expected for calcified lesions (Fig. 5–37). It is usually possible to differentiate psammomatous calcification from intratumoral or peritumoral hemorrhage. In 8 percent of meningiomas, noncontrast scan shows prominent hypodense component (Fig. 5–38); this is usually sharply marginated but may be irregularly shaped. It is believed that this hypodense component represents one or more of these pathological conditions: peritumoral cyst, intratumoral necrosis, loculated widened CSF spaces and lipomatous degeneration.[8, 9]

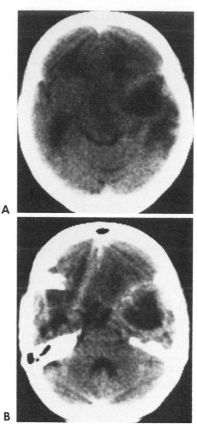

Figure 5–38. A 40-year-old woman had generalized seizure disorder of 10 years' duration. She developed right focal motor seizures. EEG showed left temporal spike discharge; isotope scan was positive. *CT findings:* left temporal-parietal hypodense lesion with marked mass effect (*A*) and irregular complex ring enhancement (*B*). A meningioma with necrotic and lipomatous degeneration was removed surgically.

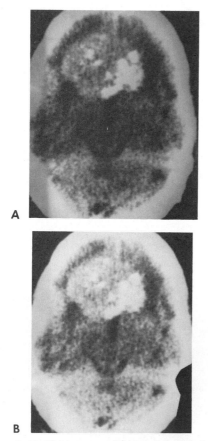

Figure 5–37. This 59-year-old man developed dementia, gait impairment and urinary incontinence. EEG showed monorhythmic frontal delta pattern; isotope scan showed bifrontal uptake. *CT findings:* bifrontal hyperdense lesion with speckled and globular components (*A*). There is dense homogeneous enhancement in a speckled hyperdense region (*B*). At surgery, a fibroblastic meningioma was removed.

Cyst formation was most common in meningiomas in a parasagittal location and those showing fibroblastic or angioblastic pathological features. Certain of these peritumoral cysts contained xanthochromic material and were believed to represent necrotic or lipomatous material, while other cysts are arachnoidal and contain CSF.[10] In some meningiomas that showed a prominent hypodense portion there were atypical findings on postcontrast CT, heterogeneous or irregular complex enhancement, and peripheral dense nodular enhancement with no enhancement in the medial cystic portion. In 4 percent of meningiomas that appeared hypodense, cellular density was very low and there was no psammomatous calcification. These hypodense meningiomas showed dense and homogeneous enhancement and their location was consistent with meningioma. Thirty percent of meningiomas appeared isodense on noncontrast scan (Fig. 5–39); however, in the majority of cases suspicion of slightly hyperdense lesion or evidence of mass effect was present (Fig. 5–40). In only very rare cases was noncontrast scan entirely normal.

In meningiomas, there may be a hypodense rim surrounding the hyperdense portion. This may represent edema fluid, widened subarachnoid spaces, or loculated CSF.[11] In meningiomas that appear hyperdense, there may be some focal interspersed hypodense regions. These represent cystic, necrotic or lipomatous change. Edema has frond-like projections extending into the white matter causing mass effect; this is usually seen with large menin-

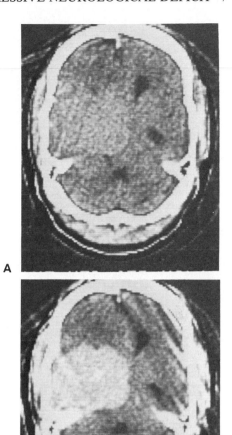

A

B

Figure 5–40. An 18-year-old man developed left-sided rubral tremor after phenothiazine treatment. EEG, skull radiogram and isotope scan were negative. *CT findings:* noncontrast scan shows a isodense (vaguely hyperdense) lesion with marked mass effect in the left middle fossa (*A*). Postcontrast scan shows a densely enhancing mass, which has extended into the cavernous sinus and suprasellar region (*B*). Operative findings confirmed the diagnosis of meningioma.

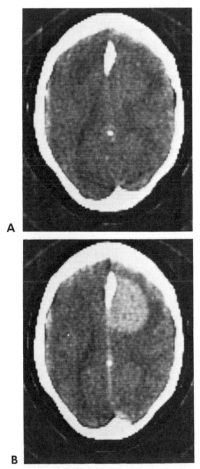

A

B

Figure 5–39. A 45-year-old woman developed left leg focal motor seizures. EEG showed left parietal spike discharge. *CT findings:* noncontrast scan shows dense anterior falx calcification (*A*) and there is dense speckled homogeneous enhancement with its base at the falx extending into the right parasagittal region (*B*). Surgical findings confirmed the diagnosis of meningioma.

giomas. Meningiomas cause less mass effect than would be predicted by the size of tumor. This is postulated as resulting from local pressure atrophy occurring at a rate that is similar to tumor growth. CT signs that are relatively specific for meningioma include thickening of the dura, attachment of the lesion to the dura (best visualized with coronal sections) and bony erosion or hyperostosis (best visualized with bone settings).

Ninety-six percent of meningiomas showed contrast enhancement. This usually appeared

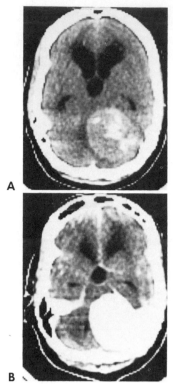

Figure 5–41. A 44-year-old woman developed gait instability and diplopia. Findings were right-sided limb ataxia and facial and abducens paresis. *CT findings*: right posterior fossa hyperdense globular and speckled mass (*A*), which densely enhances (*B*). It extends upward to the tentorium and has effaced the fourth ventricle with associated biventricular enlargement. There is a thin surrounding hypodense rim. Shape and extension are characteristic of meningioma.

as homogeneous dense and sharply marginated enhancement (Fig. 5–41). Less commonly observed enhancement patterns include (1) heterogeneous and patchy, (2) complex and irregularly shaped ring and (3) nodular. The complex ring and nodular pattern was seen most commonly in three types of neoplasms: angioblastic meningiomas, meningiomas with sarcomatous degeneration and meningiomas with more aggressive and infiltrating pathological features (Fig. 5–42). The nonenhancing meningiomas (4 percent) appeared densely calcified (globular), but angiography showed abnormal stain in these cases. It is possible that the lesions did enhance numerically; however, because of high density resulting from calcification, there was no visible evidence of enhancement (Fig. 5–43).

On the basis of the combined noncontrast and postcontrast findings, predictive accuracy

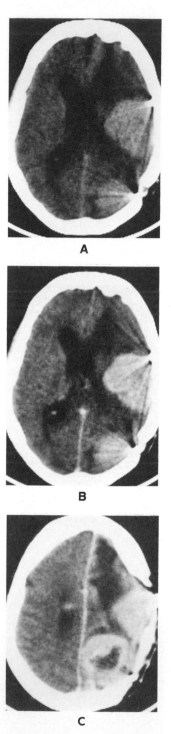

Figure 5–42. Two years following removal of a right convexity meningioma, this 45-year-old woman developed frequent seizures. *CT findings*: hyperdense right hemispheric lesion with a small hypodense component extending across the midline with marked mass effect (*A*). There is dense (*B*) and heterogeneous multifocal enhancement (*C*). The surgical clips are seen. Atypical meningioma with necrotic change and sarcomatous degeneration was removed surgically.

TABLE 5–1. Differential Consideration of the CT Features of Meningioma

Location	Noncontrast Features	Postcontrast Findings	Accuracy (%)	Differential Considerations
Supratentorial convexity-falx	Hyperdense calcified	Homogeneous enhancement	100	—
Supratentorial convexity-falx	Hyperdense noncalcified	Homogeneous enhancement	95	Glioma; metastases
Supratentorial convexity-falx	Hyperdense calcified	None	80	Oligodendroglioma; thrombosed angioma; aneurysm
Supratentorial convexity-falx	Hypodense or mixed-density noncalcified	Heterogeneous, nodular or ring	Nonspecific	Glioma; metastases; angioma
Intraventricular	Hyperdense noncalcified	Homogeneous enhancement	Nonspecific	Ependymoma; choroid plexus papilloma; glioma; metastases
Suprasellar medial sphenoid	Hyperdense noncalcified	Homogeneous enhancement	Nonspecific	Pituitary adenoma; craniopharyngioma; aneurysm
Posterior fossa	Hyperdense calcified	Homogeneous enhancement comma-shaped	90	Acoustic neuroma; aneurysm

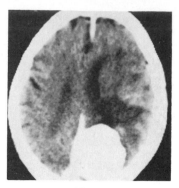

Figure 5–43. A 53-year-old woman developed sudden onset of left hemiparesis 7 years previously. Her condition has remained stable. *CT findings:* right occipital globular calcified falx nonenhancing mass. Angiogram showed a stain pattern characteristic of meningioma.

of CT was 85 to 90 percent in meningiomas. On the basis of CT findings, it is not possible to determine histological pattern. The finding of a hyperdense calcified homogeneously enhancing lesion in convexity or in the high parasagittal region is quite specific for meningiomas; however, if the lesion is hyperdense noncalcified and homogeneously enhancing, gliomas (Fig. 5–44) and metastases may have identical CT findings.[12] These malignant neoplasms may also cause dural thickening identical to meningioma. If enhancing meningioma is located directly contiguous to normal enhancing vascular structure, this may be incorrectly interpreted as an abnormal vessel due to angioma. The finding of a hypodense lesion with irregular margination or a sharply marginated hyperdense lesion with interspersed hypodense regions is seen in 7 to 15 percent of meningiomas.

Following presumed total surgical removal of meningioma, recurrence develops in 8 to 12 percent of cases. Because recurrence is most common at the site of the initial tumor, this is not believed to represent a manifestation of multiple meningiomas. Recurrence is most likely to occur in locally invasive meningiomas; however, it is not usually possible to predict which meningiomas will recur on the basis of histological features. Recurrence is most likely in meningiomas that have certain CT findings: (1) hypodense lesion with irregular margination, (2) heterogeneous (mixed-density) noncalcified appearance and (3) ring, nodular or irregular enhancement pattern. If a patient who has had meningioma surgically removed then develops recurrent symptomatology, this may represent such other diagnostic possibilities as second intracranial neoplasm, sarcomatous degeneration of meningioma or postsurgical effect, e.g., gliotic scar or porencephalic cyst.

LOCATIONS OF MENINGIOMAS

Parasagittal and Falx. Parasagittal meningiomas are attached to the superior sagittal sinus and compress the medial hemispheric surface. Falx meningiomas originate from the inferior sagittal sinus region. They may extend through the falx to become bilateral. The majority arise from the middle one third of the sagittal sinus; those originating from the anterior one third are more common than those in the posterior region. Clinical symptomatology is dependent upon location and size of meningiomas. Middle region lesions cause focal seizures and monoparesis that usually begin in the leg. Anterior lesions may grow to large size before causing intracranial hypertension, dementia, behavioral changes

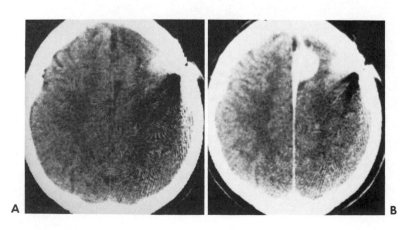

Figure 5–44. A 42-year-old woman had generalized seizure. CT and angiographic findings were consistent with meningioma; however, Grade II glioma was surgically removed. Six months later, seizures recurred. *CT findings:* hypodense falx lesion (A) with dense homogeneous enhancement and thickening of the adjacent falx (B). Operative findings confirmed the diagnosis of astrocytoma.

or disturbances to simulate normal pressure hydrocephalus, e.g., dementia, gait ataxia, incontinence. Posterior lesions cause such visual symptoms as homonymous hemianopsia. Surgical removal of these meningiomas may be complicated by several factors: large tumor size, highly vascularized tumors that cause extensive blood loss, attachment of the tumor to bone and falx, and invasion with occlusion of sagittal sinus.

CT shows a hyperdense homogeneously enhancing lesion with base (flat surface) directed toward the sagittal sinus. Certain of these lesions are hypodense with a peripheral enhancing nodule; this represents cystic meningioma. The dura is frequently thickened. These meningiomas may extend bilaterally between the hemispheres. Angiography shows mass effect and characteristic stain. Small middle one third lesions may be angiographically silent but well visualized by CT. Angiography should complement CT to provide the surgeon with information relating to tumor vascularity, patency of sinus and pattern of cortical veins. Solitary metastasis and superficial gliomas may simulate parasagittal meningiomas. If a parasagittal lesion is clinically suspected, it is important to include the high vertex region (including coronal views) or a small lesion may be missed by CT.

Convexity. These meningiomas arise in the region of the coronal suture and do not involve dural sinuses. Clinical symptoms include focal seizures and focal neurological deficit. CT shows hyperdense round or lens-shaped densely enhancing lesion located in the region of the sylvian fissure. The lesion is usually contiguous to bone. It is surrounded by a thin peripheral hypodense rim. Based upon radiographic finding of hyperostosis alone, it is not possible to determine if the meningioma is attached to bone; however, the finding of pressure erosion of bone is highly suggestive of bony attachment. Angiography defines mass effect, characteristic stain pattern and enlarged meningeal arteries that supply the meningioma.

Sphenoid Wing. Sphenoid bone separates the anterior and middle fossa. The lesser wing comprises the medial two thirds and the greater wing makes up the lateral one third to terminate in the pterion. Clinical symptoms are related to tumor shape (globular, en plaque), location (medial, lateral) and vector of extension to such contiguous structures as orbit, cavernous sinus, sella turcica, anterior

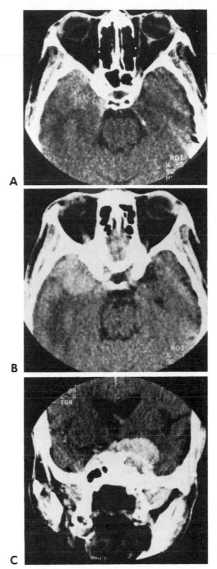

Figure 5–45. A 46-year-old woman had progressive right-sided visual loss. Findings were right optic atrophy and decreased pupillary reactivity. *CT findings:* left sphenoid left hyperdense (A) mass that enhances (B) and extends into the cavernous sinus and dorsal orbital region at reader's right (C).

and middle fossa (Fig. 5–45). Medial tumors may involve several structures: optic nerve to cause unilateral visual loss and optic atrophy, optic chiasm to cause temporal visual field defect and cavernous sinus to cause ophthalmoparesis and paresthesias in the ophthalmic branch of the trigeminal nerve. Skull radiogram may show hyperostosis of the orbital roof, anterior clinoid or medial sphenoid ridge. Angiography is important to determine if these tumors encase the cartoid, middle or anterior cerebral arteries and to exclude the presence of aneurysm.

Lateral sphenoid meningiomas may be globular in shape or spread as a sheet of tumor along the dura (en plaque). Patients with globular tumors usually present with psychomotor seizures, whereas those with en plaque tumors develop exophthalmus, ophthalmoparesis and visual loss. Skull radiogram usually shows hyperostosis of sphenoid bone. Angiography may be negative with en plaque meningiomas. CT shows hyperdense homogeneous enhancing lesion with hyperostosis of sphenoid ridge.[13]

Olfactory Groove. These arise in the midline from the floor of the anterior fossa. These tumors may grow to a large size to compress the frontal lobes. Symptoms include anosmia and Foster-Kennedy syndrome. Skull radiographic (hyperostosis) pattern, angiographic pattern (stain pattern and posterior displacement of the anterior cerebral vessels) and CT pattern (round hyperdense calcified densely enhancing bifrontal lesion) is quite specific, such that preoperative diagnosis is frequently possible.

Parasellar. These meningiomas usually arise from the tuberculum sella (Fig. 5–46). They may cause visual and endocrine symptoms. In 90 percent of cases, skull x-rays and sella tomograms show hyperostosis (blistering) of the tuberculum sella and planum sphenoidale with normal-sized sella turcica. If the lesion is small, angiography may be negative. In two patients studied with first-generation scanners, CT showed false-negative results; however, with improved contrast resolution, coronal reconstructions and intravenous contrast administration, CT has detected all parasellar meningiomas. Parasellar meningiomas had uniform appearance consisting of homogeneously speckled hyperdense round densely enhancing mass; however, this could not be reliably differentiated for other lesions, e.g., pituitary adenoma, aneurysms.

Posterior Fossa. The majority arise from posterior surface of petrous bone (40 percent), tentorium (30 percent), clivus (10 percent), foramen magnum (8 percent), and cerebellar convexity (8 per cent). Those originating from petrous bone may simulate acoustic neuroma; however, they do not initially erode the internal acoustic meatus or cause hearing loss. Tentorial meningiomas may extend supra- or infratentorially and invade contiguous venous sinuses. Initial clinical symptomatology of tentorial meningiomas includes ataxia and intra-

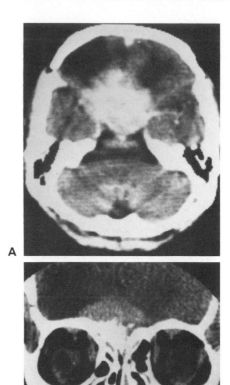

Figure 5–46. A 56-year-old man had multiple resections of parasellar meningioma. He was blind and had recently developed psychomotor seizures. *CT findings:* suprasellar enhancing mass extending into the bifrontal region (A). Bony hyperostosis is also visualized (B).

cranial hypertension; cranial nerve dysfunction develops later. Clivus meningiomas cause prominent cranial nerve abnormalities; these may clinically simulate acoustic neuromas or brain stem tumors. Skull x-ray shows bone erosion of the clivus. Foramen magnum tumors cause neck pain with subsequent development of motor dysfunction. Diagnosis is usually established by CT and vertebral angiography; however, myelography may be required for those extending to the high cervical region. CT appearance of posterior fossa meningiomas has been quite uniform. They appear as hyperdense lesions that have interspersed calcification with dense homogeneous enhancement. The finding of a heterogeneous enhancement pattern in the posterior fossa lesion is unlikely to represent meningioma.

Intraventricular. These meningiomas arise from the tela choroidea or choroid plexus most commonly in the atrium of lateral ventricles.[14] In 33 to 50 percent of cases, symptoms are episodic; this is believed to relate to intermit-tent CSF obstruction. Other symptoms relate to hydrocephalus or extension into contiguous brain parenchyma (hemiparesis, hemianes-thesia, homonymous hemianopsia). Air study demonstrates an intraventricular mass; angiog-raphy (carotid and vertebral) is necessary to define the intraventricular location of tumor and extent of blood supply. CT shows a hy-perdense noncalcified enhancing lesion. It is deeply situated and surrounded by hypodense component. If the meningioma is entirely in-traventricular, the portion of the lateral ven-tricle contiguous to the tumor is locally bal-looned; however, if tumor extends into brain parenchyma (temporal-parietal), preoperative differentiation from other deeply situated neo-plasms is not usually possible. Based upon CT findings, differentiation from other intraven-tricular tumors such as ependymomas, papil-lomas, gliomas, germinomas and metastases is not usually possible (Fig. 5–47).

MULTIPLE MENINGIOMAS

This must be differentiated from two other conditions: recurrence of meningioma, which usually is located at the site of the initial tumor resection but may be somewhat remote from this region because intradural spread had occurred, and meningiomatosis, in which there is a plethora of small meningiomas lo-cated diffusely throughout the dura. Both mul-tiple meningiomas and meningiomatosis occur most frequently in patients with von Reckling-hausen's disease; lesions occur in characteristic locations for meningiomas. The incidence of multiple meningiomas was 1 to 3 percent in the pre-CT era; however, it is 9 to 10 percent in CT series.[15]

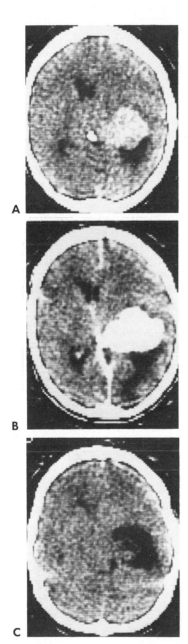

Figure 5–47. A 50-year-old woman had intermittent headache. Findings were early papilledema and left hemiparesis-hemianesthesia. Isotope scan showed right parietal uptake. *CT findings:* speckled round right hemispheric (*A*) densely enhancing lesion ex-tending to the tentorium (*B*). There is localized dila-tation of the posterior portion of the lateral ventricle with right hemispheric mass effect (*C*). *Operative finding:* intraventricular meningioma.

REFERENCES

1. Quest DO: Meningiomas: an update. Neurosurgery 3:219–225, 1978
2. Gold LH, Kieffer SA, Peterson HO: Intracranial meningiomas: a retrospective analysis of the diag-nostic value of plain skull films. Neurology 19:873–878, 1969
3. New PFJ, Aranon S, Hesselink JR: Evaluation of computed tomography in the diagnosis of intracra-nial neoplasms. Radiology 136:665, 675, 1980
4. Claveria LE, Sutton D, Tress BM: The radiological diagnosis of meningiomas, the impact of EMI scan-ning. Br J Radiol 50:15–22, 1977
5. Russell EJ, George AE, Kricheff II: Atypical com-puted tomographic features of intracranial menin-gioma. Radiology 135:673–682, 1980

6. Vassilouthis J, Ambrose J: Computerized tomography scanning appearances of intracranial meningiomas. J Neurosurg 50:320–327, 1979

7. Weisberg LA: Computed tomography in the diagnosis of intracranial meningioma. Comput Tomogr 3:115–126, 1979

8. Becker D, Norman D, Wilson CB: Computerized tomography and pathological correlation in cystic meningiomas. J Neurosurg 50:103–105, 1979

9. Kendall B, Pullicino P: Comparison of consistency of meningiomas and CT appearances. Neuroradiology 18:173–176, 1979

10. Dell S, Ganti R, Steinberger A: Cystic meningiomas; a clinicoradiological study. J Neurosurg 57:8, 1982

11. Sigel RM, Messina AV: Computed tomography: the anatomic basis of the zone of diminished density

surrounding meningiomas. Am J Roentgenol 127:139–141, 1976

12. Fink LH: Metastasis of prostatic adenocarcinoma simulating a falx meningioma. Surg Neurol 12:253–261, 1979

13. Fine M, Brazis P, Palacios E: Computed tomography of sphenoid wing meningiomas: tumor location related to distal edema. Surg Neurol 13:385–397, 1980

14. Fornari M, Savoiardo M, Morello G: Meningiomas of the lateral ventricles. J Neurosurg 54:64–74, 1981

15. Lusins JD, Nakagawa H: Multiple meningiomas evaluated by computed tomography. Neurosurgery 9:137, 1981

Glioma

Gliomas are the most common primary intracranial tumors. Pathological classification may be difficult because of the varied appearance of different regions of individual neoplasms and the finding of increasing degree of malignancy with time (Fig. 5–48). A grading system based on a single biopsy specimen may fail to indicate the actual extent of pathological heterogeneity. Gliomas have irregular and jagged-edged borders with frond-like projections. They are intra-axial tumors. These may extend into the corpus callosum, septum pellucidum, basal ganglia, thalamus and brain stem. Their gross and microscopic appearances are de-

pendent upon multiple factors, such as cellular morphology, degree of anaplasia, cellular density, neovascularity, calcification, degenerative change (cyst, hemorrhage, necrosis). In our studies we attempted to correlate CT findings in gliomas with certain pathological findings. We followed a histological grading system utilizing the classification established by Kernohan and colleagues[1]: (1) low-grade gliomas correspond to Grade I astrocytoma, (2) anaplastic gliomas include Grade II and Grade III astrocytoma, (3) glioblastoma multiforme corresponds to Grade IV astrocytoma.

Low-grade gliomas consist of astrocytes

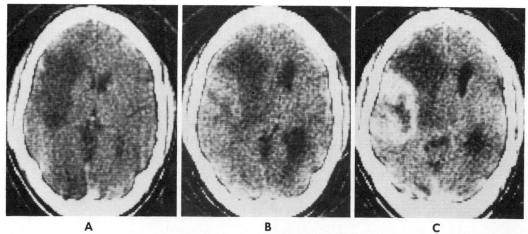

A **B** **C**

Figure 5–48. A 32-year-old man developed right focal motor seizure. Air studies and angiogram showed a temporal lobe mass. He received irradiation for presumed malignant glioma. Six months later seizures increased in frequency. *CT findings:* speckled ovoid homogeneous left hemispheric mass without enhancement (A). Surgical biopsy showed Grade I astrocytoma. Eight months later he became aphasic with right hemiparesis. *CT findings:* mixed-density lesion (B) with irregularly thick enhancement (C). This represented glioblastoma multiforme.

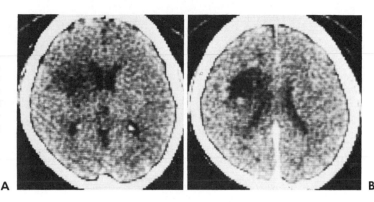

Figure 5–49. A 21-year-old man had generalized seizure; examination was normal and EEG was diffusely slow. *CT findings*: irregularly marginated hypodense left hemispheric lesion (A) with faint patchy enhancement (B). *Surgical biopsy*: Grade I astrocytoma.

showing minimal cellular anaplasia; however, there may be marked variation in degree of cellular density within the tumor. Some low-grade gliomas may be of low cellular density such that they are difficult to differentiate from areas of reactive gliosis or normal brain parenchyma. There may be cyst formation or calcification; however, other degenerative changes such as necrosis, hemorrhage and abnormal vascularity do not usually occur. Anaplastic astrocytomas have a more polymorphic histopathological appearance. Glioblastoma multiforme has variegated and polymorphic microscopic appearance with prominent degenerative (necrosis, cyst, hemorrhage) change, marked cellular anaplasia and

abnormal neovascularity. CT findings of supratentorial gliomas reflect their infiltrative and malignant pathological characteristics.[2-4] This is manifested by irregular shape with frond-like projections extending into contiguous brain parenchyma, heterogeneous density and complex irregular enhancement pattern (Table 5–2). The majority of gliomas extend deeply into hemispheric white matter; however, 5 to 10 percent are located superficially.

Low-grade gliomas usually appear hypodense on noncontrast CT, frequently with speckled (salt and pepper) pattern. They usually have irregular shape with jagged edges (Fig. 5–49); less commonly, they are round or

TABLE 5–2. CT Findings in Supratentorial Gliomas (%)

Characteristic	Low-Grade Grade I	Anaplastic Grades I & III	Glioblastoma Multiforme Grade IV
DENSITY			
Hypodense	92	52	38
Mixed			
Calcified	8	12	2
Noncalcified	–	36	60
Isodense			
MASS EFFECT			
None visualized	50	7	–
Ventricular distortion	50	23	16
Ventricular effacement	–	43	32
Ventricular displacement	–	27	52
CYST FORMATION	16	18	13
EDEMA	8	32	73
HYDROCEPHALUS	–	27	45
ENHANCEMENT	50	78	100
Homogeneous			
Nodular	–	34	9
Diffuse	100	6	4
Heterogeneous			
Multiple nodular	–	15	7
Ring-shaped	–	30	38
Garland-shaped	–	2	18
Mixed	–	13	24

ovoid with sharply marginated edges (Fig. 5–50). The hypodense region may represent the pathological features of cyst formation, central necrosis and low cellular density. Cystic gliomas contain a homogeneous central hypodense region. This has sharp margination and may show a thin peripheral enhancing rim on postcontrast scan. The cyst may show contrast fluid level.[5] It may be difficult to differentiate cystic from necrotic tumors; however, the hypodense central region of necrotic tumors is more heterogeneous in density and is surrounded by an irregularly marginated enhancing rim that has variable thickness. Mass effect is seen in 50 percent of low-grade gliomas; hydrocephalus or herniation patterns are not

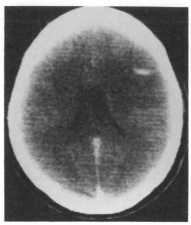

Figure 5–51. A 34-year-old man developed generalized seizures. Examination was normal. EEG showed right frontal-parietal delta pattern. *CT finding*: right frontal-parietal hypodense nonenhancing lesion with interspersed calcification. *Operative finding*: Grade I astrocytoma.

usually seen. Calcification was seen in only 8 percent of low-grade gliomas (Fig. 5–51). This is a lower incidence than pre-CT scan studies, probably reflecting earlier diagnosis with CT.[6, 7] Abnormal contrast enhancement is seen in 50 percent; it is usually diffuse and faint. Based upon CT findings, other differential diagnostic conditions are listed (Table 5–3).

Anaplastic gliomas show varied CT pattern. They have a hypodense or mixed-density pattern on plain scan. The hyperdense region may represent calcification (12 percent). This appears punctate or linear and not usually dense globular. If the calcified region is small, attenuation values may simulate hemorrhage because of partial-volume effect.[8] The hyperdense component of some gliomas may represent high cellular density; however, this is frequently diagnosed incorrectly as calcification or hemorrhage. Fifty-two percent of ana-

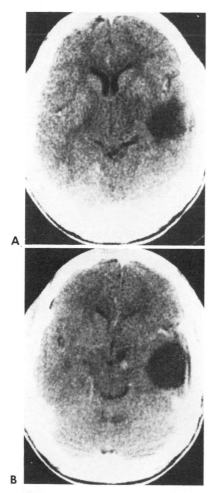

Figure 5–50. This 25-year-old man developed psychomotor seizures and intermittent psychotic behavior. EEG showed bitemporal spike discharges. *CT findings*: right temporal sharply marginated ovoid homogeneously hypodense lesion (*A*). There is a medial hypodense region with a small area of nodular enhancement (*B*). *Operative finding*: noncystic Grade I astrocytoma.

TABLE 5–3. Differential Considerations in Low-Grade Gliomas

Neoplastic
  Meningioma
  Solitary metastases
  Oligodendroglioma
Non-neoplastic
  Angioma
  Cyst—subarachnoid, epidermoid
  Cerebral infarction
  Multiple sclerosis
  Cerebritis
  Nonhemorrhagic contusion
  Reactive gliosis

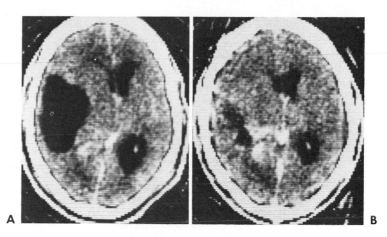

Figure 5–52. A 31-year-old man developed headache and increasing impairment of consciousness. Examination showed bilateral papilledema and dilated left pupil. *CT findings:* irregularly shaped sharply marginated hypodense (*A*) nonenhancing left temporal lesion with marked mass effect. Following surgical decompression of cystic Grade II astrocytoma, he showed clinical improvement. One month later, CT shows a small residual hypodense region with persistent mass effect and two medial enhancing areas (*B*).

plastic gliomas appear hypodense. Of these gliomas, the hypodense region represented cysts (Fig. 5–52) in 18 percent and 4 percent had prominent central necrosis. In the other 30 percent, the hypodense lesions had an irregular contour with jagged edges; these tumors had low cellular density (Fig. 5–53) but no degenerative features. Mass effect with edema is seen in 93 percent and of these, 12 percent have CT evidence of transtentorial herniation. Abnormal contrast enhancement is seen in 78 percent; it is homogeneous (diffuse or nodular) in 34 percent (Fig. 5–54) and

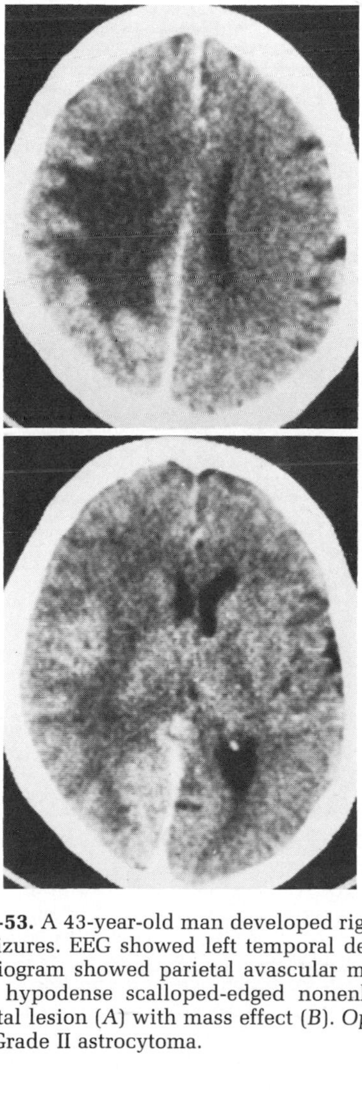

Figure 5–53. A 43-year-old man developed right focal motor seizures. EEG showed left temporal delta pattern; angiogram showed parietal avascular mass. *CT findings:* hypodense scalloped-edged nonenhancing left parietal lesion (*A*) with mass effect (*B*). *Operative finding:* Grade II astrocytoma.

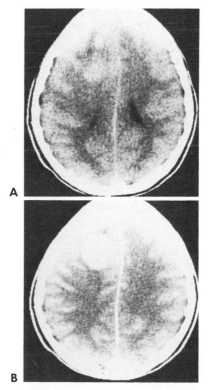

Figure 5–54. A 15-year-old girl developed headache and had generalized seizure. *CT findings:* mixed-density noncalcified left frontal lesion (*A*) with dense nodular enhancement (*B*). *Biopsy finding:* Grade II astrocytoma.

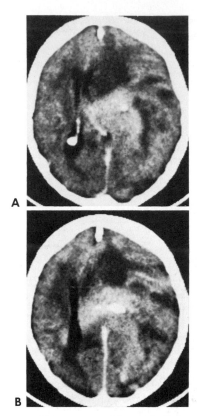

Figure 5–55. This 36-year-old man had previous resection of Grade III astrocytoma. He developed seizures and left hemiparesis. *CT findings:* right temporal mixed-density lesion with dense enhancement (A) extending across the corpus callosum (B).

heterogeneous in 44 percent (Fig. 5–55). The finding of eccentric nodular enhancement within a hypodense region is characteristic of cystic anaplastic gliomas (Fig. 5–56). Peripheral ring enhancement with complex shape and thicker portion on deeper subcortical surface is also seen. Other conditions that may simulate CT findings of anaplastic astrocytomas are listed (Table 5–4).

In patients with glioblastoma multiforme, CT findings reflect their polymorphic and var-

TABLE 5–4. Differential Considerations in Anaplastic Gliomas

Neoplastic
Metastasis
Meningioma
Sarcoma
Nonneoplastic
Reactive gliosis
Abscess
Ring-enhancing hematoma
Tuberculoma

iegated pathological characteristics; 38 percent show an irregularly marginated homogeneous hypodense lesion, whereas 62 percent appear as mixed-density heterogeneous lesions (Fig. 5–57). CT evidence of calcification is an unusual finding. Mass effect is usually present and

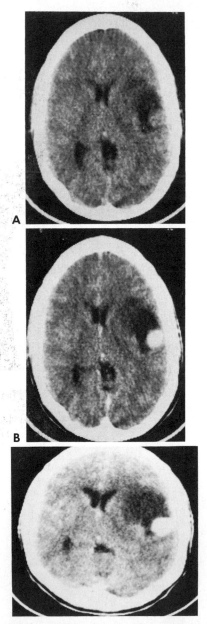

Figure 5–56. A 23-year-old man developed infrequent generalized seizures controlled on medication for seven years. He then developed an aura. CT showed right parietal hypodense lesion (A) with peripheral nodular enhancement (B). Six months later he developed hemiparesis. *CT finding:* increased size and mass effect (C) of the lesion. *Operative finding:* cystic Grade II astrocytoma.

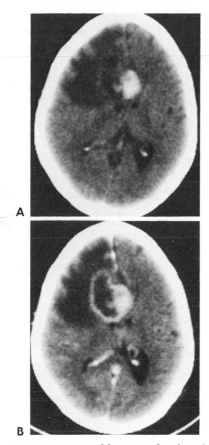

Figure 5–57. A 40-year-old woman developed rapidly worsening right hemiparesis. EEG showed monorhythmic frontal delta pattern: isotope scan showed left frontal uptake. *CT findings:* left frontal mixed-density lesion (*A*) with variable-thickness ring enhancement (*B*). *Operative finding:* glioblastoma multiforme.

TABLE 5–5. Differential Diagnostic Considerations in Glioblastoma Multiforme

Neoplastic
  Meningioma with sarcomatous degeneration
  Meningioma with atypical pathological features
  Sarcoma
  Metastasis
Non-neoplastic
  Ring-enhancing hematoma
  Brain abscess
  Reactive gliosis
  Angioma
  Tuberculoma

edema is visualized in 73 percent. Almost all glioblastomas show postcontrast enhancement (Fig. 5–58). The finding of an irregularly shaped enhancing ring of variable thickness is characteristic of malignant neoplasm; however, it is not specific for anaplastic glioma or glioblastoma multiforme (Table 5–5). The garland-shaped enhancement pattern is seen in 18 percent. This pattern is relatively specific but not unique to glioblastoma multiforme.[9]

Astrocytoma Location

Supratentorial Hemispheric Astrocytoma. Initial studies of supratentorial glioma indicated that CT was capable of earlier diagnosis than achieved by other neuroradiographic studies. The incidence of low-grade gliomas is 20 to 30 percent compared with 5 to 7 percent demonstrated in the pre-CT scan era. Moreno reported results of isotope scan in diagnosis of supratentorial glioma; Grade I was positive in

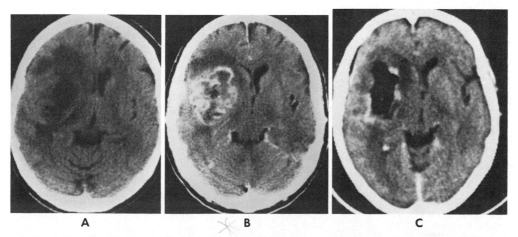

Figure 5–58. A 31-year-old woman developed right-sided weakness. EEG showed left temporal delta pattern. Angiogram showed a temporal mass with neovascularity. *CT findings:* mixed-density temporal lesion (*A*) with complex variable thickness ring enhancement (*B*). Following surgical resection of glioblastoma, CT shows air within the area of a residual-enhancing tumor (*C*).

only 50 percent, Grade II and III in 75 to 80 percent, Grade IV in 96 percent.[10] EEG shows polymorphic delta slow wave focus in 93 percent of Grade IV; spike and spike–slow wave discharges were more common in other astrocytomas. Twenty-five percent of low-grade gliomas showed radiographic calcification, whereas this was seen in only 2 percent of glioblastoma. The characteristic angiographic finding in low-grade glioma is avascular mass, usually without abnormal tumor circulation. Anaplastic astrocytoma and glioblastoma multiforme may appear as avascular masses or show extensive abnormal vascular pattern with abundant irregularly sized feeding vessels and prominent early draining veins. In certain cases the only manifestation of abnormal circulation of gliomas is the presence of an early draining vein; however, this is a nonspecific finding occurring in other conditions such as metastases, abscesses, angiomas and cerebral infarcts. In 15 percent of glioblastoma multiforme, angiography shows avascular mass only; in these cases pathological diagnosis requires surgical biopsy confirmation.[11, 12]

In 50 percent of patients with CT findings and pathological verification of Grade I gliomas, seizures were the initial symptom (Fig. 5–59). In 20 percent of patients, neurological examination was normal and angiogram showed no evidence of mass effect or abnormal vascularity; however, earlier diagnosis in neurologically intact patients has not usually resulted in improved outcome. In clinically symptomatic patients with astrocytoma, initial CT scan was negative in 2 percent. Within 4 months there was worsening of neurological symptomatology, and repeat CT showed evidence of intracranial glioma. In 6.5 percent of cases glioma was present at surgery but CT findings were most consistent with another pathological condition; in 6.4 percent CT findings were most consistent with malignant glioma but this diagnosis was not surgically confirmed.[12]

Deeply Situated Malignant Astrocytoma. The majority of these tumors are thalamic in origin; they may also originate in basal ganglia. Their peak age incidence is the second or fourth decade.[13] Clinical presenting features

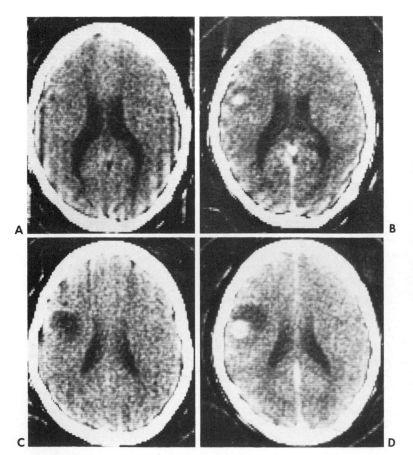

Figure 5–59. A woman patient with von Recklinghausen's disease had right focal motor seizure. EEG and isotope scan were negative. *CT findings:* left parietal isodense (*A*) region with nodular enhancement (*B*). She was asymptomatic seven months later. *CT findings:* increased size of the left parietal hypodense (*C*) lesion with nodular enhancement (*D*). Surgical biopsy showed Grade II astrocytoma.

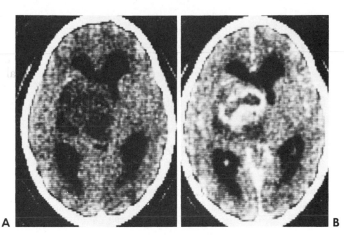

Figure 5–60. A 7-year-old girl developed headache and right arm weakness. Findings included right hemiparesis and papilledema. Angiogram showed an avascular thalamic mass. *CT findings:* left thalamic hypodense lesion effacing the third ventricle and elevating lateral ventricle (*A*). There is irregular ring enhancement (*B*). *Surgical finding:* anaplastic glioma.

include intracranial hypertension and progressive focal neurological deficit such as hemiparesis, hemianesthesia and ataxia. The diagnosis of thalamic glioma is difficult to establish by noninvasive neurodiagnostic studies: (1) EEG shows focal slowing in 25 percent but is normal or shows bilateral abnormalities in 75 percent, (2) isotope scan is positive in 25 percent and (3) skull x-ray usually shows no abnormalities. The diagnosis has usually been established by air studies; these have shown thalamic mass that elevated third ventricle. Angiography is sometimes necessary to exclude the presence of such vascular lesions as angioma, which may simulate clinical features of thalamic glioma.

CT has been quite sensitive in detecting thalamic gliomas. These lesions usually appear hyperdense (56 percent); others appear hypodense (32 percent) or isodense (12 percent). If the lesion is densely calcified, this is more consistent with oligodendroglioma. All thalamic gliomas enhance, with the exception of calcified lesions and certain cystic tumors. The enhancement pattern is usually an irregularly shaped and variable-thickness ring (Fig. 5–60) or a nodular pattern (Fig. 5–61). Mass effect is manifested by elevation and contralateral displacement of the third ventricle. The detection of thalamic mass is established at an earlier stage by CT than is possible with air studies, but CT findings do not always permit specific pathological diagnosis. Angiography is necessary to exclude vascular malformation; however, certain cryptic angiomas appear as avascular masses. The prognosis is best for patients with thalamic gliomas who have irradiation without prior surgical biopsy, tumor debulking or shunting.[14]

Brain Stem Glioma. Clinical course may be characterized by either deterioration or rapid worsening; this later course may be due to

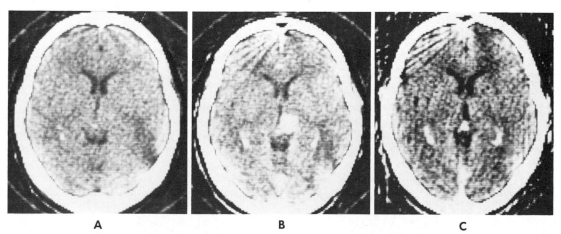

Figure 5–61. A 50-year-old man developed left arm clumsiness and numbness. EEG and isotope scan were negative. *CT findings:* right thalamic isodense lesion (*A*) with dense nodular enhancement (*B*). The lesion is causing elevation of third ventricle. Following irradiation (6 months later) he was neurologically asymptomatic; CT shows no abnormality (*C*).

anaplastic transformation within the tumor.[15] Pathological evidence of calcification, hemorrhage or cyst formation is uncommon in these tumors. Primary intramedullary brain stem gliomas usually cause brain stem enlargement. When tumor expands the brain stem, the fourth ventricle appears flattened. The fourth ventricle has widened transverse diameter and is displaced posteriorly; the pontine and interpeduncular cisterns are narrowed. These tumors appear isodense or hypodense on noncontrast scan.[16] Fifty to sixty percent show contrast enhancement; this may be localized to the small nodular region or be more extensive. Bilaniuk reported that hypodense lesions were highly anaplastic and mixed-density lesions were low-grade in their histopathological appearance[17]; however, our findings are not concordant with these findings.[16]

Surgery for confirmation of brain stem gliomas is not usually done because of their location. Surgical exploration would be of potential benefit if a large intratumoral cyst was causing significant brain stem compression or hydrocephalus. The presence of this cyst is reliably detected by CT. CT is effective in defining several characteristics of brain stem glioma that affect treatment planning: extension into the midbrain, thalamus and posterior third ventricle; the presence of a large exophytic portion of tumor; subarachnoid seeding or extension into cisterns; the presence of intratumoral hemorrhage or cyst formation and change in size, density and enhancement pattern of the neoplasm after treatment. Radiotherapy is primary treatment modality for brain stem gliomas. Most patients show initial clinical improvement but their condition subsequently deteriorates. In patients with CT evidence of brain stem glioma, clinical deterioration developed most rapidly in those patients who had initial surgical exploration and biopsy. There is a correlation of survival with histopathological grade of brain stem gliomas. Most patients with anaplastic tumors die within 18 months and 66 percent do not clinically improve despite irradiation. The most consistent CT finding correlating with poor clinical outcome was complex ring enhancement; this represented glioblastomatous transformation.

Cerebellar Astrocytoma. These tumors arise in the vermis or lateral cerebellar hemisphere. They are of four types: solid, cystic with mural nodule, solid with interspersed cystic and necrotic regions, and calcified. The protein content of tumor cyst may be high enough so that density appears visibly different from that expected for CSF.[18] Large cystic tumors have most benign histological features. These are usually located in cerebellar hemispheres. Those tumors that were entirely solid with small cystic or necrotic component are midline or paramedian in location and had more malignant histopathological characteristics. Those neoplasms with large solid or necrotic components were more likely to recur after surgical removal and irradiation. The cerebellar astrocytomas are of variable size (2.0 to 6.0 cm); clinical outcome does not correlate with lesion size. The best outcome occurred in patients with cerebellar astrocytomas that had these CT features: hypodense nonenhancing lesion, hypodense lesion with small eccentrically located enhancing mural nodule, and densely calcified nonenhancing lesions. Recurrence was seen in 30 percent of patients with these two CT patterns: heterogeneous mixed-density lesion with ring enhancement and mixed-density lesion with diffuse enhancement. The tumor recurs within 36 months of initial surgery, and patients with CT evidence of recurrence developed clinical deficit. CT findings of tumor recurrence were similar to that seen on initial scan; however, enhancement pattern frequently shows complex-shaped and variable-thickness ring enhancement. It is important to differentiate postoperative and postradiation change from tumor recurrence.[19] This may not always be possible on the basis of CT findings only; however, in our experience tumor recurrence does not develop without clinical deterioration. Zimmerman[18] has reported that CT evidence of recurrence may precede clinical worsening.

Other Primary Malignant Intracranial Neoplasms

Oligodendroglioma. These account for 5 to 7 percent of intracranial gliomas. They are usually located in the cerebral hemispheres with the majority in the frontal lobes. These tumors usually grow slowly. Some patients may have seizures as the only clinical manifestation for many years prior to diagnosis. Other tumors grow rapidly to cause acute neurological deterioration resulting from intratumoral hemorrhage or glioblastomatous transformation. There is little correlation between clinical symptoms or neurological findings and histological features of oligodendroglioma. The characteristic pathological finding is prominent calcification (Fig. 5–62). Calcification is usually related to blood vessel wall and occurs at the peripheral part of tumor. Other pathological features include central necrosis, cystic degeneration, gelatinous mucoid change and intratumoral hemorrhage. Microscopically, oligodendrogliomas are highly cellular and uniform in appearance unless glioblastomatous transformation has occurred.

The characteristic CT finding is calcification (90 percent), which has patterns that are (1) peripheral, linear or shell-like or (2) central, dense nodular or globular. The finding of a hyperdense noncalcified portion sometimes showing fluid level is consistent with intratumoral hemorrhage. In all oligodendrogliomas there is a hypodense component surrounding calcified lesion. In one study 66 percent of oligodendrogliomas showed postcontrast enhancement.[20] The calcified portion and enhanced rim may outline the periphery of the neoplasm. If there has been glioblastomatous degeneration, the enhancement pattern is that of an irregularly shaped ring of variable thickness (Fig. 5–63). Surgical removal of oligodendrogliomas is the treatment of choice, and these neoplasms are not usually radiosensitive. There has been no CT verification that operative intervention accelerates rate and growth of tumor. The relationships of calcification,

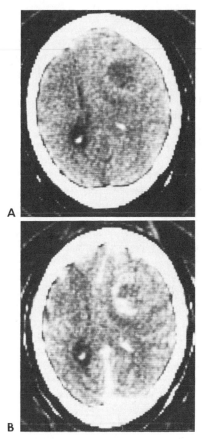

A

B

Figure 5–63. A 42-year-old woman developed rapidly progressive left-sided paralysis. EEG showed right temporal delta focus; isotope scan was negative. *CT findings:* right parietal hypodense lesion with surrounding hyperdense rim (A) with irregular variable-thickness ring enhancement, which is thickest on the medial wall (B). *Operative findings:* oligodendroglioma with glioblastomatous features.

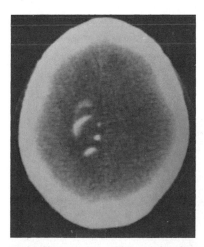

Figure 5–62. This 40-year-old man developed right focal motor seizures; examination was entirely normal. Isotope scan and skull radiogram were negative. *CT findings:* parietal linear calcified bands with surrounding hypodense nonenhancing region. Angiogram showed an avascular mass. *Operative finding:* oligodendroglioma.

cyst, hemorrhage and enhancement pattern to prognosis have not been established.[21]

Ependymomas. These constitute 6 percent of all intracranial gliomas. Sixty percent originate below the tentorium and 40 percent are supratentorial in location. They are predominantly tumors of childhood and originate most commonly from the floor of the fourth ventricle, whereas those occurring in adults are located in cerebral hemispheres. The ependymomas that originate from the fourth ventricle may project into and occlude this cavity and may also extend outward through the foramina of Luschka and into the posterior fossa cisterns—that is, the cerebellopontine angle cistern or foramen magnum. Pathological characteristics of posterior fossa ependymomas are calcification, cyst formation, intratumoral hemorrhage and central necrosis. On the basis of CT findings, differentiation from other posterior fossa tumors (medulloblastoma, astrocytoma, hemangioblastoma) is not always possible. These tumors are highly cellular; they are low in malignant potential but may sometimes undergo malignant degeneration.

CT findings are dependent upon location of tumor and pathological features. Those located within the fourth ventricle may extend through lateral recesses into the cerebellopontine cisterns or through the vallecula into the cisterna magna. The intraventricular component of tumor appears round or oval in shape. On noncontrast scan ependymomas have mixed-density heterogeneous characteristics that may represent cysts, central necrosis or calcification. Following contrast medium administration, they usually enhance with a heterogeneous ring-like pattern; however, certain ependymomas show dense homogeneous enhancement. Cerebral hemispheric ependymomas have CT characteristics that simulate malignant gliomas. Tumors in this location may calcify but do sometimes show intratumoral hemorrhage. On noncontrast scan they appear as mixed-density lesions with irregularly shaped ring enhancement of variable thickness on postcontrast scan (Fig. 5–64).

Medulloblastomas. In children, these neoplasms usually originate in the vermis of the cerebellum, invade the floor of the fourth ventricle and may extend into cisternal spaces, whereas in adolescents and young adults, neoplasms originate in lateral cerebellar hemispheres. Medulloblastomas are usually solid and highly cellular neoplasms that rarely undergo hemorrhage, calcification or cystic

degeneration. On noncontrast CT, these tumors appear as round or pyramidal-shaped lesions that are central in location and that expand the fourth ventricle. On noncontrast scan they appear isodense or hyperdense, usually without evidence of calcification. There is usually dense homogeneous enhancement on postcontrast scan. These tumors characteristically metastasize by spreading along the subarachnoid spaces; this occurrence correlates with CT evidence of basal cisternal enhancement. In older children and young adults these tumors (desmoplastic medulloblastoma, cerebellar sarcoma) are located in lateral cerebellar hemispheres. They are homogeneously dense lesions with dense contrast enhancement; in rare cases they appear hypodense with ring enhancement of variable thickness.

Ganglioglioma. These tumors occur most commonly in children and young adults. The most characteristic location is the floor of the third ventricle but these also occur in temporal lobe. They are slow-growing lesions with hamartomatous features and they rarely undergo malignant transformation. When ganglioglioma is located in the floor of the third ventricle, diabetes insipidus and hypopituitarism usually result, whereas those located in temporal lobe cause psychomotor seizures. The lesions located in cerebral hemispheres frequently calcify but this finding is rare in third ventricular lesions. In the past, air studies were usually necessary to detect the presence of third ventricular-hypothalamic gangliogliomas, but diagnosis is now reliably established by CT. CT findings are similar to those of hypothalamic gliomas or craniopharyngiomas. These include a hypodense suprasellar mass with an irregularly shaped enhancing ring of variable thick-

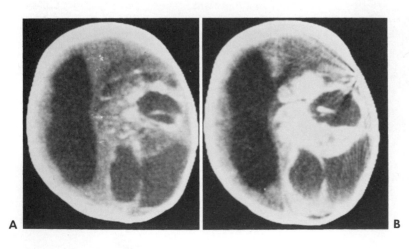

A **B**

Figure 5–64. A 12-year-old child had prior surgery and irradiation of cerebral hemispheric ependymoma. *CT findings:* right hemispheric mixed-density calcified lesion (*A*) with dense heterogeneous enhancement (*B*).

ness. The CT finding of hemispheric lesions is that of round heterogeneous mixed-density lesion with varible-thickness ring enhancement (Fig. 5–65). CT shows evidence of calcification, but this is usually not seen by skull radiogram.

Neuroblastoma. These neoplasms may be of two types: (1) primary intracranial lesions located in the cerebral hemispheres (Fig. 5–66) and (2) metastatic craniocerebral lesions. These involve the orbit, skull base and calvarium and may extend to the epidural and subdural spaces (Fig. 5–67). The primary cerebral neuroblastomas occur in the first decade of life and may originate in any part of cerebral hemispheres. These tumors are rapidly growing neoplasms that are intraparenchymal and sharply delineated from surrounding brain.

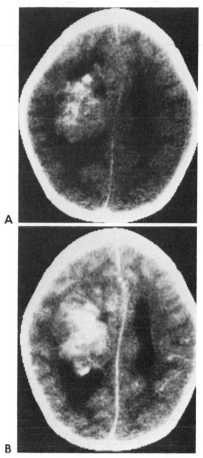

Figure 5–66. A 1-year-old child developed right-sided hemiplegia. Skull x-ray was negative; EEG showed left parietal delta activity. *CT findings:* left parietal, thalamic and intraventricular mixed-density lesion with interspersed calcification (A) and heterogeneous enhancement (B). *Operative finding:* neuroblastoma.

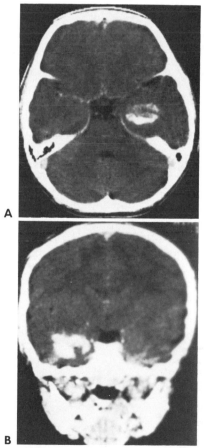

Figure 5–65. An 8-year-old boy developed partial complex seizures. EEG showed right medial temporal spike focus; skull radiogram showed no calcification. *CT findings:* irregular hyperdense calcified medial-inferior temporal heterogeneous lesion with enhancement (A). This lesion is well visualized on coronal scan (reader's left) (B). *Operative finding:* ganglioglioma.

The tumor is usually multilobulated with prominent hemorrhage, necrosis and mucoid gelatinous cystic degeneration. CT findings reflect presence of these pathological characteristics.[22]

Metastatic neuroblastoma to skull and orbit occurs in 25 percent of cases and may be the initial clinical manifestation of neuroblastoma. Early skull involvement is reliably detected by isotope bone scan. Skull radiogram usually shows bone thickening, multiple osteolytic lesions, suture separation and periosteal reaction. The tumor elevates the periosteum to cause fine radial bone spiculation ("hair-on-end" periosteal reaction). CT may show these abnormalities: bony erosion of both inner and outer tables of skull, subperiosteal masses

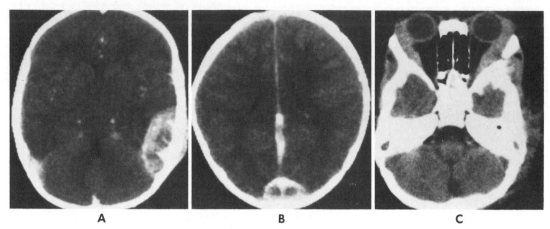

Figure 5–67. A 17-month-old girl became increasing lethargic and irritable. Examination showed nuchal rigidity and left hemiparesis. *CT findings:* right temporal (*A*) and occipital enhancing epidural lesion with overlying soft tissue involvement (*B*). There is nonfilling of the sagittal sinus consistent with sinus thrombosis by tumor. Bilateral lateral rectus enlargement is consistent with orbital extension (*C*). *Biopsy findings:* neuroblastoma (metastatic from abdomen).

involving orbit and facial bones, and epidural tumor.

Gliosis of Unknown Etiology

Supratentorial. Intracranial gliosis is nonspecific reactive tissue response to surgical intervention, trauma, infection, neoplasms, demyelination and vascular lesions; in rare cases this may develop spontaneously. Areas of reactive gliosis may occur at the periphery of tumors; that is, metastases, meningiomas or in association with zones of demyelination in multiple sclerosis, progressive multifocal leukoencephalopathy or acute necrotizing leukoencephalopathy. In certain cases, diagnosis of "gliosis of unknown etiology" is made on the basis of limited surgical biopsy and may not be representative of pathology of the entire lesion. Certain low-grade gliomas may be pathologically difficult to differentiate from reactive gliosis, but the clinical course usually shows evidence of increasing size or neoplasia in malignant gliomas. In rare cases final diagnosis of "reactive gliosis" is established definitively by necropsy findings.

In patients with "gliosis of unknown etiology," clinical findings included focal neurological deficit without intracranial hypertension and altered consciousness or seizures. The onset was sudden in 33 percent and gradual in 67 percent. In one half of cases, neurological deficit worsened over an interval of one to five weeks. EEG usually showed focal slowing and isotope scan showed abnormal uptake in 25 percent. Carotid angiography revealed supratentorial avascular mass in all cases.[23]

CT findings showed a variable pattern, including hypodense ovoid nonenhancing lesion (Fig. 5–68), mixed density noncalcified lesion with nodular or ring enhancement (Fig. 5–69) and isodense lesion with serpiginous enhancement. CT evidence of edema and mass effect was present in one third of cases but was not prominent (Table 5–6). In only 8 percent (one case) did subsequent studies show evidence of an underlying etiology (metastatic neoplasm). In all cases diagnosis was established by pathological findings with adequate follow-up interval (up to 4 years) for the underlying etiology to be detected. On the basis of CT findings, initial presumptive diagnosis was intracranial neoplasm; however, irradiation without initial surgical biopsy is a dangerous and unwarranted approach.

TABLE 5–6. Differential Diagnostic Considerations in Supratentorial Gliosis

Pattern	Differential Diagnosis
Hypodense nonenhancing	Nonneoplastic cyst Low-grade glioma Solitary metastasis Cystic angioma Nonhemorrhagic contusion Focal encephalitis Cerebritis
Mixed-density enhancing (ring or nodular)	Anaplastic glioma Solitary metastases Cerebritis-abscess Ring-enhancing hematoma
Isodense enhancing (serpiginous)	Enhancing infarct Angioma

Figure 5–68. A 34-year-old woman developed headaches with vomiting; examination was normal. CSF showed normal pressure and fluid content. *CT findings:* right parietal hypodense nonenhancing lesion (*A*). Angiogram showed parietal avascular mass. Biopsy showed encephalomalacia with marked gliosis; bacterial cultures were negative. Four weeks later she developed left hemiparesis. *CT findings:* right parietal-occipital hypodense lesion with ring enhancement (*B*), which represented an encapsulated abscess that had developed as a complication of initial surgery.

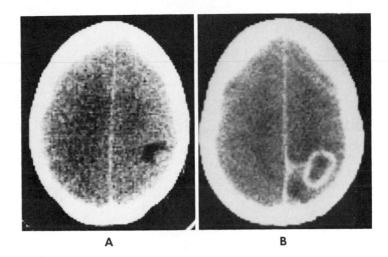

A   B

Infratentorial. In posterior fossa, non-neoplastic simple (gliotic) cerebellar cyst may occur spontaneously or develop as a delayed complication of surgical removal or irradiation of a tumor. Five patients with gliotic cerebellar cyst showed typical clinical features, including progressively worsening gait with evidence of gait and limb ataxia. In cases in which air studies are performed, these show a vermian mass; vertebral angiogram usually shows an avascular mass without tumor stain or abnormal vessels.[24] The characteristic CT finding is that of a hypodense ovoid sharply marginated lesion (Fig. 5–70). The fourth ventricle is sometimes poorly visualized; however, it was not always possible to determine if it is effaced from mass effect by cyst or whether the fourth ventricle has been volume-averaged with cyst, thereby making its delineation from cyst quite difficult. If there is definite fourth

Figure 5–69. A 48-year-old man suddenly developed left hemiparesis-sensory syndrome. Isotope scan was negative. *CT findings:* irregularly shaped isodense (*A*) ring-enhancing lesion with minimal effect (*B*). He showed slight clinical improvement and repeat CT five weeks later showed a hyperdense (*C*) lesion with enhancement (*D*). Isotope scan was positive; angiogram showed parietal avascular mass. At operation a firm gray-whitish mass was removed, which represented gliosis without neoplasia. He was clinically asymptomatic 4 years later.

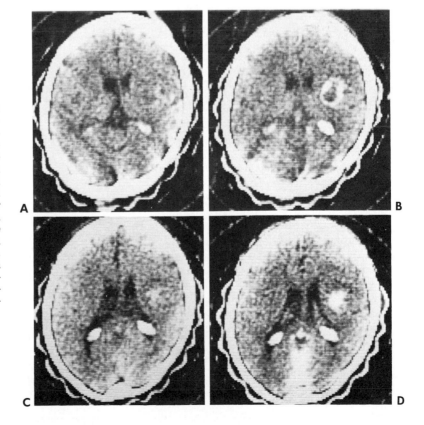

A   B

C   D

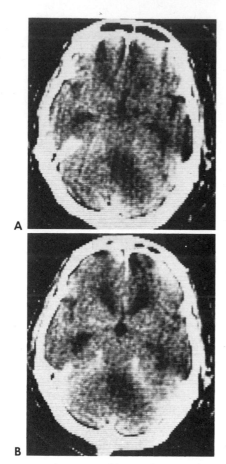

Figure 5–70. A 50-year-old man developed gait instability; examination showed gait and right-sided limb ataxia. *CT findings:* right cerebellar hemispheric ventricle (A) and biventricular enlargement. The enhancement at the periphery represents normal tentorium (B). *Operative finding:* simple cerebellar cyst.

ventricular mass effect, there is accompanying biventricular enlargement. In those patients who had a cerebellar astrocytoma surgically removed one to two decades previously, an area of enhancement contiguous to a hypodense region was sometimes seen on postcontrast scan (Fig. 5–71). It is important not to confuse normal vermian (nodular in shape) or tentorial (ring-like in shape) enhancement located at the periphery of the hypodense region with abnormal tumor enhancement. In two patients who had surgically proved gliotic cerebellar cyst, paucity of mass effect (midline enlarged fourth ventricles, prominent folial pattern) was a reliable finding to differentiate gliotic cyst from recurrent neoplasm. Other pathological conditions that have similar CT appearance to simple cerebellar cysts include hemangioblastoma, metastasis, subarachnoid

cyst, cerebellar infarction and entrapped fourth ventricle.[25]

Gliomatosis Cerebri. This condition is characterized by diffuse and widespread infiltration of the brain by neoplastic glial cells of astrocytoma series.[26, 27] There is marked diffuse astrocytic infiltration in both supra- and infratentorial regions. This is most prominent in the brain stem, cerebellum and subcortical white matter with less involvement of cerebral cortex. There is preservation of neuronal elements in involved regions, and it is not possible to differentiate normal from involved regions. Presenting clinical features are varied and include (1) prominent mental deterioration with minimal focal deficit, (2) signs of

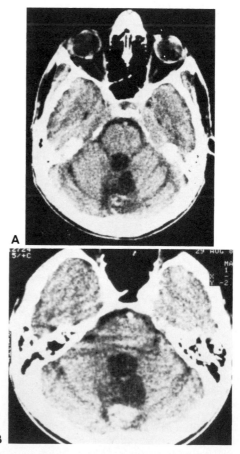

Figure 5–71. This 30-year-old man had had a cerebellar astrocytoma surgically removed two decades previously. Over the last six months he felt increasingly unsteady; however, examination showed no interval change. *CT findings:* hypodense lesion located posterior to the enlarged fourth ventricle and a prominent folial pattern (A). There is a small nodular enhancing area (B). Repeat CT (2 years later) showed no interval change. This is believed to represent reactive gliosis rather than recurrent neoplasm.

Figure 5–72. A 12-year-old developed ptosis and diplopia. Findings were oculomotor paresis. EEG showed right hemispheric delta pattern; isotope scan was negative. Angiogram showed diffuse hemispheric mass effect. *CT findings:* irregularly marginated hypodense nonenhancing right hemispheric lesion (A) with marked mass effect (B). *Operative finding:* gliomatosis cerebri.

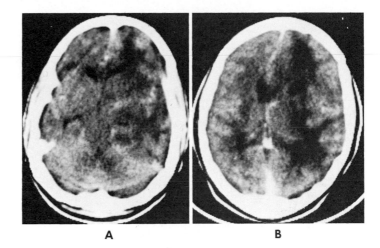

A   B

intracranial hypertension and (3) ataxia and cranial nerve dysfunction. Seizures are uncommon, reflecting less severe cerebral cortical involvement. Intracranial hypertension is caused by diffuse tumor overgrowth rather than ventricular obstruction; herniation syndrome may occur. Air study and angiography are frequently normal; CSF shows elevated pressure but negative cytology. EEG shows bilateral diffuse abnormal pattern. CT may show these abnormalities: (1) hypodense lesions with irregular frond-like projections in subcortical white matter and sparing gray matter, (2) widespread cerebral hemispheric involvement frequently with both cingulate and transtentorial herniation (Fig. 5–72), (3) marked mass effect with extension across corpus callosum, and (4) minimal contrast enhancement. Although brain stem and cerebellar white matter are involved by tumor infiltration, CT may show no abnormalities. Periventricular enhancement may indicate subependymal tumor spread; however, this did not correlate with cellular malignancy.

REFERENCES

1. Svien HJ, Mabon RF, Kernohan JW: Astrocytomas. Proc Staff Meetings Mayo Clinic 24:54–64, 1949
2. Thompson JLA: CT and the diagnosis of glioma. Clin Radiol 27:431–441, 1976
3. Tchang S, Scotti G, Terbugge K: Computerized tomography as a possible aid to histological grading of supratentorial gliomas. J Neurosurg 46:735–739, 1977
4. Weisberg, LA: Cerebral computed tomography in the diagnosis of supratentorial astrocytoma. Comput Tomogr 4:87–105, 1980
5. Afra D, Norman D, Levin VA: Cysts in malignant gliomas: identification by computerized tomography. J Neurosurg 53:821–825, 1980
6. Kalen C, Burrows, EH: Calcification in intracranial gliomata. Br J Radiol 35:589–596, 1962
7. Gouliamos AD, Jimenez JR, Goree JA: Computed tomography and skull radiography in the diagnosis of calcified brain tumor. Am J Roentgenol 130:761–764, 1978
8. Dohrmann GJ, Greehr RB, Robinson F: Small hemorrhages versus small calcifications in brain tumors: difficulty in differentation by computed tomography. Surg Neurol 10:309–312, 1978
9. Steinhoff H, Lanksch W, Kozner E: Computed tomography in the diagnosis and differential diagnosis of glioblastomas. Neuroradiology 14:193–200, 1977
10. Moreno JB, Deland FH: Brain scanning in the diagnosis of astrocytomas of the brain. J Nuclear Med 12:107, 1971
11. Joyce P, Bentson J, Takahashi M: The accuracy of predicting histologic grades of supratentorial astrocytomas on the basis of computerized tomography and cerebral angiography. Neuroradiology 16:346–348, 1978
12. Kendall B, Jakubowski J, Pullicon P: Difficulties in diagnosis of supratentorial gliomas by CAT scan. J Neurol Neurosurg Psychiat 42:485–492, 1979
13. Cheek WR, Taveras JM: Thalamic tumors. J Neurosurg 24:505–513, 1966
14. Weisberg LA: Thalamic gliomas: clinical and computed tomographic correlations. Comput Radiol 7:210, 1983.
15. Panitch HS, Berg BD: Brain stem tumors of childhood and adolescence. Am J Dis Child 119:465–472, 1970
16. Weisberg LA: Computed tomography in the diagnosis of brain stem gliomas. Comput Tomogr 3:145, 1979
17. Bilaniuk LT, Zimmerman RA, Littman P: Computed tomography of brain stem gliomas in children. Radiology 134:89–95, 1980
18. Zimmerman RA, Bilaniuk LT, Bruno L: Computed tomography of cerebellar astrocytoma. Am J Roentgenol 130:929–933, 1980
19. Weisberg LA: Computed tomographic findings in cerebellar astrocytoma. Comput Tomogr 6:137, 1982
20. Vonofakos D, Marcu H, Hacker H: Oligodendrogliomas: CT patterns with emphasis on features indicating malignancy. J Comput Asst Tomogr 3:783–788, 1979
21. Lilja A, Bergstrom K, Spannare B: Reliability of

computed tomography in assessing histopathological features of malignant supratentorial gliomas. J Comput Asst Tomogr 5:625–636, 1981

22. Zimmerman RA, Bilaniuk LT: CT of primary and secondary neuroblastoma. Am J Neuroradiol 1:431–434, 1980
23. Weisberg LA: Computed tomographic findings in intracranial gliosis. Neuroradiology 21:253–257, 1981
24. Silverberg DH: Non-neoplastic cerebellar cyst. J Neurosurg 35:320, 1971
25. Weisberg LA: Non-neoplastic gliotic cerebellar cyst. Neuroradiology 23:300, 1982
26. Couch JR, Weiss SA: Gliomatosis cerebri. Neurology 24:504, 1974
27. Hayck J, Valavanis A: CT of gliomatosis cerebri. Comput Radiol 6:93, 1982

Chapter 6

RAPID ONSET OF NEUROLOGICAL DEFICIT (STROKE SYNDROMES)

Cerebral Ischemia and Infarction

Cerebrovascular accidents result from thromboembolism causing abrupt decrease in cerebral perfusion with cerebral infarction or intracerebral hemorrhage with brain parenchymal bleeding. *Stroke syndrome* is defined as an episode in which focal neurological deterioration suddenly occurs and deficit becomes maximal within minutes to several hours. Clinical classification is based upon temporal and spatial pattern. *Transient ischemic attacks (TIA)* are episodes of rapidly developing neurological deficit localized to the carotid territory (hemiparesis, hemianesthesia, aphasia, amaurosis fugax [transient monocular blindness]) or vertebral-basilar territory (vertigo, diplopia, ataxia, drop-attacks, bilateral visual disturbances). They characteristically persist for 2 to 30 minutes and then resolve spontaneously and completely; however, they may be more prolonged, extending for as long as 24 hours before resolving. These attacks may be recurrent; sometimes they are harbingers of completed stroke.

The term *completed stroke* is used to define acutely developing neurological deficit that rapidly stabilizes without subsequent worsening. Neurological deficit may be submaximal (hemiparesis rather than hemiplegia), or spatial distribution (monoplegia rather than hemiplegia) may not be complete in patients with "completed stroke." *Stroke in evolution (SIE)* or *progressing stroke* refers to a disorder in which patients show sudden onset of neurological deficit and the clinical condition worsens over minutes to several hours before reaching maximal severity. Twenty percent of patients with stroke syndromes suffer subsequent delayed neurological deterioration. During the period of progression it is believed that the underlying pathological process, which may involve ischemia, infarction, edema and hemorrhage, is actively extending. Worsening may continue for 96 hours in some patients with progressing stroke. In patients with carotid ischemia, 24 hours of stabilization suggests that further progression is unlikely; for vertebral basilar territory, 72 hours of stabilization is sufficient to expect no further progression.[1] Neurological deficit may worsen in the gradual progressive pattern, the stepwise or stuttering pattern and the fluctuating-severity pattern. Common etiologies for strokes that show progressive worsening include (1) lacunar infarcts, (2) cerebral embolism, (3) brain stem ischemic episodes such as basilar artery occlusion, lateral medullary syndrome due to vertebral artery occlusion, (4) progressive internal carotid artery stenosis or occlusion, (5) cerebral hemorrhages and (6) intracranial mass lesions which mimic cerebrovascular lesions. Although the majority of strokes in evolution are caused by cerebral infarctions, it has been reported that 10 to 18 percent of cerebral hemorrhages have a progressive or stuttering course.[2] When focal neurological deficit develops rapidly and persists for longer than 24 hours but less than one week, this is defined as "reversible ischemic neurological deficit" syndrome (Fig. 6–1). The mechanism of this clinical syndrome is believed to be reversible but prolonged focal cerebral ischemia; however, necropsy

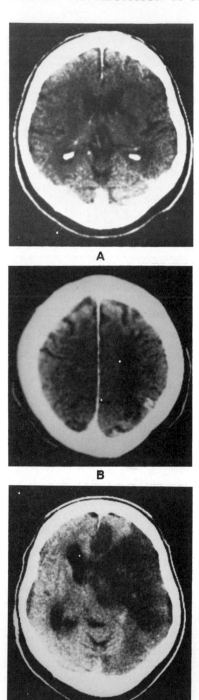

Figure 6–1. This 46-year-old woman had five TIA episodes. She subsequently developed right hemiparesis and transcortical motor aphasia, which cleared in 6 days. *CT findings:* left ganglionic hypodense lesion (*A*) with parietal gyral enhancement (*B*). Two weeks later, she developed severe headache and became obtunded with right hemiplegia. *CT findings:* extensive right hemispheric hypodense lesion with mass effect (*C*). Angiogram showed carotid artery occlusion.

and CT studies have shown that the syndrome may be caused by cerebral embolism, lacunar infarcts or watershed infarcts due to severe stenosis of the carotid artery.

Although the majority of clinically diagnosed stroke syndromes are due to cerebrovascular disease, episodes of rapid neurological deterioration may be caused by neoplasm, abscess, subdural hematoma or demyelinating disorder.[3] In these patients, rapid clinical deterioration may be caused by sudden shifts in intracranial pressure, mechanical compression by the mass to cause venous infarction, peritumoral hemorrhage and sudden paroxysmal electrical activity (seizures, demyelination). If neoplasms simulate stroke syndrome, the patient frequently exhibits prodromal symptoms such as headache, vomiting, altered mentation and behavioral change. In patients with stroke syndromes caused by cerebrovascular disease, there is usually no further progression after 96 hours; whereas in patients with nonvascular disorders there may be subsequent worsening. In patients with hemorrhagic neoplasm, there may be initial clinical improvement as hemorrhage resolves, but following continued tumor growth and edema, worsening subsequently occurs.

In the pre-CT era, the incidence of incorrect diagnoses in stroke syndromes was 2 to 4 percent. Bull et al. assessed the accuracy of clinical diagnosis of "acute stroke syndrome" by performing angiography on 80 consecutive patients; two neoplasms (glioma, metastases) were visualized. In both patients initial clinical improvement occurred with later neurological worsening.[4] Angiography defined the location of the vascular occlusive process in 40; avascular mass that represented intracerebral hematoma was seen in 20; angiography was normal in 18. Dalsgaard-Nielson demonstrated that necropsy diagnosis in stroke patients was frequently discordant with clinical impression. Clinical diagnosis of cerebral hemorrhage was confirmed at necropsy in 65 percent and cerebral infarction was confirmed in only 57 percent.[5]

Several groups of investigators have classified clinical and necropsy diagnosis in stroke syndrome: (1) cerebral embolism, 3 to 15 percent; (2) intracerebral hemorrhage, 8 to 15 percent; (3) cerebral thrombosis, 52 to 72 percent; (4) clinically unsuspected mass lesions, 2 to 4 percent and (5) aneurysms and arteriovenous malformations, 5 to 7 percent. In one prospective study utilizing CT and angiography, incidence of each type of stroke

TABLE 6–1. Incidence of Findings in Each Type of Stroke (%)

Finding	Large-Artery Thrombo-embolism	Lacune	Embolism (cardiac)	Small Superficial Cerebral Ischemia-Infarction	Intra-cerebral Hematoma
Seizure	2	0	24	25	14
Headache	18	10	10	2	58
Vomiting	6	0	2	0	50
Altered consciousness					
Mild	14	0	10	0	40
Severe	12	0	8	0	20
Bloody CSF	2	0	2	0	20
Prodromal TIA	0	0	10	46	58
Course					
Progressive	30	33	5	30	20
Nonprogressive	70	67	95	70	80

was determined: thrombosis of large artery, 34 percent; lacunar infarcts, 19 percent; intracerebral hemorrhage, 10 percent; aneurysm and arteriovenous malformation, 6 percent and embolism, 31 percent. A higher percentage of embolism reflects inclusion of embolic strokes caused by carotid occlusive disease combined with those of cardiac source.[6] Of 111 patients with stroke syndromes studied with CT, Kinkel reported cerebral infarction (90) and intracerebral hemorrhage (21). In 58 patients, initial clinical diagnosis had been thrombotic stroke based on the features of prodromal TIA, normal consciousness at onset of focal neurological deficit and nonbloody CSF. CT findings confirmed the diagnosis of cerebral infarctions in 42, whereas CT showed intracerebral hemorrhage in 11 and was negative in 5. Twenty-one patients were initially clinically diagnosed as having intracerebral hemorrhage based on these features: no prodromal TIA, prominent headache, vomiting, apoplectic nonprogressive focal deficit and altered mentation. CT showed ICH in 12 and cerebral infarction in 9. Thirty-two patients were clinically diagnosed as having TIA; however, CT showed cerebral infarction in 9 patients.[7]

In our prospective analysis of 100 patients with carotid TIA, CT showed lesions in 20 percent. These abnormalities included: (1) malignant astrocytoma, (2) subdural hematoma, (3) cerebral infarction (hypodense nonenhancing lesion), (4) ischemic lesion (isodense enhancing lesion), (5) intracerebral hematoma and (6) hemorrhagic cerebral infarction due to cerebral embolism from a cardiac source. Those patients who had CT evidence of cerebral ischemia had prolonged TIA lasting 6 to 24 hours. In patients with TIA, CT should

complement angiography if anticoagulation or carotid surgery are considered. If patients have TIA and CT shows recent infarction, surgical restoration of blood flow may precipitate hemorrhagic infarction.

In our series of 100 consecutive patients with clinical diagnosis of completed stroke, there were five neoplasms; however, only one was hemorrhagic. Forty of these patients had CT findings consistent with cerebral infarction; five of these lesions were small deep lacunes. Certain clinical findings in patients with nonhemorrhagic cerebral infarction were unexpected; headache was initial symptom in 33 percent, seizures were present in 25 percent and altered consciousness was observed in 25 percent. In 10 other cases, CT showed hemorrhagic infarction. Subsequent cardiovascular assessment (ECG, Holter monitor, echocardiogram), detected cardiac abnormalities including arrhythmia, myocardial infarction and valvular heart disease in all patients. In only one patient with hemorrhagic cerebral infarction was CSF bloody or xanthochromic. Since the risk of recurrence of embolism is 45 to 60 percent and this complication is most likely to occur within the first month after initial stroke, anticoagulation therapy is initiated if the infarction is nonhemorrhagic; however, there is potential risk of subsequent deterioration with anticoagulation if CT or CSF examination shows evidence of recent hemorrhage.[8] In 45 patients with completed stroke, CT showed evidence of intracerebral hemorrhage (ICH). Locations were putamen (25), thalamus (10), lobar (7), cerebellum (2) and brain stem (1). Forty-six percent of these patients were hypertensive, and no etiology for stroke was defined in 54 percent. Clinical findings of ICH included: (1) premonitory transient ischemic episodes were seen in 20 percent, (2) stuttering or fluctuating onset was characteristic in 30 percent, (3) classic symptoms of intracerebral hemorrhage such as headache, seizures, vomiting and altered consciousness were present in only 67 percent, (4) CSF was bloody or xanthochromic in 52 percent. Angiography was performed in 15 patients suspected of having underlying aneurysm or angioma; it did not show underlying vascular lesion, and mass effect caused by hematoma was seen in only 5 cases. Mortality of these 45 patients was 20 percent.

In 50 consecutive patients with clinical diagnosis of progressive stroke, CT findings included intracerebral hemorrhage (10), mass lesion (12) and cerebral infarction (28). In evaluation of patients with progressing stroke, CT should be performed immediately. This will exclude cerebral hemorrhage and most neoplasms if performed in the initial 72 hours after the stroke; however, it may be negative in 20 to 50 percent of cerebral infarcts. If progression was stepwise, CT showed cerebral infarction in all cases; if clinical deficit progressed more gradually over 12 to 96 hours, all patients had CT findings of nonvascular mass lesion. If maximal deficit developed in less than 12 hours, CT showed infarction or hemorrhage. In patients with progressing stroke, angiography is indicated in these circumstances: (1) if CT shows a lesion such as neoplasm that requires further delineation, e.g., abnormal circulation; (2) if clinical features suggest increasing carotid stenosis or ulcerated plaque (amaurosis fugax, carotid bruit, retinal emboli) and (3) if progressing

stroke cannot be differentiated from prolonged TIA. If CT is negative, angiography is usually not necessary immediately as initial CT may not always detect cerebral infarct. Angiography is not indicated if the patient has: (1) CT evidence of hemorrhage or infarction with edema and mass effect, (2) clinical findings of impaired consciousness or severe focal deficit, (3) an evident source of cardiac embolism or (4) acute myocardial infarction.

Management of patients with progressive stroke is determined by clinical, CT and angiographical findings. If CT shows evidence of intracranial hemorrhage, anticoagulation should be avoided. In patients with progressing stroke who are diagnosed as having nonhemorrhagic cerebral infarction, CT may show these abnormalities: (1) edema that is sometimes extensive enough to cause significant mass effect, (2) isodense enhancing ischemic lesion, (3) lacunar infarct and (4) hypodense infarct without edema or mass effect. Since edema is maximal in the initial 96 hours and usually resolves spontaneously, the beneficial effect of corticosteroids and hyperosmolar agents is controversial. In most patients who die in first week of progressive stroke, edema and herniation invariably occur; however, it is not possible to predict development of this complication. If patients with progressing stroke have normal CT scan or show small superficial infarct, anticoagulants should probably be utilized; if CT shows small deep (lacunar) infarct, the value of anticoagulation is less clearly established.

The development of delayed neurological worsening that occurs later than 96 hours after

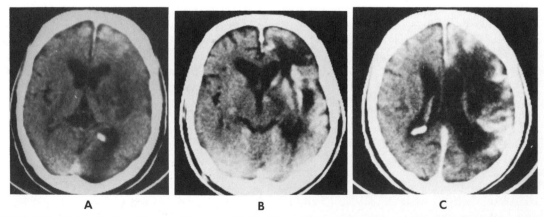

Figure 6–2. The patient, a 70-year-old man with bladder carcinoma, became unable to express himself and could not walk. Findings were nonfluent aphasia and right hemiparesis. *CT findings:* left hemispheric wedge-shaped nonenhancing lesion with minimal mass effect (A). One week later, he showed no clinical improvement. *CT findings:* hypodense lesion with dense ganglionic (B) and dense gyral enhancement (C) but resolution of mass effect.

the initial clinical episode does not represent SIE (Fig. 6–2). This is important because anticoagulation may be beneficial in progressive stroke but not in delayed deterioration unless recurrent cerebral embolism is suspected. In cases of delayed deterioration CT may show: (1) intracerebral hemorrhage with intraventricular extension that developed after the initial scan, (2) a separate noncontiguous hypodense lesion presumed caused by recurrent cerebral embolism, (3) enlargement of a hypodense region with marked mass effect, e.g., herniation. In 50 percent of patients with delayed neurological deterioration, CT showed no interval change. The mechanism of neurological worsening in these patients may be local or systemic metabolic factors. Recurrent stroke within two weeks of initial episode is uncommon, especially if the patient receives anticoagulation.

CT FINDINGS OF ISCHEMIC STROKE

In early studies of CT in cerebral infarction, Paxton and Ambrose reported positive findings in 27 of 55 cases.[9] CT was positive in 8 to 15 patients studied in the initial 7 days following clinical ictus, 8 of 17 studied at 7 to 21 days, and positive in only 4 of 23 scanned after 3 weeks. Initial CT abnormalities usually consist of evidence of edema as manifested by effacement of cortical sulcal spaces or ventricular compression. This may precede development of nonhomogeneous speckled (salt and pepper) hypodense lesion.[10] This lesion, representing infarction, is triangular, rectangular, trapezoid, round or oval in shape, has sharp margination and is confined to specific vascular territories. It shows minimal evidence of mass effect and no abnormal enhancement. The most common pattern is a wedge-shaped hypodense lesion that extends to the cortical surface; its apex is directed toward the ventricles. It is believed that the hypodense region represents cerebral edema. This is based on findings of edema in experimental models of acute stroke that begins 8 to 24 hours after ictus and is maximal 72 to 96 hours later.[11] The edema resolves spontaneously, and there should be no evidence of edema and mass effect in infarcts by the third week after clinical ictus. Despite invariable development of edema in patients with acute ischemia and infarction, only 20 percent show CT evidence of mass effect with prominent ventricular distortion or herniation.[12, 13] Other early pathological changes in cerebral infarction include tissue hyperemia caused by dilatation and congestion of subpial vessels, petechial hemorrhages and early tissue necrosis. It is possible that these factors contribute to the speckled heterogeneous appearance of predominantly hypodense-appearing infarct.

CT may show no abnormality for several days after clinical ictus. Our earliest detectable abnormality was seen 12 hours after clinical ictus, and the longest interval between clinical onset and visualization of a hypodense lesion was 72 hours (Fig. 6–3). Those infarcts that are visualized within 12 hours after onset of clinical deficit represent large lesions. With high-resolution scanners 50 to 75 percent of

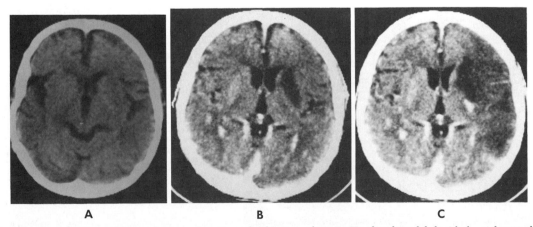

A   **B**   **C**

Figure 6–3. A 60-year-old man had nephrectomy for hypernephroma. He developed left-sided weakness that became maximal in 6 hours. Initial CT showed no abnormality (A). Repeat scan 18 hours later showed large ganglionic nonenhancing lesion (B). One week later, he showed slight clinical improvement. CT shows an extensive wedge-shaped hypodense lesion with slight ganglionic enhancement and no mass effect (C).

infarcts are detected within the initial 36 hours. The initial CT findings are effacement of cortical sulcal spaces and ventricular compression ipsilateral to the infarct, although the hypodense component and enhancement that develop later are not seen at this early phase. In patients in whom CT evidence of cerebral ischemia is an isodense enhancing lesion, scan may remain normal for 10 days after the ictal event. Within the first week, serial scans may show progressive enlargement of hypodense regions resulting from increasing edema or necrosis.

By the beginning of the second week, changes in the CT appearance include (1) reduction in the amount of mass effect and edema, (2) more sharp delineation and margination of the hypodense lesion from surrounding normal brain parenchyma, (3) more homogeneous appearance of the hypodense lesion and (4) abnormal contrast enhancement. The lesion usually appears hypodense; however, it may be isodense because of "fogging effect." This refers to an increase in density that occurs during the second and third weeks. This causes a hypodense lesion to appear isodense on noncontrast scan.[14] It may occur uniformly throughout the lesion or in one or several isolated areas only. When fogging effect occurs, abnormal contrast enhancement is usually present but mass effect is not seen. Because of fogging effect, false-negative results may be obtained unless the initial scan had been performed in the first week and had showed hypodense lesion, or postcontrast scan is performed on patients with isodense appearance. The fogging effect should not be confused with the false-negative scan that occurs when hypodense infarct enhances sufficiently on postcontrast scan to become isodense. This isodense lesion would not be detected if only postcontrast scan is performed

and there is, therefore, no initial noncontrast scan for comparison (Fig. 6–4).

During the stage of resorption (7th to 42nd days), there is resolution of edema and lesion size further decreases. Phagocytic macrophages migrate into the infarcted region to remove necrotic tissue. At this time, infarcts appear hypodense or isodense. By the end of the third week, phagocytized necrotic material changes to neutral fat (fatty macrophages or gitter cells). This contributes to the hypodense appearance of the infarct at this stage. Cyst formation and gliosis begin during the fifth week. Infarcted areas appear hypodense; cyst-filled CSF spaces are usually visualized by CT. Pathological studies have shown that cavities one centimeter in diameter require two months to form; larger cavities may not be complete by four months. There is usually no further change in size or appearance of infarcts after 8 to 12 weeks. Large infarctions cause loss of normal brain parenchyma, and this may result in dilatation of contiguous ventricle and cisternal spaces. In certain cases, hypodense infarcts appear to extend to contiguous ventricle. This creates the impression of abnormal communication with ventricles (porencephalic cyst). However, these lesions do not actually communicate with ventricles—this has been confirmed by air studies, metrizamide cisternography, and necropsy findings.[15]

On the basis of density characteristics, enhancement pattern and effect of tissue change on contiguous structures (mass effect, atrophy), it is not always possible to approximate age of infarcts; however, with serial scans the significance of sequential changes is better appreciated than with single scan.

Early CT studies did not emphasize the importance of contrast enhancement in cerebral ischemia. Yock and Marshall reported contrast enhancement in 25 percent of cases;

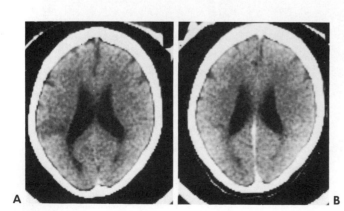

Figure 6–4. A 42-year-old man developed right hemiparesis and sensory deficit one week previously. EEG and isotope scan were negative. CT findings: hypodense left parietal lesion (A) that becomes isodense on postcontrast scan (B).

A   B

this enhancement pattern was most prominent 7 to 18 days after clinical ictus.[16] Wing and colleagues reported that 60 percent of patients with infarcts who were scanned between the end of the first and fourth week showed enhancement; in 10 percent lesions appeared isodense on noncontrast scan.[17] Masdeu et al. reported that the most frequently observed enhancement pattern was a diffuse, patchy or peripheral rim within hypodense lesion.[18] In our studies we observed enhancement in 65 percent of patients with cerebral infarcts if we utilized the drip infusion technique; however, bolus administration of contrast showed enhancement in only 35 percent of cases of infarction. This difference in results with these

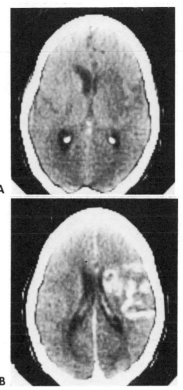

Figure 6–6. A 60-year-old woman became unable to use her left arm. Examination showed left hemiparesis and sensory deficit with anosognosia. Isotope scan showed right parietal uptake. *CT findings:* trapezoid-shaped sharply marginated right ganglionic parietal lesion with mass effect (*A*). There is superficial gyral and ganglionic enhancement (*B*).

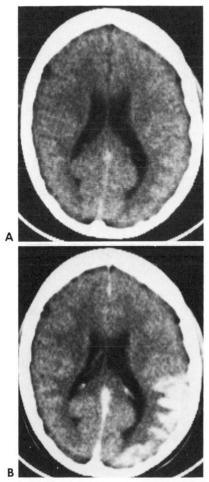

Figure 6–5. A 27-year-old man awakened from general anesthesia with left-sided numbness and visual blurring. Examination showed dense left homonymous hemianopsia. *CT findings:* isodense (*A*) right parietal-occipital lesion with dense gyral enhancement (*B*). Angiogram showed no evidence of vascular malformation.

two different techniques has not been confirmed by other studies.[19]

Abnormal enhancement was maximal between the end of the first and fourth week after clinical ictus. Follow-up studies performed later showed marked decrease in extent and intensity of enhancement. Of patients who had enhancing lesions, noncontrast scan showed isodense lesion in 26 percent (Fig. 6–5) and hypodense lesion in 74 percent (Fig. 6–6). Three postcontrast patterns were specific for infarcts: (1) linear or tubular bands of dense enhancement with interspersed low-density sulcal regions, (2) single or multiple crest-shaped densely enhancing regions conforming to superficial gyral pattern and (3) dense enhancement in subcortical nuclear (caudate, putamen, thalamus) gray matter structures. Enhancement is usually confined to gray matter zones; however, there may be thin strands of enhancement extending across white mat-

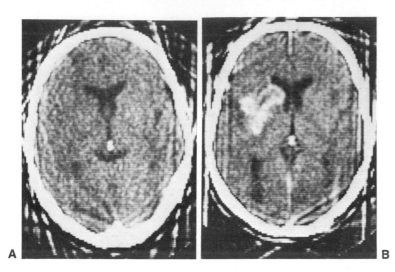

Figure 6–7. A patient with lymphosarcoma and low platelet count became dizzy and unable to express himself. Findings were nonfluent aphasia and right hemiparesis. Initial CT was normal (A). Ten days later CT shows enhancing caudate and putaminal enhancing lesion with linear bands of enhancement extending across the internal capsule (B).

ter, e.g., internal capsule (Fig. 6–7). Paucity of enhancement in white matter creates a heterogeneous appearance; this is sometimes incorrectly diagnosed as neoplasm or angioma. Other patterns included peripheral rim and diffuse and nodular enhancement (Fig. 6–8). Enhancement is believed to be caused by hypoxia and regional vascular dysautoregulation. This consists of two components: intravascular due to hyperperfusion (luxury perfusion) and extravascular due to defective blood-brain barrier with contrast extravasation.[20] Jacobs and colleagues reported that lesions that were isodense and showed gray matter enhancement represented ischemia without infarction, whereas hypodense lesions with gray matter enhancement represented infarction.[21] Several patients who had clinical transient

ischemic attacks that were prolonged were reported to have gray matter enhancement; this enhancement did not occur in patients in whom the attack lasted less than 30 minutes.

Study of the relationship of contrast enhancement to clinical outcome in patients with cerebral infarction has yielded contradictory findings. Pullicino and Kendall reported that clinical outcome was worse in patients with evidence of enhancing lesions; however, in all cases these lesions were hypodense and larger lesions enhanced more frequently than small infarcts.[22] In our series prognosis for functional recovery was better in these patients who showed enhancement. The clinical recovery was best in patients who showed isodense enhancing lesion consistent with findings reported by Jacobs and colleagues.[21]

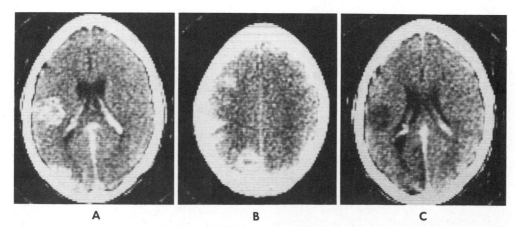

Figure 6–8. This 54-year-old man developed right-sided numbness and weakness. Examination showed right hemiparesis and sensory deficit and homonymous hemianopsia. Isotope scan showed two areas of uptake. *CT findings*: left parietal (A) and occipital (B) isodense gyral- and ring-enhancing lesions. Six weeks later he was clinically improved. CT showed parietal and occipital hypodense nonenhancing lesions (C).

SMALL DEEP CEREBRAL INFARCTS

Cerebral lacunes are defined as small infarcts located in the deep central region (basal ganglia, internal capsule, thalamus, basis pontis). They result from primary arteriopathy in small penetrating intracranial arteries.[23] They are most common in hypertensive patients. The lacunes have been reported to cause characteristic clinical syndromes: (1) pure motor hemiparesis (PMH) due to an internal capsule lesion (Fig. 6–9) or a basis pontis lesion, (2) pure sensory stroke due to a posterior thalamic lesion, (3) dysarthria–clumsy hand syndrome due to a pontine lesion and (4) homolateral ataxia-crural paresis due to a capsular–corona radiata lesion.

The uniqueness of lacunes for causing these specific classic syndromes has been recently challenged. Chokroverty and Rubino demonstrated that causes of pure motor hemiplegia (PMH) included frontal-parietal metastases, carotid occlusion or medullary pyramid infarction.[24] Positive isotope scan findings in one third of patients with pure motor hemiparesis indicated that larger lesions may also cause these syndromes.[25] In the pre-CT era, lacunar infarcts were diagnosed on a clinical basis. These were usually not confirmed by diagnostic studies because of their small size. In our series of patients with PMH, CT showed small ganglionic hematomas, solitary metastasis, subdural hematoma, demyelinating disorder, and anterior and middle cerebral artery occlu-

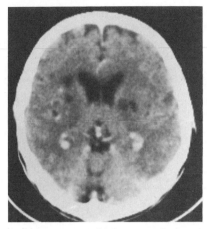

Figure 6–10. A 39-year-old hypertensive man awakened unable to use his right arm. Examination showed right hemisparesis with bilateral Babinski signs and pseudobulbar palsy. *CT finding:* multiple bilateral hypodense lacunar infarcts.

sion.[26] The role of bilateral lacunar infarcts in multi-infarct dementia is not established (Fig. 6–10). Small lacunes may cause no symptomatology and are detected only by CT; these previously have been diagnosed only at autopsy.

Utilizing CT, we have demonstrated high accuracy in detecting cerebral lacunes. This is especially true since the availability of high-resolution CT technology.[27, 28] In early CT studies we were able to detect larger giant lacunes. These were usually caused by occlusion of the largest lateral lenticulostriate arteries to involve the putamen, internal capsule (genu, posterior limb) and caudate region with vertical extension to the corona radiata. These lesions were seen on two contiguous 13 mm sections; however, we were not able to detect more typical small lacunar infarcts (0.5 to 15 mm). With high-resolution CT we have been able to detect lacunes that had a measured diameter of 8 to 10 mm and were seen on only one scan section. These smaller lacunes are probably caused by involvement of medial lenticulostriate vessels. We have detected multiple lacunes and those occurring in neurologically asymptomatic patients. It is unlikely that lacunes less than 6 mm in size are detected because of partial volume averaging. It would be possible to detect brain stem lacunes if 4 mm scan sections were utilized; however, "noise level" would probably produce obscuring artifact that would cause false-positive results.

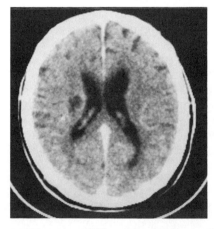

Figure 6–9. A 52-year-old hypertensive man suddenly began dropping things. Examination showed pure motor right hemiparesis. EEG and isotope scan were negative. *CT finding:* left capsular lacunar infarct.

Cerebral lacunes have a characteristic CT appearance as hypodense round or oval lesions. These are sharply marginated and nonenhancing; they cause no mass effect. In symptomatic patients, lacunes were visualized on initial scan with earliest scan being performed within 12 hours of clinical ictus. Follow-up scans showed no change in appearance of the lesion. Scans that were performed 12 months later showed no resolution of hypodense lesion or enhancement. Certain congenital intracranial cysts have similar CT appearance; however, they are usually located in cerebral hemispheres.

On the basis of retrospective necropsy studies, almost all patients with lacunar infarcts were hypertensive, whereas in CT studies 47 to 65 percent have been hypertensive. Three unexpected clinical findings were: (1) 20 percent had prodromal TIA, (2) 33 per cent showed clinical progression lasting as long as 96 hours and (3) 14 percent had resolution of neurological deficit in 48 hours. In patients with lacunar infarcts, 25 to 33 percent had significant angiographical evidence of carotid stenosis. This finding of carotid lesions raises two significant issues. First, certain patients who present with prolonged TIA or RIND syndrome may have CT evidence of lacunar infarct; this CT finding may preclude the need for angiography. Second, carotid endarterectomy may be a risk in patients with TIA symptoms who have a remediable carotid lesion but also have CT evidence of recent lacunar infarct. However, it may be that lacunar infarcts are an important sign of more proximal large vessel disease. Angiography should be performed to determine the presence of carotid or proximal middle cerebral artery stenosis that may cause recurrent stroke. If proximal large-vessel disease is present, CT may show lacunar infarct only or lacune plus superficial cortical lesions (see Fig. 6–1). The lenticulostriate vessels are end-arteries, but superficial cortical vessels may have adequate collateralization so that this cortical region is spared.

SMALL SUPERFICIAL NONHEMORRHAGIC VASCULAR LESIONS

These superficial vascular (ischemic, infarction) disorders represent a subgroup of stroke

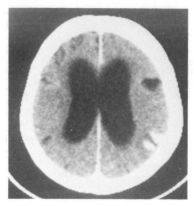

Figure 6–11. This 65-year-old hypertensive woman suddenly appeared confused. She had fluent aphasia with severely impaired comprehension and right homonymous hemianopsia. *CT findings:* posterior parietal isodense lesion with single gyral enhancement with marked cerebral atrophy.

syndromes with common clinical and CT findings.[29] Prior studies have reported seizures infrequently in nonhemorrhagic cerebral infarction. However, we have found that 25 percent of patients with small superficial vascular lesions initially presented with seizures. Forty-five percent of these patients had pure motor deficit (hemiparesis) to simulate lacunar infarct; 20 percent had monoparesis or homonymous hemianopsia only. One third of patients had more extensive clinical deficit (hemiparesis–hemisensory syndrome, hemiparesis-aphasia) to suggest a larger lesion. It is possible that CT visualized only a portion of the ischemic lesion.

CT finding included hypodense small round or wedge-shaped superficial nonenhancing lesion, isodense gyral (single) enhancing lesion (Fig. 6–11) and hypodense oval or wedge-shaped lesion with gyral or nodular enhancement (Fig. 6–12). Because enhancement was sometimes quite dense and serpiginous, angiography was sometimes performed to exclude angioma or neoplasm. Angiography was performed in 30 percent of patients. This showed carotid stenosis in 33 percent, intracranial branch occlusion in 33 percent and no abnormality in 33 percent. Isotope scan was positive in only 5 percent of patients with CT evidence of superficial vascular lesion. All patients with isodense enhancing gyral lesions had good recovery, whereas those with small superficial hypodense lesions showed slower and less complete recovery.

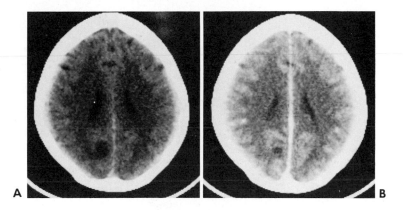

Figure 6–12. A 58-year-old woman with atrial fibrillation noted flashing lights on the right side. Examination showed right homonymous hemianopsia. EEG and isotope scan were negative. *CT findings*: hypodense left occipital (A) lesion with slight enhancement such that the lesion appears decreased in size (B).

SPECIFIC VASCULAR ISCHEMIC LESIONS

Anterior Cerebral Artery (ACA). This vessel is divided into three major divisions: (1) medial lenticulostriate arteries including the artery of Huebner and basal branches, (2) pericallosal and callosomarginal arteries and (3) medial hemispheric branches.[30] The artery of Huebner supplies the anterior portion of the caudate, putamen and internal capsule. The clinical syndrome of infarction includes paralysis of the face, arm and shoulder without sensory loss. Basal branches supply the hypothalamus; clinical symptoms are rare. Cerebral embolism *rarely* involves the ACA territory, and therefore hemorrhagic infarcts are uncommon in the frontal region. However, frontal hematomas resulting from venous sinus and cortical vein thrombosis may develop. Hemispheric branches of ACA supply the medial surface of the frontal lobe and paracentral lobule; infarction results in contralateral motor deficit involving the leg with sparing of the arm and face (Fig. 6–13). Bilateral ACA occlusion causes altered mentation and motor activity (akinetic mutism). If a lesion seen in the frontal region represents ischemia (Fig. 6–14) or infarction (Fig. 6–15), the hypodense area is confined to specific vascular boundaries and is sharply demarcated from surrounding normal brain.

Middle Cerebral Artery (MCA). This is the terminal portion of the internal carotid artery. The MCA consists of three divisions: (1) superior ascending frontal complex (orbital-frontal, operculofrontal, central sulcal), (2) horizontal complex (posterior parietal, angular), and (3) temporal (inferior) complex with branches supplying the anterior and posterior temporal region. It is sometimes difficult to differentiate internal carotid artery occlusion from proximal MCA occlusion on a clinical basis. However, in ICA occlusion CT shows involvement of both ACA and MCA territories

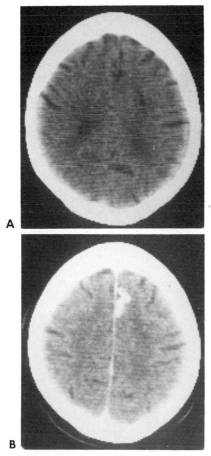

Figure 6–13. A 38-year-old man developed left foot drop and was unable to walk. EEG and isotope scan were negative. *CT findings*: right frontal parasagittal isodense (A) enhancing lesion (B).

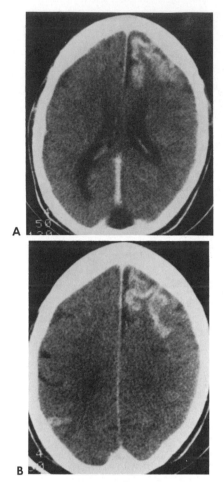

causes cortical blindness with some patients being unaware of visual impairment (Anton's syndrome). The anterior temporal artery supplies the inferior portion of the anterior temporal lobe; the posterior temporal artery supplies the temporal-occipital cortex. Involvement of these vessels may result in homonymous hemianopsia. Hippocampal branch ischemia may cause transient global amnesia if there is bilateral involvement. Occlusion of the thalamogeniculate perforating vessels (Fig. 6–19) supplying the posterior thalamus may cause "thalamic pain syndrome." This is characterized by burning dyaesthetic pain that develops after hemiparesis-hemianesthesia has partially resolved. Because of the variability in vessel supply and collateral circulation, there may be little correlation between clinical, CT and angiographical findings in PCA

Figure 6–14. A 54-year-old man developed sudden onset of left leg paresis. EEG showed monorhythmic frontal delta activity; isotope scan was negative. *CT findings*: isodense frontal superficial gyral-enhancing lesion (*A, B*) consistent with ACA territory ischemia.

(Fig. 6–16). Because of the marked variability of collateral circulation, CT findings cannot be used to predict the precise location of an occluded vessel without angiography.

Posterior Cerebral Artery (PCA). These paired vessels are terminal branches of basilar artery. PCA has multiple divisions, including paramedian and median midbrain branches, perforating branches to the thalamus (premammillary, thalamoperforators, thalamogeniculate, posterior choroidal), and cortical branches (anterior and posterior temporal, hippocampal, calcarine, parieto-occipital). The calcarine branch supplies the medial occipital surface (Fig. 6–17). The clinical finding of PCA occlusion includes contralateral homonymous hemianopsia (Fig. 6–18); bilateral involvement

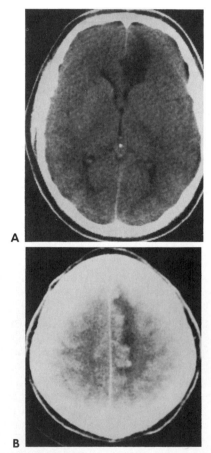

Figure 6–15. A 56-year-old man became unable to walk. Findings were left leg paresis and gait ataxia. *CT findings*: hypodense right frontal and parasagittal lesion (*A*) with interspersed parasagittal enhancement. (*B*).

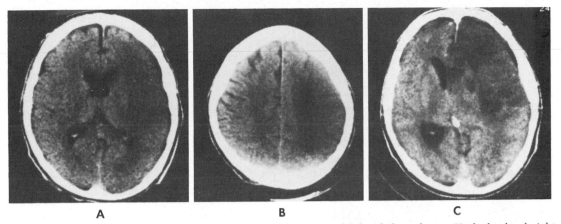

A   **B**   **C**

Figure 6–16. A 48-year-old hypertensive man had sudden onset of left-sided weakness. He had a loud right carotid bruit. *CT findings*: hypodense sharply marginated lesion in MCA distribution (*A*) with cortical sulcal space effacement (*B*) and no enhancement. Angiogram showed right carotid occlusion. Following endarterectomy he became obtunded. *CT findings*: hypodense nonenhancing lesion involving MCA and ACA distribution with mass effect (*C*).

occlusive vascular disease.[31, 32] CT usually shows hypodense occipital, inferior temporal or thalamic lesion. An occipital lesion usually appears ovoid in shape with flat base directed medially. The enhancing portion may be quite serpiginous and extend to the temporal and posterior thalamic regions.

Cerebellar Infarcts. There are no clinical featurs that permit differentiation of cerebellar infarction from hemorrhage. Two clinical courses of cerebellar infarction have been de-

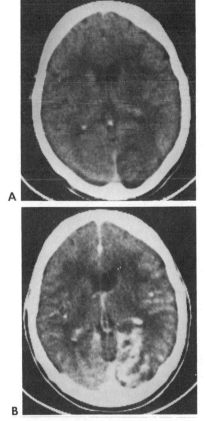

A

B

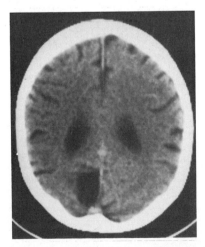

Figure 6–17. A 58-year-old man awakened with blurred vision bilaterally. Examination showed right homonymous hemianopsia. *CT findings*: left occipital hypodense ovoid nonenhancing lesion consistent with infarction in PCA distribution.

Figure 6–18. This 48-year-old man developed headache and visual blurring. The finding was left homonymous hemianopsia. EEG showed a right delta slow wave pattern. *CT findings*: hypodense right occipital lesion (*A*) with gyral and ring enhancement (*B*).

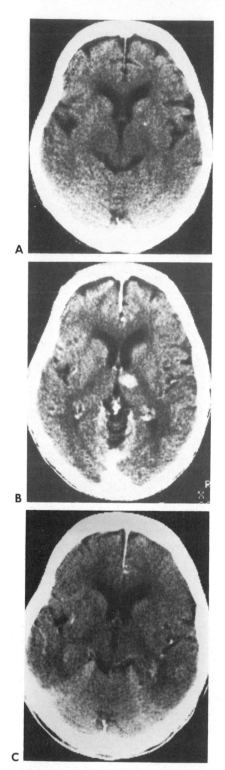

scribed. In the first of these, following rapid onset of posterior fossa symptomatology the patient's condition stabilizes and improves. In the second, following rapid onset of cerebellar and brain stem dysfunction, there is progressive deterioration including altered consciousness that may subsequently worsen to coma, miotic but reactive pupils and impaired eye movements. These findings are indicative of brain stem compression. When progressive deterioration occurs, the possibility of posterior fossa tumor must be considered. CT provides an accurate method to define ischemic lesions. In patients with suspected cerebellar infarction CT is important to differentiate infarction from hemorrhage and to delineate mass effect and hydrocephalus. The rationale for surgical decompression and shunting in cerebellar infarction is to prevent brain stem compression.[33] The CT appearance of cerebellar infarct is a hypodense, sharply marginated lesion. This may be triangular, rectangular or oval in shape (Fig. 6–20). On the basis of the location of the hypodense lesion, the presence of an occluded vessel can sometimes be predicted; however, many cases do not show isolated specific vascular lesions and others show border zone infarcts (lesions crossing between the superior cerebellar and the posterior inferior cerebellar arteries). Superior cerebellar artery infarctions are localized to the superior vermis and cerebellar hemisphere. Anterior inferior cerebellar artery in-

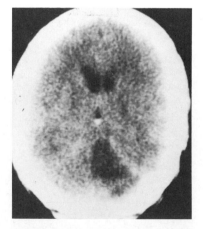

Figure 6–19. A 70-year-old woman awakened with left-sided numbness. Examination showed left pure hemisensory syndrome. *CT findings*: right thalamic (medial to internal capsule) isodense (A) lesion with nodular enhancement (B). Six weeks later CT showed no enhancement (C).

Figure 6–20. A 50-year-old man developed headache and vomiting and became unable to walk. Examination showed right-limb ataxia and facial paresis. *CT findings*: sharply marginated hypodense cerebellar lesion extending upward to the tentorium consistent with cerebellar infarction.

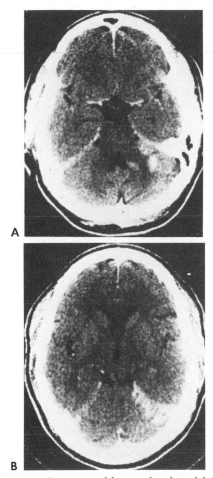

Figure 6–21. A 48-year-old man developed left arm tremor and clumsiness. Examination showed right-limb ataxia and horizontal nystagmus. *CT findings*: Plain scan shows normal-sized fourth ventricle with no abnormal density. Contrast study shows right cerebellar hemispheric gyral (*A*) and linear enhancement (*B*). This is consistent with cerebellar infarction.

(Fig. 6–21) than in supratentorial infarctions. The pattern in which the enhancement occurs in linear distribution to outline the cerebellar folia is highly suggestive of cerebellar infarction (Fig. 6–22). Other conditions that may simulate cerebellar infarction include cerebellar astrocytoma, arachnoid cyst, epidermoid cyst, cerebellar metastases and nonneoplastic cerebellar cyst.

Brain Stem Infarcts. Occlusion of branches of the basilar artery may cause abrupt onset of clinical symptoms. These may stabilize and subsequently exacerbate several days later. Clinical differentiation from other posterior fossa vascular disorders such as pontine hem-

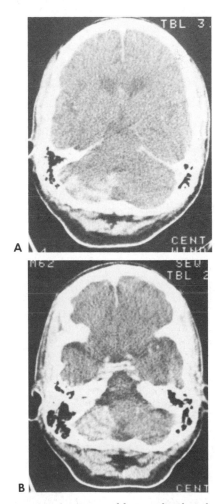

Figure 6–22. A 51-year-old man developed sudden onset of gait instability and dizziness. This worsened over a 10-day interval. Findings were gait and left-limb ataxia and right horizontal nystagmus. *CT findings*: isodense vermian and left cerebellar hemisphere (*A*) lesion with round and linear (*B*) enhancement. The fourth ventricle is not seen. *Operative finding*: cerebellar infarction.

farctions involve the lateral pons and anterior-inferior cerebellar hemisphere.[34] Most posterior inferior cerebellar artery infarcts involve the tonsils and inferior vermis.

Large lesions result in mass effect. This causes the fourth ventricle to be displaced and compressed. There may be accompanying third and lateral ventricular enlargement. In other cases the fourth ventricle is not visualized because of cerebellar infarction; however, the posterior fossa cisterns are not compressed and other ventricles are not dilated in these cases. It is possible that failure to visualize the fourth ventricle is a result of partial volume averaging and not mass effect in these cases. Enhancement is less common in infratentorial

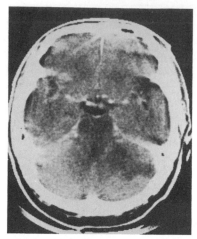

Figure 6–23. A 48-year-old man developed gait unsteadiness and vertigo. Examination showed left-limb ataxia, bilateral Babinski signs, and right facial and abducens pareses. *CT findings:* cerebellar and brain stem hypodense nonenhancing lesion with nonvisualization of the fourth ventricle. *Necropsy finding:* nonhemorrhagic infarct.

orrhage, cerebellar infarction and hemorrhage is not always possible. Vertebral angiography may be necessary to define the location of vascular occlusion. CT findings were initially limited to larger brain stem infarcts that also involved the cerebellum (Fig. 6–23); however, with new scanners we have delineated hypodense lesions confined to the brain stem (Fig. 6–24). Despite improvement in resolution and detectability, CT does not confirm diagnosis

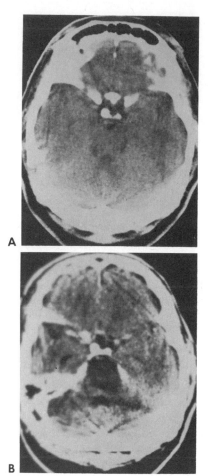

Figure 6–25. A 56-year-old hypertensive man developed vertigo, diplopia and difficulty walking. He had gait ataxia, nystagmus and bilateral abducens paresis. Initial CT shows no abnormality (*A*). Two days later, he became dysarthric. CT showed extensive hypodense brain stem lesion (*B*). He died of pulmonary embolism. Necropsy showed brain stem infarct due to basilar artery occlusion.

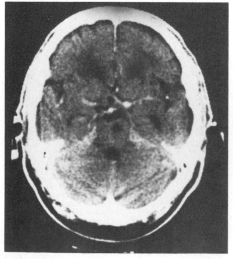

Figure 6–24. This 62-year-old man developed dysarthria and right-limb ataxia. Findings were consistent with dysarthria–clumsy hand syndrome. *CT finding:* small hypodense round nonenhancing brain stem infarct.

in one half of patients with brain stem infarcts. In patients with basilar artery occlusion, CT has remained negative for five days before showing hypodense brain stem lesion (Fig. 6–25). This hypodense brain stem lesion may not usually distort or efface the fourth ventricle or basilar cisterns (Fig. 6–26). Three of 15 patients with CT evidence of brain stem infarct showed contrast enhancement and two of these lesions were isodense on noncontrast scan (Fig. 6–27). Differential considerations for enhancing brain stem lesions include glioma, metastasis, demyelinating disorder, vascular malformation and abscess. Paucity of mass effect and spontaneous clinical remission is characteristic of brain stem ischemic lesions.

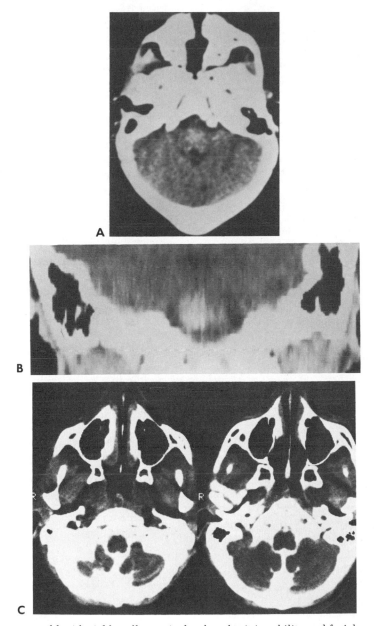

Figure 6–26. An 18-year-old with sickle cell anemia developed gait instability and facial paresis. Findings were bilateral abducens and facial pareses and gait ataxia. *CT findings:* isodense enhancing brain stem lesion (*A*). This is well visualized on sagittal section (*B*). Normal position and size of the fourth ventricle and the basal cisterns is seen on metrizamide cisternogram (*C*), which excludes brain stem tumor.

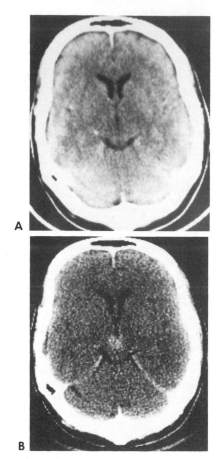

Figure 6–27. This 56-year-old man developed diplopia, eyelid drooping and gait ataxia. Findings were bilateral oculomotor paresis, left limb ataxia, bilateral Babinski sign. Initial CT showed no abnormalities (A). One week later, CT shows isodense midbrain and posterior thalamic enhancing lesion (B). Four-vessel angiography showed no abnormalities.

SPECIAL CLINICAL PROBLEMS

Cerebral Embolism. These may originate from carotid stenosis or from a cardiac source such as atrial fibrillation, myocardial infarction, valvular disease or bacterial endocarditis. However, in one third of cases of cerebral embolism, the precise source of embolism is not defined. Those originating from the heart may cause hemorrhagic infarct in 60 to 80 percent of cases. These are most common in the distal superficial branches of the MCA. The initial pathological event is ischemic infarct. This may become hemorrhagic because of re-establishment of blood flow through damaged blood vessels that have impaired autoregulatory capability. There are multiple superficial petechial hemorrhages that may coalesce to form one large hemorrhage. Embolus may be dislodged from occluded blood vessel with clot dispersal. Subsequent local metabolic factors lead to regional vasodilatation to subject the infarcted region to increased local cerebral flow. This may result in hemorrhagic infarction 48 to 96 hours after the initial embolism.[35] Factors that may increase the tendency to hemorrhagic infarct include large size of infarction, arterial hypertension and hyperperfusion. The incidence of hemorrhagic infarction was reported to be 18 percent in a series of necropsy studies of cerebral infarction and 21 to 23 percent in a CT series.[35, 36] CT findings include evidence of hypodense lesions confined to specific vascular territory with a hemorrhagic region located centrally or blood in sulcal spaces. Multiple infarctions are frequently seen; however, usually only one of these shows hemorrhagic component.[37]

Anticoagulation should be considered if the cerebral embolus originates from the heart. The benefit of anticoagulation in preventing recurrence must be weighed against the risk of precipitating hemorrhagic infarction. Angiography may be necessary to differentiate intracerebral hematoma (showing localized mass effect) from hemorrhagic infarct (showing occluded vessel caused by embolus). Hayman et al. have reported a characteristic enhancement pattern that was helpful in predicting later development of hemorrhagic infarction if double-dose (80 grams iodide) and delayed (3 hours later) scans were utilized. The enhancement was nodular or gyral. This was best seen on delayed scan. This enhancement is believed to represent vasogenic edema, and its occurrence predicted subsequent development of hemorrhagic infarction (Fig. 6–28). Utilization of hyperosmolar contrast material was not believed to worsen neurological function; however, because angiographical studies have shown extravasation of contrast medium, it should be considered a definite risk in patients with cerebral embolism.

We believe that anticoagulation should be performed in the early stage following cerebral embolism under these conditions: (1) CT shows no evidence of hemorrhage at 72 hours after clinical ictus, (2) hypodense lesion is small and there is no mass effect, (3) level of consciousness is normal and (4) CSF is nonbloody. Because the risk of recurrent cerebral embolism is very high, there is some justification for anticoagulation even in the presence of hemorrhagic infarction.

Hypertensive Encephalopathy. This is defined as an acute clinical condition resulting from sudden and pronounced increase in arterial blood pressure.[38] Symptoms include

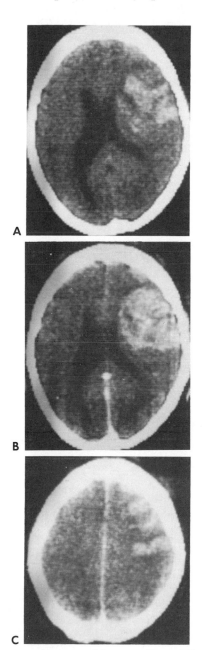

Figure 6–28. A 40-year-old man with atrial fibrillation developed left-sided weakness. CSF showed several hundred red blood cells. *CT findings:* hypodense right frontal-parietal lesion with interspersed hemorrhage and gyral blood (*A*). There is diffuse (*B*) and gyral enhancement (*C*). *Necropsy finding:* hemorrhagic cerebral infarction.

headache, visual blurring, nausea, vomiting, altered mentation and seizures. In some cases focal neurological dysfunction is present. Funduscopic examination usually shows retinal arteriolar spasm, hemorrhages, exudates and disc margin blurring. Hypertensive crisis is believed to result from impairment of cerebral autoregulatory mechanisms. Pathological findings include cerebral edema, petechial hemorrhages and ischemic brain injury. This is a potentially reversible condition, with resolution of clinical symptoms in response to rapid reduction of elevated blood pressure. If blood pressure does not decrease or if symptoms do not resolve, two possibilities must be considered. The first is incorrect clinical diagnosis, including posterior fossa neoplasms that may present with symptoms simulating hypertensive encephalopathy (headache, vomiting, papilledema, confusion). The second is development of the complicating factor of hypertensive crisis, e.g., intracerebral hematoma or infarction.

If a patient with hypertensive encephalopathy has focal neurological deficit, CT should be performed prior to initiation of vigorous antihypertensive therapy. If CT shows infarction, rapid lowering of blood pressure to normotensive levels may significantly decrease cerebral perfusion to cause extension of infarction. This occurs because perfusion pressure may be higher in hypertensive patients than in normotensive patients. The expected CT finding in hypertensive encephalopathy is generalized cerebral edema and mass effect, which then resolved following successful lowering of blood pressure. In certain patients bilateral visual blurring occurs, and in patients studied with this finding CT showed isodense bioccipital gyral enhancing lesions that were seen two to five days after onset of visual symptoms and resolved within seven days of successful lowering of blood pressure.

Aphasia Localization. Isotope brain scan studies have correlated nonfluent aphasic disturbances with lesions located anterior to the Rolandic fissure and fluent aphasic disturbances with posterior lesions. In several CT studies investigators have attempted to establish correlations of lesion location with clinical types.[39–41] However, following stroke, aphasic deficit and cerebral localization of the lesion may evolve such that clinical language findings in the first and fourth week after stroke may be quite different.

The nonfluent aphasias include global

aphasia, Broca's aphasia and transcortical motor aphasia. In global aphasia, patients have extensive lesions involving the entire perisylvian region including the posterior frontal and superior temporal region. *Broca's aphasia* patients have lesions involving the frontal opercular region or insular-lenticular region. The lesions do not extend posteriorly to the temporal region. Patients with *transcortical motor aphasia* have frontal regions involving the centrum semiovale or lenticular region.

The fluent aphasias include Wernicke aphasia, conduction aphasia, anomic aphasia and transcortical sensory aphasia. *Wernicke aphasia* patients have lesions extending from the temporal-occipital border to the posterior border of the frontal operculum, which is spared. In *conduction aphasia*, lesions involve the inferior parietal region and supramarginal gyrus. Some patients with *anomic aphasia* have small lesions involving Broca's areas and others have lesions in both the anterior and posterior speech areas. *Transcortical sensory aphasia* patients have lesions in the posterior-occipital region that may be in the posterior cerebral artery distribution (located medial, inferior, posterior) or in the watershed region between the posterior and middle cerebral arteries (located lateral, superior, anterior). Most patients with aphasia have cortical lesions; however, some patients with aphasia have subcortical lesions involving the capsular-putaminal region, with extension into the periventricular white matter.[42] There is good correlation between aphasia and location of hypodense lesion if the scan is performed in the second week after stroke; however, enhancement pattern is not helpful in establishing clinical-CT correlation.

Watershed Infarctions. These result from decreased perfusion in the terminal branches of contiguous arterial territories. This decrease may be caused by lessening of perfusion in adjacent cerebral arteries, especially under the circumstance of decreased cardiac output or because of stenosis or occlusion of the carotid artery.[43] The watershed infarctions may occur in several characteristic arterial locations—anterior and middle cerebral arteries and middle and posterior cerebral arteries. CT may show hypodense lesions in several locations; (1) the triangular region in the frontal-parietal region, (2) the head of the caudate nucleus, (3) the linear band in the periventricular and supraventricular region (Fig. 6–29), (4) the triangular region in the temporo-occipital region and (5) the linear band over the convexity in the frontal region.

REFERENCES

1. Millikan CH, McDowell FH: Treatment of progressing stroke. Stroke 12:397–409, 1981
2. McKissock W, Richardson A: Primary intracerebral hemorrhage. Lancet 2:221, 1959
3. Weisberg LA, Nice CN: Cerebral neoplasms simulating stroke syndromes: early diagnosis with cerebral CT. Am J Med 63:517–526, 1977
4. Bull JD, Marshall, Shaw DA: Cerebral angiography in the diagnosis of acute stroke. Lancet 1:562, 1960
5. Dalsgaard-Nielson T: Some clinical experience in the treatment of cerebral apoplexy. Acta Psychiatr Scand (suppl) 108:101, 1956
6. Mohr JP, Caplan LR, Melski JW: The Harvard cooperative stroke registry: a prospective study. Neurology 28:754–762, 1978
7. Kinkel WR, Jacobs L: CT in cerebrovascular disease. Neurology 26:924, 1976
8. Carter AB: Prognosis of cerebral embolism. Lancet 2:514–519, 1965
9. Paxton R, Ambrose J: EMI scanner: brief review of the first 650 cases. Br J Radiol 47:530, 1974
10. Davis KR, Taveras JM, New PFJ: Cerebral infarction diagnosis by computerized tomography. Am J Roentgenol 124:643, 1975
11. Drayer BP, Dujovny M, Bochnke M: The capacity for computed tomography diagnosis of cerebral infarction. Radiology 125:393–402, 1977
12. Drayer BP, Rosenbaum AE: Brain edema defined by cranial computed tomography. J Comput Assist Tomogr 3:317–323, 1979
13. Wall SD, Brant-Zowadzki M, Jeffry RB: High frequency CT findings within 24 hours after cerebral infarction. Am J Neuroradiol 2:553–557, 1981
14. Becker H, Desch H, Hacker H: CT fogging effect

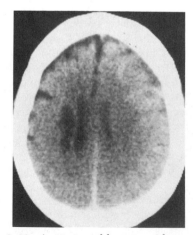

Figure 6–29. A 60-year-old man with myocardial infarction developed congestive heart failure. He developed right hemiparesis. *CT findings:* hypodense left paraventricular sausage-shaped lesion representing watershed infarct.

with ischemic cerebral infarcts. Neuroradiology 18:185–192, 1979

15. Ramsey RG, Huckman MS: CT of porencephaly and other CSF-containing lesions. Radiology 123:73–77, 1977.

16. Yock DA, Marshall WH: Recent cerebral ischemic brain infarctions at computed tomography. Radiology 117:599, 1976

17. Wing SD, Norman D, Pollock JA: Contrast enhancement of cerebral infarcts in CT. Radiology 21:89, 1976

18. Masdeu JC, Azar-kia B, Rubino FA: Evaluation of recent cerebral infarction by CT. Arch Neurol 34:417–421, 1977

19. Weisberg LA: Computer tomography enhancement patterns in cerebral infarction. Arch Neurol 37:21–25, 1980

20. Inoue Y, Takemoto K, Miyamoto T: Sequential CT scans in acute cerebral infarction. Neuroradiology 135:655–662, 1980

21. Kinkel WR, Jacobs L, Kinkel PR: Gray matter enhancement: a CT sign of cerebral hypoxia. Neurology 30:810–819, 1980

22. Pullicino P, Kendall BE: Contrast enhancement in ischemic lesions. Neuroradiology 19:235–239, 1980

23. Fisher CM: Lacunes, small deep cerebral infarcts. Neurology 15:774–784, 1965

24. Chokroverty S, Rubino FA: Pure motor hemiplegia. J Neurol Neurosurg Psychiat 38:896, 1975

25. Richter RW, Brust JCM, Bruun B: Frequency and course of pure motor hemiparesis. Stroke 8:58, 1977

26. Weisberg LA: Computed tomography and pure motor hemiparesis. Neurology 29:490–495, 1979

27. Weisberg LA: Lacunar infarcts: clinical and CT correlations. Arch Neurol 39:37, 1982

28. Pullicino P, Nelson RF, Kendall BE: Small deep infarcts diagnosed on computed tomography. Neurology 30:1090–1096, 1980

29. Weisberg LA: Small superficial cerebrovascular lesions. Comput Radiol (in press)

30. Berman SA, Hayman AL, Hinck VC: Correlation of

CT vascular territories with function. 1. Anterior cerebral artery. Am J Neuroradiol 3:259–263, 1981

31. Hayman AL, Berman SA, Hinck VC: Correlation of CT cerebral vascular territories with function. II. Posterior cerebral artery. Am J Neuroradiol 2:219–225, 1981

32. Goto K, Tagawa K, Uemura K: Posterior cerebral artery occlusion: clinical, computed tomographic and angiographic correlation. Radiology 132:357–368, 1979

33. Scott G, Spinnler H, Steizi R: Cerebellar softening. Ann Neurol 8:133–140, 1980

34. Weisberg LA: Cerebellar infarction: clinical and CT correlations. Comput Tomogr 6:155, 1982

35. Easton JD, Sherman DG: Management of cerebral embolism of cardiac origin. Stroke 11:433–442, 1980

36. Hayman AL, Evans RA, Baston FA, et al: Delayed high dose contrast CT: identifying patients at risk of massive hemorrhagic infarction. Am J Neuroradiol 2:139–147, 1981

37. Yock DH: CT demonstration of cerebral emboli. J Comput Assist Tomogr 5:190–196, 1981

38. Gifford RW, Westbrook E: Hypertensive encephalopathy. Prog Cardiovasc Dis 17:115, 1974

39. Hayward RW, Naesser MA, Zatz LM: CT in aphasia: correlation of anatomical lesions with functional deficits. Radiology 123:653, 1977

40. Kertesz A, Harlock W, Coates R: CT localization, lesion size and prognosis in aphasia and nonverbal impairment. Brain Language 8:34, 1979

41. Mazzocchi F, Vignolo LA: Localization of lesions in aphasia: clinical-CT correlation in stroke patients. Cortex 15:627, 1979

42. Naeser M, Alexander MP, Helm-Estabrooks N: Aphasia with predominantly subcortical lesion sites. Arch Neurol 39:4, 1982

43. Wodarz R: Watershed infarctions and computed tomography. A topographical study in cases with stenosis or occlusion of the internal carotid artery. Neuroradiology 19:245, 1980

Intracerebral Hemorrhage

Before the development of CT, antemortem diagnosis of intracerebral hemorrhage (ICH) was established in patients who developed sudden onset of neurological deficit and had bloody CSF with angiographical evidence of avascular mass. However, necrospy examination demonstrated that many intracerebral hemorrhages were not detected utilizing these diagnostic criteria. Since the introduction of CT it appears that the incidence of ICH in these pre-CT era stroke studies was underestimated. CT has been highly reliable for detecting ICH. There have been no reports of

clinically symptomatic acute hematomas that have not been detected by CT. Furthermore, small hematomas have been demonstrated in patients without fixed neurological deficit.

Isotope scan is positive in only 50 to 60 percent of patients with ICH. This abnormal uptake is seen as round in shape and is not confined to specific arterial vascular territories. There is no flow abnormality demonstrated on dynamic scan. In patients with ICH, isotope scan is positive immediately after the ictal episode, and this uptake usually persists longer than uptake due to cerebral in-

TABLE 6–2. Etiologies of 300 Intracranial Hemorrhages

Etiology of Hemorrhage	Thalamic-Ganglionic	Brain Stem	Lobar	Location Cerebellar	Subarachnoid	Intraventricular
Angioma	2	1	5	1		2
Aneurysm	2		5		12	2
Coagulopathy	2		2			
Blood dyscrasia	2		2			
Anticoagulants	1		5			
Neoplasm	1		4	1		
Mycotic aneurysm	0		2			
Hypertension	162	6	8	9		2
Spontaneous	35	4	12	5		3

farction. EEG may show focal hemispheric delta activity in lobar hematoma; however, in hematomas in other areas such as ganglionic, thalamic and posterior fossa, EEG may show only diffuse slowing or be normal. Angiography may show avascular mass, but was reported as negative in 15 to 35 percent in ICH in the era before the development of CT.[1]

The incidence of false-negative angiograms in ICH is probably higher; however, angiography is less commonly performed in cases in which diagnosis of ICH is established by CT unless an underlying lesion such as an angioma, neoplasm, aneurysm or vasculitis is suspected. In pre-CT era studies, patients with ICH had bloody or xanthochromic CSF in 80 percent of cases; however, in cases diagnosed by CT, CSF showed evidence of blood in less than 50 percent.[2]

The clinical course of ICH is usually characterized by sudden development of neurological deficit.[3] There is maximal deficit at onset (34 percent) or gradual progression over a several-hour interval (66 percent). The neurological deficit may progress; however, fluctuation between normal and abnormal does not usually occur. In patients with ICH, blood leaks from small penetrating arterioles into the brain parenchyma over a period of several minutes to hours; continued active bleeding does not occur.[4] If CT is performed immediately after the development of neurological deficit, there may sometimes be evidence of continued active bleeding.[5] However, repeated CT scans performed 2 to 14 days after initial ICH have not shown increased size of hematoma unless hemorrhage is caused by ruptured berry aneurysm. Follow-up CT studies in patients with ICH who have progressive neurological worsening may show an increase in surrounding edema and mass effect, intra-

ventricular extension of hemorrhage or no change in scan appearance.

In the acute phase, these hemorrhages appear as round or irregularly shaped hyperdense noncalcified lesions. It is believed that the hyperdense portion is related to protein content of hemoglobin. Hematomas usually have smooth margination, but this may be irregular or jagged-edged. The central portion of hematoma may be denser and more homogeneous than the peripheral region. Hematomas are usually surrounded by hypodense vasogenic edema with frond-like projections extending into white matter. Large hemorrhages cause mass effect as manifested by midline shift and displacement of ventricles (Fig. 6–30). Some of these hemorrhages have small surrounding lucent collars and cause minimal mass effect (Fig. 6–31). Some hema-

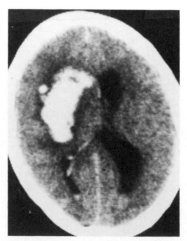

Figure 6–30. A 48-year-old man developed severe headache and rapidly developed right hemiplegia. CSF was bloody. *CT findings:* ganglionic hematoma with surrounding edema causing marked ventricular mass effect.

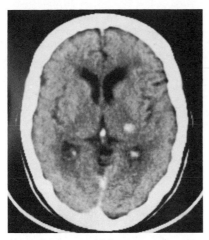

Figure 6–31. A 62-year-old hypertensive woman suddenly developed left-sided weakness. Examination showed left hemiparesis–sensory syndrome. EEG, isotope scan and CSF were normal. *CT findings:* small right posterior thalamic hematoma without mass effect. The surrounding hypodense region is posterior capsular region and not edema.

pattern. This decrease in density of hematoma is visually evident within seven days after hemorrhage and may continue for several months. This decrease in density is usually associated with reduced hematoma size; however, it is possible for the hematoma to become isodense or hypodense with minimal reduction in size.[6] As hematoma "ages," it may become hypodense and cystic, usually with ipsilateral ventricular dilatation; or it may become isodense and indistinguishable from normal brain parenchyma. Larger hematomas usually appear hypodense, whereas smaller hematomas are likely to be either hypodense or isodense.

Between the beginning of the second and sixth week following clinical ictus, ICH may show peripheral ring enhancement. This occurs in 20 to 25 percent of ICH of hypertensive, traumatic and spontaneous etiologies.[7–9] Enhancement is more common with cerebral hemispheric lobar hematomas (Fig. 6–33) than with ganglionic-thalamic (Fig. 6–34) or cerebellar hemorrhages. A peripheral rim is seen on postcontrast scan and the rim may be faintly seen on plain scan. The central region that represents degenerating hematoma may be isodense or hyperdense. Density of the central region is determined by extent of hematoma resolution. Mass effect and edema caused by ICH have usually resolved when enhancement occurs; however, in certain cases mass effect is still prominent.

Following contrast infusion, the characteristic finding is a thin (less than 3 mm) homogeneous and regular-shaped peripheral enhancing rim (Fig. 6–34). If peripheral ring-enhancing hematoma is associated with significant mass effect, differentiation from other

tomas may extend into ventricles; however, there is usually no CT evidence of cisternal blood in nonaneurysmal ICH. Ventricular extension is not related to hematoma size. In the acute stage (the first five days after the clinical ictus), ICHs do not usually show visual evidence of contrast enhancement unless there is an underlying lesion such as neoplasm, aneurysm or angioma (Fig. 6–32).

Repeat CT shows change in morphology, density, mass effect and enhancement characteristics of ICH with time. Because there is phagocytosis of blood pigment, necrotic tissue and xanthochromic fluid, CT density changes from hyperdense to isodense or hypodense

Figure 6–32. This 34-year-old normotensive man had two episodes of left-sided numbness and subsequently became obtunded with left hemiplegia. CSF was bloody; isotope scan was negative. *CT findings:* right thalamic hyperdense lesion distorting the third ventricle (*A*) and diffuse enhancement (*B*). Angiogram showed thalamic AVM.

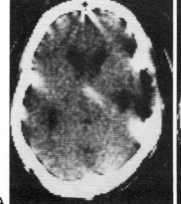

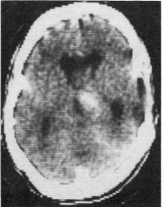

A

B

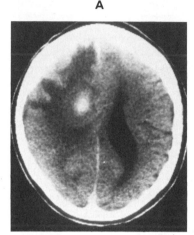

A

B

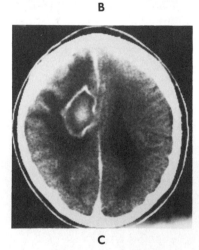

C

Figure 6–33. A 52-year-old hypertensive man awakened with right-sided weakness. Examination showed right hemiparesis–sensory syndrome. *CT findings:* left parietal lobar hematoma with sharp margination and irregular shape and surrounding edema (*A*). Three weeks later, he showed clinical improvement. *CT findings:* decreased size and density of hematoma with faint hyperdense rim (*B*), which is better visualized on postcontrast scan as peripheral enhancement (*C*).

TABLE 6–3. Differential Diagnostic Considerations for Peripheral Rim Enhancement

Neoplastic
  Glioma
  Metastasis
  Lymphoma
Non-neoplastic
  Abscess
  Aneurysm
  Gliotic reaction
  Angiomas

mass lesions may be difficult unless *serial* scans are available (Table 6–3). This typical sequence is (1) the initial finding in the first week is hyperdense hematoma with surrounding edema and mass effect but no enhancement; (2) in the second to fourth week there is a decrease in density of the hematoma, resolution of edema and mass effect, evidence on postcontrast scan of peripheral rim enhancement and (3) after one month the hematoma appears as an isodense or hypodense lesion with no evidence of mass effect and decreased intensity of enhancement. Peripheral enhancing rim associated with neoplasms is usually more irregular in shape and has variable thickness. This hyperdense rim of neoplasm may be well visualized on *noncontrast* scan, whereas this finding is not usually seen with spontaneous ICH. In neoplasms, enhancement occurs when there is significant edema and mass effect; in spontaneous ICH, enhancement usually develops as edema and mass effect are resolving. Rim enhancement of brain abscess appears thicker and denser on the superficial cortical surface, and satellite rings or nodular enhancement are seen contiguous with abscess rim. Thrombosed aneurysms and angiomas that have not recently bled may cause peripheral enhancement. The presence of calcification or ring-like structures resembling vessels suggests these vascular lesions; however, angiography is usually necessary to distinguish these vascular malformations. Ring-enhancing hematomas may occur in patients who have angiomas or aneurysms that have blood. In several cases of gliosis (pathologically confirmed), peripheral rim enhancement was present.

In rare instances the central portion of spontaneous ICH appears to enhance. This usually occurs at the stage when ICH has decreased to barely visible hyperdense or has reached isodense appearance (Fig. 6–35); that is, three

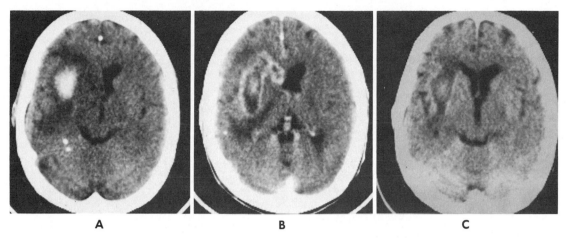

Figure 6–34. A 48-year-old normotensive man awakened with headache and right arm weakness. Findings were confusion and right hemiparesis–anesthesia. He improved following treatment with corticosteroids. *CT findings:* left ganglionic hematoma with mass effect (A) with complex ring enhancement (B). Three weeks later, he had minimal motor dysfunction. *CT findings:* marked reduction in hematoma size and density, mass effect and enhancement (C).

to six weeks after the bleeding episode. This enhancement usually disappears within two months. If CT is performed several weeks after the ictal episode, it is necessary to perform both plain and contrast infusion study. If only postcontrast scan is performed, hyperdense enhancing lesion may be incorrectly interpreted as hyperdense nonenhancing hematoma.

The mechanism of enhancement in ICH is not clearly established. Enhancement that occurs within the initial three to four weeks after hemorrhage is believed to be caused by impaired blood-brain barrier. This enhancement may be decreased by corticosteroids. After the

third week, enhancement is believed to result from hypervascularity of granulation tissue surrounding the hematoma. This is not modified by corticosteroids. It has been reported that degree of functional recovery in patients with ICH who show rim enhancement is better than in those patients with hematomas of similar size without evidence of enhancement. Follow-up CT in patients with ICH that has shown peripheral enhancing rim subsequently indicates resolution to an isodense nonenhancing region (75 percent) or appears hypodense (25 percent). It is possible that hypervascular granulation tissue that may result in rim enhancement may cause the lesion to appear

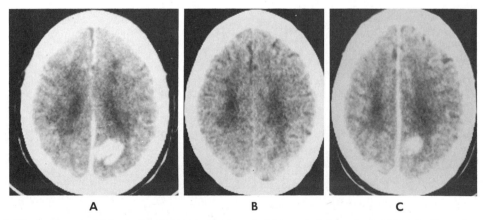

Figure 6–35. A 65-year-old hypertensive man developed right occipital headache. Examination showed left homonymous hemianopsia. *CT findings:* right medial occipital hematoma (A). Angiogram showed no abnormalities. Three weeks later, he was neurologically asymptomatic. *CT findings:* isodense (B) nodular enhancing lesion (C).

isodense. Therefore, hypodense cystic lesions would be expected to have a paucity of granulation tissue.

Intracerebral hematomas are located in characteristic locations (Table 6–4).

BASAL GANGLIONIC HEMATOMA

The putamen (lateral ganglionic region) is most frequent site of hypertensive ICH (Fig. 6–36). Previous studies have described two clinical syndromes: (1) lateral ganglionic hemorrhage in which patients present with headache, mild impairment of consciousness, hemiparesis (with early development of spasticity), hemianesthesia but usually no hemianopsia; (2) medial ganglionic hemorrhage in which

TABLE 6–4. Distribution of 300 Intracranial Hemorrhages Visualized by CT

Location	No. of Cases
Ganglionic	157
Thalamic	75
Temporal	13
Frontal	15
Unilateral	11
Bilateral	4
Occipital	6
Parietal	6
Posterior fossa	4
Intraventricular	7
Subarachnoid	12
Multiple intracerebral	5

patients present with more severe deficit, including marked alteration in consciousness, flaccid hemiplegia, hemianesthesia and conjugate lateral-gaze palsy. In patients with lateral ganglionic hematoma, CSF is frequently clear or shows only a small number of red blood cells. Prognosis for spontaneous recovery is usually better with lateral ganglionic lesions. Medial ganglionic hematomas usually result in blood CSF. They are more likely to rupture into ventricles and spread throughout the white matter. These may cause transtentorial herniation. The prognosis for recovery is worse for medial ganglionic hematomas.

It is important to delineate certain lateral ganglionic hematomas because if consciousness normalizes but motor weakness persists, some of these patients may benefit from surgical evacuation. On the basis of the vector of displacement of lenticulostriate vessels as determined by angiographical analysis, ganglionic hematoma may be detected as avascular mass; however, these findings may underestimate lesion size compared with surgical or necropsy findings. This difference in size has been explained by the continued enlargement of hematoma or edema that may develop after angiography; but continued bleeding or rebleeding does not usually occur in nonaneurysmal hemorrhage.

In patients with CT evidence of ganglionic ICH, seven characteristics have been delineated: (1) Eighty-three percent of patients were 40 to 60 years old. (2) Eighty-one percent had been previously diagnosed as having systemic arterial hypertension and had significantly elevated blood pressure immediately following the clinical ictus. (3) The neurological deficit became maximal in less than 4 hours in 86

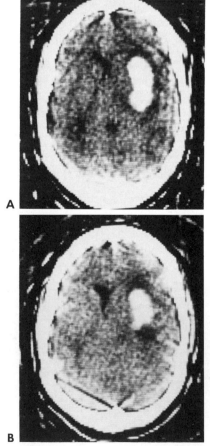

Figure 6–36. This 23-year-old woman developed frontal headache and was unable to use her left arm and leg. CSF was bloody. Angiogram showed an avascular ganglionic mass. *CT findings:* right medial ganglionic hematoma with marked mass effect (*A*). Following surgical evacuation of the hematoma, CT showed reaccumulation of the hematoma (*B*).

percent of patients, and in 14 percent progression to maximal deficit occurred in 6 to 24 hours. (4) Sixty-five percent of patients reported headache as the initial symptom. (5) Twenty-two percent of patients had seizure, and this occurrence correlated with lateral ganglionic hematoma that extended to the cortical region or into the ventricles. (6) Sixty-three percent of patients had bloody or xanthochromic CSF. (7) Thirty percent of patients were stuporous or comatose. Of patients who had CT scan performed within 7 days after ictal episode, 37 percent had intraventricular extension of hemorrhage. Mortality was 58 percent if there was intraventricular extension, but only 20 percent of patients without intraventricular blood subsequently died.

With the ability to localize hematoma in the ganglionic region, we have become aware of an increasingly wide clinical spectrum.[10] If hematoma involves the anterior limb of the internal capsule, motor deficit may be prominent but frequently is reversible. Lateral hematomas extending to the insula may cause aphasia. In hematomas involving the genu and anterior two thirds of the posterior capsular region, motor and sensory deficit are most severe. If hematoma extends into the posterior capsular region with dissection in occipital lobe white matter, visual field defect with minimal motor or sensory defect may be seen. Lateral-gaze paresis is seen with large ganglionic hemorrhages, irrespective of location. Bilateral motor dysfunction in patients with putaminal hemorrhage correlated with poor clinical outcome.

In patients with ganglionic hematoma, plain CT shows hyperdense putaminal mass. This may extend across the internal capsule and into the thalamus, ventricles or cortical region. If CT shows blood in the subarachnoid space or extension of hematoma across the sylvian fissure, this is highly suggestive of an aneurysmal etiology. Despite the large size of ganglionic and thalamic hematomas, edema is less prominent than with cerebral hemispheric (lobar) hematomas. Postcontrast scan is not usually necessary in most patients with ganglionic hematomas in the acute phase but may be performed for the following indications: (1) the patient is younger than 40, (2) there is no adequate documentation of systemic arterial hypertension, (3) neurological deficit progressed to maximal deficit over an interval longer than four hours or there had been prodromal transient neurological symptomatology, (4) the patient has a complicating condition such as neoplasm, blood dyscrasia, vasculitis or bacterial endocarditis and (5) CT appearance of ganglionic hematoma is atypical or subarachnoid blood is visualized.

Neurological deficit in putaminal hemorrhage correlates with hematoma size and location and intraventricular extension. Mortality was highest with hemorrhages that had a maximal diameter of 4.0 cm and extended into ventricles. Severity of permanent residual neurological deficit did not correlate with hematoma size. Of patients studied with lateral ganglionic hematoma who survived, good functional recovery frequently was seen: 60 percent had mild spastic hemiparesis, 20 percent had flaccid hemiplegia and 20 percent were functionally normal. In patients with medial ganglionic hematoma, recovery was less complete: 50 percent had flaccid hemiplegia, 35 percent had spastic hemiparesis and 15 percent were normal. Seizures initially occurred in 22 percent but persisted in only 5 percent and subsequently developed at a later phase in 10 percent. Lateral-gaze palsy was present in 40 percent; this correlated with hematoma size. Consciousness was impaired in 55 percent. Thirty percent of these patients were stuporous or comatose; this correlated with two factors—lesion size larger than 3.3 cm and intraventricular extension. Fourteen percent of patients with ganglionic ICH had progression of neurological deficit for 12 hours after the initial ictus. In 3 percent of patients, delayed neurological deterioration occurred 1 to 7 days after patients had initially stabilized. In patients with delayed deterioration, repeat CT frequently showed no change in size of hematoma or mass effect; however, in some patients intraventricular extension was visualized.

In patients who survived acute ICH and had serial scans, resolution of hematoma and mass effect was seen. The ganglionic region showed residual hypodense (40 percent) or isodense (60 percent) lesion. Functional neurological recovery was better in those patients who had ring enhancement and in whom hematoma subsequently appeared isodense after the hypodense portion resolved. Surgical evacuation was carried out in selected cases of lateral ganglionic hematoma without recurrence of hematoma; however, recurrence of hematoma was documented by CT in several surgically treated patients with ganglionic hematoma (Fig. 6–36).

THALAMIC HEMATOMA

Thalamic hemorrhage represented 10 to 15 percent of hypertensive hemorrhages in the pre-CT era. These account for 25 percent of hemorrhages demonstrated by CT.[11] The clinical syndrome of thalamic hemorrhage may include sudden onset of headache followed by focal motor weakness and numbness; findings are altered mentation, hemiparesis, hemianesthesia, impaired upward gaze with downward eye deviation, and small and poorly reactive pupillary light response. Small thalamic hematomas may cause hemiparesis-hemianesthesia without altered consciousness (Fig. 6–37). Aphasia rarely occurs with thalamic hematomas. In 60 percent of thalamic hematomas, CSF shows blood or xanthochromia. EEG shows focal slowing in 20 percent and bilateral slowing in 50 percent; it was normal in 30 percent. Isotope scan showed abnormal uptake in only one third of cases. The angiographical finding of avascular mass effect was seen only if hematoma was larger than 2.0 cm.

In the acute state, the CT appearance of thalamic hematoma is that of a hyperdense, irregularly contoured, round or oval-shaped lesion. These ranged in size from 1.0 to 7.0 cm. If the hematoma was larger than 2.0 cm, the third ventricle was usually distorted or displaced. Indications for postcontrast scan in patients with thalamic ICH are the same as for ganglionic hematomas. Peripheral ring en-

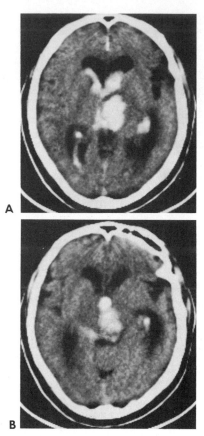

Figure 6–38. A 50-year-old hypertensive man became unresponsive and stiff. Findings were coma, downward deviation of eyes, dilated and fixed right pupil, and quadriplegia. *CT findings*: large right thalamic hematoma (A) with intraventricular extension and ventricular enlargement. A solid clot was present at the intraventricular foramina (B).

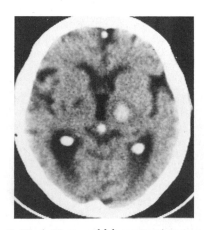

Figure 6–37. A 60-year-old hypertensive man developed slurred speech and began to drop things from his left hand. He had dysarthria–clumsy hand syndrome. *CT findings*: right small thalamic hematoma with slight surrounding edema but no mass effect. Left nonhemorrhagic lacunar infarct is also seen.

hancement was rarely seen in thalamic hematomas. Larger thalamic hematomas sometimes extended into ventricles, putamen, midbrain and cerebral hemispheric white matter. If the hematoma ruptured into the third ventricle or occipital horns, hydrocephalus was invariably seen. If the thalamic hematoma caused intraventricular extension and ventricular dilatation, mortality was 75 to 90 percent (Fig. 6–38). In those patients who survived ICH with intraventricular extension, the ventricles subsequently decreased in size as blood resolved. Mortality was 10 percent if hematoma was confined to the thalamic region. We have observed four patients with small thalamic hematomas who had TIA symptoms and no fixed neurological deficit.

CEREBRAL HEMISPHERIC HEMORRHAGE

In 15 to 25 percent of cases of nontraumatic ICH, lesions are located in cerebral hemispheric white matter (lobar hematoma). This finding should prompt thorough investigation for angioma, aneurysm, neoplasm, blood dyscrasia, collagen vascular disease, cortical vein or dural sinus thrombosis. In McCormick and Rosenfield's series of patients with brain hemorrhage, only 4 of 37 hypertensive patients had lobar hematoma.[12] In two thirds of patients with lobar hematoma, specific etiologies for ICH were identified. In this series, 40 percent of patients with presumed hypertensive hematomas were found to have other etiological factors for hemorrhage; however, this represents carefully selected rather than randomly selected patients. In our series of lobar hematomas diagnosed by CT, specific etiologies were identified in only 10 percent. In 40 percent, patients had established arterial hypertension; however, 50 percent of lobar hematomas occurred in normotensive patients. Location of lobar hematomas in our series included frontal (38 percent), occipital (15 percent), temporal (32 percent), parietal (15 percent).

The CT finding of a hyperdense nonenhancing lesion located in cerebral hemispheric white matter is characteristic. Large hematomas may have extensive surrounding edema, cause significant mass effect or extend into ventricles. Small hematomas usually had minimal surrounding edema. Small subcortical slit-like hematomas may appear to dissect along white matter as linear hyperdense bands and have minimal surrounding edema. Within the second to fourth week, peripheral ring enhancement occurred in 60 percent of lobar hematomas. On the basis of CT findings it may be difficult to differentiate lobar hematoma from hemorrhagic infarction. However, hemorrhagic infarction shows these CT findings: (1) a sharply marginated wedge or rectangularly shaped hypodense region conforming to vascular territory and (2) a central round hyperdense or linear gyral hyperdense component that represents blood. Lobar hematomas are frequently caused by anticoagulants; hemorrhagic infarcts are frequently caused by cerebral embolism and may subsequently require anticoagulant therapy.

Ninety percent of patients with lobar hematoma initially presented with headache. This was followed by rapid development of focal neurological dysfunction. This became maximal within four hours of onset and did not subsequently progress. The level of consciousness sometimes deteriorated later; this occurrence correlated with intraventricular extension. Ten percent of patients initially presented with seizures.[13] This was most common with slit-like subcortical hematomas. Lobar hematomas showed a characteristic clinical pattern dependent upon location.

FRONTAL HEMORRHAGE

Those of spontaneous or hypertensive etiology were usually unilateral; however, in cases caused by ruptured aneurysm, hemato-

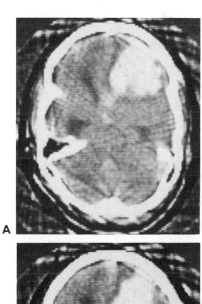

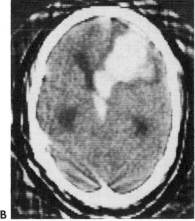

Figure 6–39. A 32-year-old woman suddenly developed headache and became obtunded. Findings were obtundation, lateral gaze preference to the right, left hemiplegia. CSF was bloody. *CT findings:* right frontal hematoma (A) pointing toward and extending into the lateral ventricles (B). Angiogram showed a right frontal avascular mass.

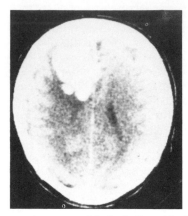

Figure 6–40. A 48-year-old alcoholic with thrombocytopenia developed headache and a right arm weakness with numbness. Findings were pure right hemiparesis. *CT findings*: left superior frontal hematoma with surrounding edema.

mas were unilateral or bilateral. Patients with unilateral frontal hematomas may present with these clinical patterns: (1) inferior frontal hematomas cause impaired consciousness, lateral-gaze palsy and hemiparesis; these may stimulate ganglionic hematoma (Fig. 6–39). (2) Superior frontal hematomas (Fig. 6–40) cause initial monoparesis that rapidly progresses to hemiparesis with normal consciousness. This may simulate pure motor hemiparesis caused by lacunar infarcts. Inferior hematomas appeared wedge-shaped (with base being superficial and apex directed toward ventricles), oval or round; superior hematomas were ovoid or round in shape. Twenty percent of frontal hematomas extended into ventricles; one half of these patients died.

TEMPORAL HEMORRHAGE

These patients usually presented with altered mentation (confusion, obtundation). If ICH involved the dominant temporal lobe, aphasia was a prominent and consistent finding; motor and sensory deficits were less common (Fig. 6–41). Hemiparesis is usually caused by transtentorial herniation or ventricular extension of hematoma. CT shows a round temporal hyperdense nonenhancing hematoma. Intraventricular extension into the temporal horn (Fig. 6–42) and early transtentorial herniation may develop. Follow-up CT showed hematoma resolution with a residual small hypodense lesion or isodense region and temporal horn dilatation with signs of trans-

tentorial herniation. Early surgical evacuation of temporal ICH may be necessary in some cases. If temporal hematoma extends across the sylvian cistern, ruptured aneurysm is most likely (Fig. 6–43). Only 5 percent of patients with temporal lobe hematoma died.

PARIETAL HEMORRHAGE

These patients rapidly developed hemiparesis-hemianesthesia deficit, usually with normal level of consciousness. Other findings included homonymous hemianopsia and anosognosia. CT showed a round superficial parietal hyperdense lesion. This developed most commonly in the posterior parietal region. There was usually spontaneous CT evidence of resolution of hematoma and good clinical outcome.

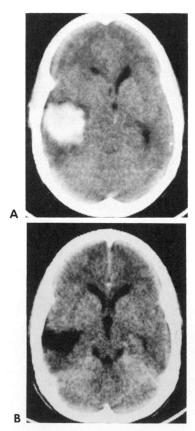

Figure 6–41. A 13-year-old girl developed headache and neck pain and became confused. Findings were fluent aphasia and right homonymous hemianopsia. *CT findings*: left temporal hematoma with ventricular compression (*A*). Angiography showed a temporal intracerebral mass. Following surgical evacuation of the hematoma, CT showed a hypodense region (*B*) and marked temporal horn enlargement.

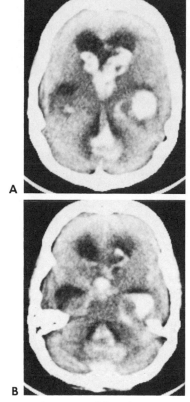

Figure 6–42. A 48-year-old cirrhotic with portocaval shunt suddenly vomited and became unresponsive. Findings included coma, dilated right pupil, quadriparesis with bilateral Babinski sign. *CT findings:* right temporal hematoma (A) with blood–CSF fluid level in temporal horn (B) and marked intraventricular blood and ventricular enlargement.

OCCIPITAL HEMORRHAGE

These patients presented with severe headache. This was frequently localized to the neck or orbital region. These patients complained of blurred vision. Findings were homonymous hemianopsia, usually with normal level of consciousness and minimal motor and sensory deficit. CT showed round or ovoid hematoma. Extension into the occipital horn occurred in 10 percent of cases. All patients recovered; however, visual field deficit persisted in 50 percent.

MULTIPLE INTRACEREBRAL HEMORRHAGE

In patients with systemic arterial hypertension, the finding of recurrent ICH of different times of onset is not an unusual event; however, simultaneous multiple hemorrhages are rare (Fig. 6–44). Multiple spontaneous hemorrhages occur usually with identifiable etiology. These include blood dyscrasias, neoplasms (primary or metastatic), vasculitis, venous sinus thrombosis and herpes simplex encephalitis. Bacterial endocarditis may cause septic emboli, which usually result in multiple hemorrhagic cerebral infarctions.

In 3 percent of our patients with ICH, CT showed multiple hematomas.[14] In these cases underlying etiology was not found despite angiography and necropsy findings. The majority of patients with multiple ICH were normotensive. Two thirds had lobar hematomas and one third had the following combi-

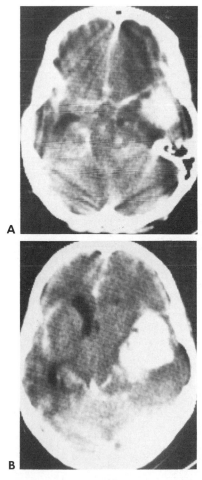

Figure 6–43. A 42-year-old woman suddenly collapsed. Findings were left hemiparesis and right pupillary dilatation. *CT findings:* right temporal hematoma (A) extending across the sylvian cistern with cisternal and intraventricular extension (B). Angiogram showed carotid artery aneurysm.

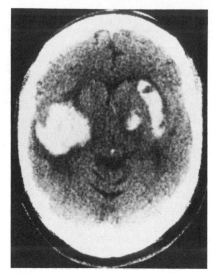

Figure 6–44. A 33-year-old drug addict suddenly developed severe headache and right-sided weakness. Findings were lethargy, right hemiplegia and bilateral Babinski signs. *CT findings*: bilateral ganglionic hematomas.

nations: lobar-ganglionic (Fig. 6–45), thalamic-cerebellar (Fig. 6–46), bilateral cerebellar hematomas. One half of patients with multiple ICH presented with headache, altered mentation and nuchal rigidity. In these patients without localizing neurological findings, CSF was bloody; initial diagnosis was aneurysmal SAH. In the other half of patients with multiple ICH, there was focal deficit that was caused by the largest of multiple hematomas. Diagnosis of multiple ICH was established by CT. Angiography usually defined the presence of large hematoma; however, neither angiography, EEG nor isotope scan suggested the presence of *multiple* hematomas. CT findings were characteristic of multiple recent hemorrhages. Attenuation values of the hematomas were similar; this suggested that they had developed at the same time. In one patient with multiple ICH, CT showed one hyperdense hematoma and another was a ring-enhancing isodense hematoma; angiography,

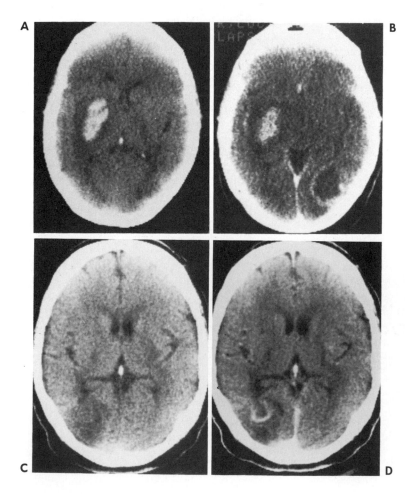

Figure 6–45. A 52-year-old woman developed headache and right arm numbness. Findings were aphasia with right hemiparesis with sensory deficit. *CT findings*: left hyperdense ganglionic hematoma (*A*) and right occipital hypodense lesion with ring enhancement (*B*). Angiogram showed a left ganglionic avascular mass. Two months later there had been excellent clinical recovery. *CT findings*: occipital hypodense lesion (*C*) with a small area of incomplete occipital ring enhancement (*D*).

Figure 6–46. A 45-year-old hypertensive woman suddenly collapsed. Findings were stupor, quadriplegia, absent caloric response and miotic but reactive pupils. CT *findings:* left cerebellar and brain stem (A) and thalamic hematoma with intraventricular extension (B). Necropsy showed three separate areas of hemorrhage.

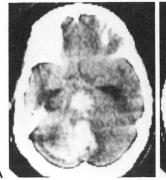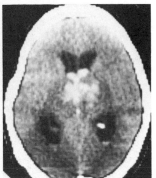

A   B

follow-up CT and clinical course were consistent with multiple spontaneous hematomas (Fig. 6–45).

If CT shows multiple hyperdense nonenhancing lesions, other diagnostic entities must be considered. Metastatic neoplasms may show CT evidence of multiple hyperdense nonenhancing lesions, but in most cases metastatic neoplasms densely enhance on postcontrast scan. In rare instances, metastatic neoplasms appear as hyperdense enhancing lesions. This pattern may represent peritumoral hemorrhage or high cellular density of neoplasms without hemorrhage. Multiple meningiomas may appear as hyperdense (calcified or noncalcified) lesions, but these usually enhance densely. Multicentric gliomas may have a hyperdense component; however, the appearance of mixed-density lesion with irregular margination and complex enhancement is characteristic of malignant gliomas. Multicentric AVM are quite rare. CT may show multiple hematomas with abnormal vessels on postcontrast CT; however, this diagnosis is established only by angiography.[15]

POSTERIOR FOSSA HEMORRHAGE

Ten to fifteen percent of spontaneous intracranial hemorrhage occur in posterior fossa. Utilizing CT, accurate localization within the posterior fossa (brain stem, fourth ventricle, cerebellum) and precise pathological delineation (hematoma, infarction) is possible. Rapid diagnostic assessment is important because certain lesions require immediate surgical intervention. In several studies it was reported that surgical intervention is potentially lifesaving in patients with cerebellar hemorrhage. This is frequently successful if surgery is performed before brain stem compression occurs. Cerebellar hemorrhage may follow several clinical courses. In the acute form, initial symptoms include headache, vomiting, dizziness and gait instability. Patients become unable to walk and level of consciousness may rapidly deteriorate. Examination shows signs of brain stem compression such as miotic pupil, lateral gaze palsy, 6th and 7th nerve paresis (ipsilateral to hematoma) and bilateral Babinski signs. There is rapid progression to coma with signs of lower brain stem compression unless immediate surgical intervention is performed.

CT usually shows large cerebellar hematoma with obstructive hydrocephalus. The fourth ventricle and basal cisterns are usually effaced. In other patients with cerebellar hemorrhage, the course is more subacute, with the predominant abnormality being gait instability. Examination shows gait or limb ataxia or both with few or no signs of brain stem compression. CT shows smaller cerebellar hematoma with less marked mass effect.

In rare instances, neurological deficit develops more slowly over several weeks. Clinical features of impaired level of consciousness (lethargy, confusion), gait instability and incontinence may develop. This pattern may simulate normal pressure hydrocephalus or neoplasm. CT may show a cerebellar mass of variable density (hyperdense, isodense or hypodense) usually without enhancement. There usually is obstructive hydrocephalus.

The diagnosis of cerebellar hemorrhage is very difficult to establish on a clinical basis alone. Differentiation from other conditions, including cerebellar infarction, pontine hematoma, ruptured intracranial aneurysm and supratentorial mass lesion with brain stem compression, is not always possible based upon clinical findings alone.

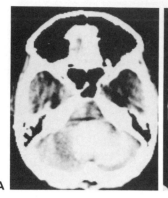
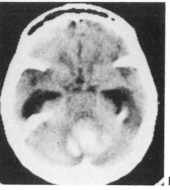

Figure 6–47. This 48-year-old man developed headache, became unable to walk and collapsed. Findings were consistent with brain stem compression. *CT findings:* bilobulated cerebellar hematoma (*A*) that had compressed the fourth ventricle and caused marked obstructive hydrocephalus with massive temporal horn dilatation (*B*).

In patients with cerebellar hemorrhage, bleeding frequently originates from the region of the superior cerebellar artery. Hemorrhage may be located in the vermis and extend into the cerebellar hemisphere, brain stem, or fourth ventricle. CSF examination usually shows bloody or xanthochromic fluid with elevated pressure. If the hematoma is small and confined to the cerebellar hemisphere, CSF may be clear. In the pre-CT era, Fisher believed that diagnosis of cerebellar hemorrhage could be suggested on clinical basis such that posterior fossa exploration may be warranted; however, air studies and vertebral angiography were usually performed.[16] Angiographical findings of cerebellar hematoma is based upon demonstration of cerebellar mass effect; that is, forward displacement of basilar artery, stretching of posterior inferior and cerebellar arteries and exclusion of such causal vascular lesions as aneurysm and angioma. Before the development of CT, angiography was positive in 81 percent; however, ventriculography was also used to define the presence of cerebellar hematoma.

CT has changed our approach to diagnosis and management of patients with cerebellar hemorrhage. On the basis of CT findings these patients with cerebellar hemorrhage have been divided into two clinical categories. In one group, patients show rapid neurological deterioration with early evidence of brain stem compression (Fig. 6–47). All these patients were hypertensive on admission to the hospital. Despite vigorous attempts to control elevated blood pressure with antihypertensive medication, this reduction in blood pressure was poorly achieved. Ninety percent of these patients had been treated with antihypertensive medication for less than two years and had no evidence of accelerated atherosclerosis such as myocardial infarction, transient ischemic attacks or peripheral vascular disease. In these cases, CT shows large cerebellar hematoma—greater than 3 cm. There is marked fourth ventricular mass effect and ventricular enlargement caused by obstructive hydrocephalus. These hematomas cause "tight" posterior fossa in which case there is nonvisualization of fourth ventricle posterior

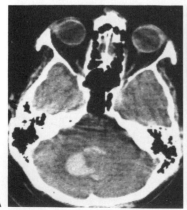
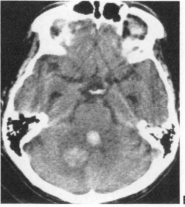

Figure 6–48. A 52-year-old hypertensive man developed headache and gait instability. *CT findings:* cerebellar hematoma (*A*) with intraventricular extension (*B*). The posterior fossa cisterns are well visualized. He recovered clinically without surgery. Follow-up CT (not shown) showed resolution of blood.

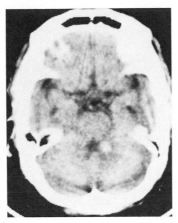

Figure 6–49. An elderly man developed gait instability. Findings were right limb ataxia, right gaze nystagmus and facial paresis. CSF was xanthochromic with elevated protein content. *CT findings:* small right cerebellar hematoma contiguous with the fourth ventricle.

fossa subarachnoid spaces. Intraventricular extension was seen in only 10 percent and was seen in occipital horns or posterior third ventricle. Blood was not seen in the compressed fourth ventricle. Surgical evacuation was necessary in these patients. Mortality was 35 percent; however, all patients who were comatose on admission died.

In the second group of patients with cerebellar hemorrhage, clinical features included prominent cerebellar dysfunction with less severe impairment of consciousness and minimal brain stem dysfunction. In these cases, CT showed a hematoma that was less than 3.0 cm in size. These caused less mass effect, and ventricles were not dilated. Hematoma may be decompressed by extending into the fourth ventricles, and in these cases posterior fossa cisterns are usually visualized. Intraventricular extension into the fourth ventricle was seen in one half of cases. These patients frequently recover without surgery (Fig. 6–48) and serial CT may show hematoma resolution. All patients with smaller hematomas (less than 1.2 cm) recovered without surgery.[17–19] In those patients with small cerebellar hematomas, indications for surgery may need to be reassessed in light of the more benign outcome that may occur spontaneously (Fig. 6–49).

BRAIN STEM HEMORRHAGE

These hemorrhages usually occur in the pons at the junction of the basis pontis and

tegmentum.[20] Pathological studies have defined four categories of brain stem hemorrhage: (1) large hematomas with ventricular extension, (2) encapsulated hematoma located within brain stem parenchyma, (3) secondary petechial brain stem hemorrhages secondary to mass effect and herniation and (4) traumatic brain stem contusions. Patients with primary brain stem hemorrhage present with a relatively characteristic clinical pattern.[21] This includes rapid onset of coma, quadriplegia, bilateral Babinski signs, miotic pupils that retain light reactivity, absent horizontal eye movements and caloric response and irregular respiratory pattern. CSF shows blood or xanthochromia in 90 percent of cases. The etiology is most commonly arterial hypertension (Fig. 6–50), but other etiologies include vascular malformation (Fig. 6–51) and basilar aneurysm. Prognosis is poor and most patients die within 48 hours. Utilizing CT, it is clear that the clinical spectrum is more variable

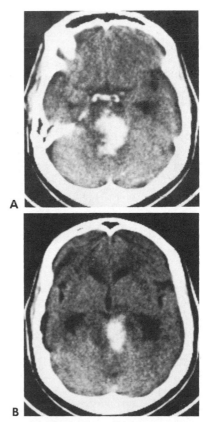

Figure 6–50. This 46-year-old hypertensive suddenly collapsed. Findings were coma, quadriplegia, miotic pupils and absent caloric response. *CT findings:* extensive brain stem hematoma (A) extending to the posterior thalamic region (B).

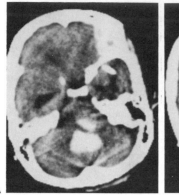
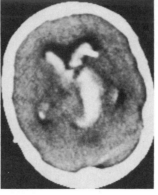

A

B

Figure 6–51. A 30-year-old woman with brain stem telangiectasia developed severe headache and became comatose, with irregular respirations. *CT findings:* extensive brain stem hematoma (A) extending to the thalamus with intraventricular extension (B).

than previously appreciated. Some patients may make good functional recovery (Fig. 6–52).

CT usually shows a hyperdense brain stem lesion representing the hematoma. This is maximal in size in the pontine region; however, it may extend upward into the midbrain-thalamic region or downward into the medullary region. Hematomas may extend into the fourth ventricle; however, there is no correlation of size with presence of ventricular extension. Brain stem hematomas may be smaller and remain localized to the pontine or midbrain region. There was no correlation of hematoma size with clinical outcome. Clinical outcome was best in patients with these findings: (1) no history of arterial hypertension, (2) preserved horizontal eye movements, (3) minimal alteration in level of consciousness, and (4) CSF was not bloody.

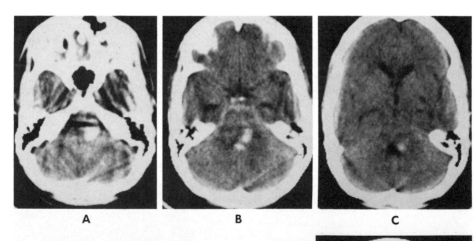

A

B

C

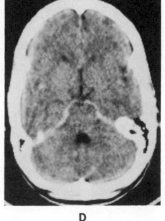

D

Figure 6–52. A 29-year-old woman developed headache and collapsed. Findings were right hemiplegia and right oculomotor and left gaze palsy. CSF was bloody. *CT findings:* right intrapontine hematoma (A) with fourth ventricular and cisternal blood (B). One week later she regained consciousness. *CT findings:* decreased size in a pontine hematoma (C). Four-vessel angiogram was negative. One month later she was ambulating independently. *CT finding:* complete resolution of hematoma (D).

INTRAVENTRICULAR HEMORRHAGE

This may result from intracerebral hematoma that extends through ependymal lining (secondary), or rupture of abnormal blood vessels located within the ventricular wall or choroid plexus (primary). Primary intraventricular hemorrhage (Fig. 6–53) may develop in patients with choroid plexus hemangioma, saccular aneurysm, arteriovenous malformation, or rarely with malignant neoplasms.[22] Clinical findings in patients with primary intraventricular hemorrhage have included seizures, altered level of consciousness, nuchal rigidity, high fever, extensor spasms and bilateral Babinski signs. However, with CT, we are becoming aware that the clinical spectrum may be quite diverse. In some cases, patients have meningeal signs but are neurologically intact; however, CT may show extensive intraventricular blood with markedly dilated ventricles. In other cases patients are comatose and quadriplegic, with miotic reactive pupils and absent caloric response; CT shows a less extensive amount of intraventricular blood. The clinical condition does not correlate with the amount of ventricular blood or ventricular size.

In patients who have primary ICH, delayed neurological deterioration may occur as hemorrhage dissects into the ventricles (secondary intraventricular hemorrhage). It has been speculated that extension of hematoma into the ventricles may reduce local parenchymal pressure. Utilizing CT, the incidence of intraventricular extension of ICH is much higher than previously suspected by clinical and necropsy studies. The mortality rate of patients with ICH that has extended into ventricles is 40 percent. This is much lower than reported before the development of CT scanning. Development of hydrocephalus that follows intraventricular hemorrhage is due to impaired flow at level of intraventricular foramina or aqueduct of sylvius; however, it may also be extraventricular, resulting from basal cisternal bleeding.[23]

In patients with intraventricular hemorrhage, CT shows a hyperdense cast outlining the ventricular system. Blood-cerebrospinal fluid levels may be visualized within ventricles. Blood is frequently initially seen in the occipital horns. If ventricular blood has resulted from extension of primary ICH, hemorrhage may be localized to the ipsilateral ventricle, and parenchymal hematoma is identified. Blood is rarely visualized in the temporal horns unless there is temporal lobe hematoma. Some small caudate or thalamic hematoma may cause extensive ventricular hemorrhage (Fig. 6–54). It may be difficult to identify small parenchymal hematoma as distinct from ventricular blood-filled cast. Triventricular hemorrhage usually results from anterior cerebral artery aneurysms. If hemorrhage is confined to the fourth and third ventricles, this is usually caused by ruptured posterior fossa aneurysm. In certain cases of posterior fossa hemorrhage, blood is seen only in the occipital horns. The CT finding of hyperdense mass located at intraventricular foramina may represent hemorrhage from ruptured aneurysm of the anterior cerebral and the anterior communicating artery. This may be incorrectly diagnosed as colloid cyst. It is

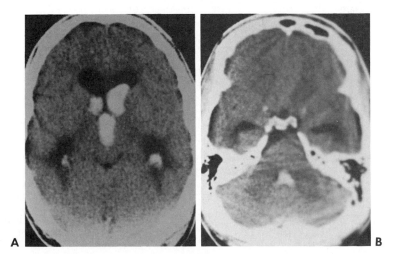

Figure 6–53. A 26-year-old man had generalized seizure and remained comatose. CSF was bloody. *CT findings:* ventricular hemorrhage (*A*) including the fourth ventricle (*B*). Angiogram showed anterior cerebral–anterior communicating artery aneurysm.

A   B

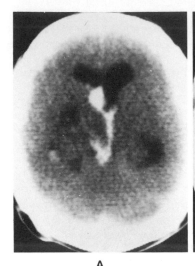
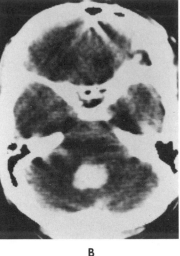

A   **B**

Figure 6–54. A 53-year-old hypertensive woman developed headache and became obtunded. Findings were right hemiparesis, gaze paresis to the right side and miotic pupils. *CT findings:* small left ganglionic (caudate region) hematoma (*A*) with marked intraventricular extension of blood (*B*).

not always possible to differentiate solid from liquefied intraventricular hematoma. As intraventricular clot ages, attenuation values of hematoma may be isodense; however, the mass does not always decrease in size and localized ventricular dilatation may persist because of the lesion. In this case diagnosis of persistent intraventricular mass is established by air or metrizamide ventriculography.

HEMORRHAGE CAUSED BY CEREBRAL NEOPLASM

In one reported series of ICH in which etiologies were verified, 10 percent were caused by either primary or metastatic neoplasms. In randomly selected cses of ICH, one to two percent of ICH are caused by neoplasms.[24] Metastatic neoplasms that most commonly cause intracranial hemorrhage include melanoma, hypernephroma, choriocarcinoma and lung carcinoma. Primary intracranial neoplasms include glioblastoma, oligodendroglioma, angioblastic meningioma and pituitary adenoma. Mechanism of hemorrhage within neoplasm includes multiple factors: (1) systemic complications such as arterial hypertension and coagulation disorders, (2) rupture of pathological vessels including neovascularity of glioblastoma and (3) rapid growth of neoplasm such that it outgrows vascular supply, as in metastatic neoplasms.[25] In one half of patients with hemorrhagic neoplasms, the apoplectic event was the initial symptom. All patients with hemorrhage neoplasms presented with sudden onset of focal neurological deficit and altered level of consciousness. Hemorrhagic neoplasms were intracerebral or intracerebellar; intraventricular extension may also occur. CT findings were quite characteristic. Noncontrast scan shows single or multiple hyperdense mass(es) with a single large hemorrhagic region or multifocal hemorrhagic areas. There may be fluid level because of liquefied hemorrhage. Hematoma may be seen at the interface between the neoplasm and the edematous brain. Following contrast infusion, there is usually enhancement in neoplasm surrounding the hemorrhagic component. If hemorrhage is extensive, no visual enhancement may be seen within the tumor, and differentiation from spontaneous ICH is not possible. In certain patients with intracranial metastases who also develop coagulopathy, multiple nonenhancing hemorrhagic neoplasms may be detected by CT.

REFERENCES

1. Huckman MS, Weinberg PE, Kim KS: Angiographic and clinicopathologic correlates in basal ganglionic hemorrhage. Radiology 95:79, 1970
2. Weisberg LA: Computed tomography in intracranial hemorrhage. Arch Neurol 36:422–426, 1979
3. Caplan L: Intracerebral hemorrhage. *In* Tyler HR, Dawson DM (eds): Current Neurology, vol 2. Boston, Houghton-Mifflin, 1979, pp. 185–205
4. Herbstein DJ, Schaumberg HH: Hypertensive intracerebral hematoma. Arch Neurol 30:412, 1974
5. Kelley RE, Berger JR, Scheinberg P: Active bleeding in hypertensive intracerebral hemorrhage: computed tomography. Neurology 32:852, 1982
6. Messina AV, Chernik NL: The resolving intracerebral hemorrhage. Radiology 118:609, 1975

7. Weisberg LA: Peripheral rim enhancement in supratentorial intracerebral hematoma. Comput Tomogr 4:145, 1980
8. Laster DW, Moody DM, Ball MR: Resolving intracerebral hematoma: alteration of the ring sign with steroids. Am J Roentgenol 130:935–939, 1978
9. Zimmerman RD, Leeds NE, Naidich TP: Ring blush associated with intracerebral hematoma. Radiology 122:707, 1977
10. Hier DB, Davis KR, Richardson EP: Hypertensive putaminal hemorrhage. Ann Neurol 1:152, 1977
11. Walshe TM, David KR, Fisher CM: Thalamic hemorrhage: computed tomographic—clinical correlations. Neurology 27:217, 1977
12. McCormick WF, Rosenfield DB: Massive brain hemorrhage. Stroke 4:946, 1973
13. Ropper AH, Davis KR: Lobar cerebral hemorrhages: acute clinical syndromes in 26 cases. Ann Neurol 8:141–147, 1980
14. Weisberg LA: Multiple spontaneous intracerebral hematomas; clinical–computed tomographic correlations. Neurology 31:897–900, 1981
15. Schlacter LB, Fleischer AS, Faria M: Multifocal intracranial arteriovenous malformations. Neurosurgery 7:444, 1980
16. Fisher CM, Picard EH, Polak A: Acute hypertensive cerebellar hemorrhage. J Nerve Ment Dis 140:38–57, 1965
17. Little JR, Tubman DE, Ethier R: Cerebellar hemorrhage in adults. J Neurosurg 48:575–579, 1978
18. Weisberg LA: Cerebellar hemorrhage in adults. Comput Radiol 6:75, 1982
19. Heiman TDF, Satya-Murti S: Benign cerebellar hemorrhages. Ann Neurol 3:366–368, 1978
20. Goto N, Kaneko M, Hosaka Y: Primary pontine hemorrhage: clinicopathological correlations. Stroke 11:84–90, 1980
21. Weisberg LA, Bryan R: Prolonged survival with good functional recovery in patients with brain stem hemorrhage. Comput Radiol 6:43, 1982
22. Little JR, Blomquist GA, Ethier RA: Intraventricular hemorrhage in adults. Surg Neurol 8:143–150, 1977
23. Graeb DA, Robertson WD, Lapointe JS: Computed tomographic diagnosis of intraventricular hemorrhage. Radiology 143:91, 1982
24. Scott M: Spontaneous intracerebral hematoma caused by cerebral neoplasms. J Neurosurg 42:338–342, 1975
25. Little JR, Dial B, Belanger G: Brain hemorrhage from intracranial tumor. Stroke 10:283–287, 1979

Aneurysmal Subarachnoid Hemorrhage

ANEURYSMS

These represent abnormal dilatations of blood vessel walls. Aneurysms are of the following five types: (1) saccular, congenital defects occur in the media and internal elastic layers to cause localized dilatation of major arterial trunks; (2) fusiform aneurysm is caused by atherosclerosis with loss of elasticity to result in tortuosity of elongated arterial segments; (3) mycotic, infectious-inflammatory process causes arteritis to result in localized vessel wall weakening and dilatation; (4) miliary, hypertensive disease causes degenerative change in the muscular and elastic lamina of penetrating vessels supplying the basal ganglia, thalamus, brain stem and cerebellum; (5) traumatic injury can cause aneurysm.

SACCULAR (BERRY) ANEURYSM

These occur at bifurcation of large intracranial vessels located in subarachnoid spaces. Ninety percent occur in the anterior circle of Willis; those involving the anterior cerebral–anterior communicating, internal carotid–posterior communicating, trifurcation of the middle cerebral artery are most common. Ten percent originate from vertebral-basilar arteries. Those that arise at the rostral basilar artery tip or posterior inferior cerebellar-vertebral artery junction are most common. Aneurysms appear as round or oval-shaped lobulated arterial dilatations. These have narrow (pedunculated) or wide (diffuse) neck. Multiple bleeding points may be identified pathologically. Small aneurysms (3 to 10 mm in diameter) are likely to bleed, whereas larger (giant) aneurysms are less likely to cause hemorrhage but more likely to compress contiguous structures and act as mass lesions. Multiple aneurysms are present in 20 percent of cases.

Of patients with aneurysmal subarachnoid hemorrhage (SAH), 30 to 40 percent have a "warning sign" resulting from small hemorrhage. Severe headache may be the only symptom of this prodromal phase. This may be incorrectly identified as an initial "migraine" attack or as being part of a systemic infectious disorder. If the aneurysm bleeds directly into subarachnoid spaces, initial symptoms are caused by meningeal irritation: headache, back pain, stiff neck and vomiting. One half of patients have altered consciousness with the headache.

Patients with aneurysmal SAH are classified by clinical grades: Grade I, alert with no neurological deficit; Grade II, alert with stiff neck and minimal neurological deficit or oculomotor nerve palsy; Grade III, drowsy or confused, stiff neck with or without neurological deficit; Grade IV, marked impairment of consciousness with or without neurological deficit; Grade V, comatose and decerebrate. Immediately following aneurysmal SAH, poor neurological condition suggests a complicating process such as intercerebral, subdural or intraventricular hemorrhage or hydrocephalus or edema.

Diagnostic evaluation of aneurysmal SAH has been modified by CT. Clinical staging may be correlated with CT evidence of complicating pathological disturbances such as hematoma, edema, infarction and hydrocephalus. These are more accurately delineated by CT than by angiography, isotope scan, EEG or CSF findings. In patients with headache and stiff neck only, the initial study should be lumbar puncture to confirm the presence of subarachnoid blood and exclude other diagnostic entities such as meningitis and hypertensive crisis. CT is indicated in patients in good clinical condition with aneurysmal SAH to determine these parameters: (1) baseline ventricular size, (2) presence and location of intracranial blood and (3) presence of clinically unsuspected complications. If CT shows diffuse or localized subarachnoid blood, this confirms aneurysmal SAH. Angiography is not necessary at this time unless early surgery is contemplated.

Some patients with intracerebral or intraventricular hematoma are in good clinical condition; they are alert and have no abnormal neurological findings. However, most patients with good clinical condition following aneurysmal SAH have normal CT, and diagnosis of SAH is established by CSF findings. In patients with suspected aneurysmal SAH who have poor neurological condition, i.e., altered mentation, focal neurological deficit and intracranial hypertension, CT scan should be the *initial* procedure because of the risk of precipitating herniation with lumbar puncture. In some of these patients immediate angiography may be performed. Emergency surgery may be carried out to remove complicating pathological processes such as intracerebral hematoma and to clip the aneurysm before the time when vasospasm develops. CT pattern of the hemorrhage may suggest which aneurysm has bled and indicate which vessel should be initially studied angiographically. Because mortality in the initial 24 hours after aneurysmal SAH is related to such complicating factors as localized hematoma, cerebral edema and hydrocephalus, CT may define the need for surgical evacuation or intracranial pressure monitoring. It is possible that patients with large, thick collections of subarachnoid blood are at increased risk for subsequent development of vasospasm, and therefore early surgical clipping is indicated despite poor clinical condition.

Angiography is performed to define the nature of the vascular lesion (aneurysm, angioma) and to determine size and patency of intracranial vessels which may be modified by vasospasm. It is believed that the largest and multilobulated aneurysm has most likely bled, and this aneurysm may be surrounded by vasospasm. The bleeding aneurysm is usually contiguous with CT evidence of blood, mass effect and ischemia-infarction. If angiography demonstrates multiple aneurysms or aneurysm with associated angioma, CT frequently correctly predicts most probable source of this bleeding episode.

In some patients with aneurysmal SAH, initial angiographical studies do not demonstrate a bleeding source. False-negative results may be caused by two factors: First, focal vascular spasm that impedes flow through the aneurysm and second, clot that forms within the aneurysmal sac to render the aneurysm angiographically invisible. If the initial angiogram is negative, the patient is usually restudied 7 to 14 days later. If the aneurysm is completely thrombosed, angiography may show an avascular mass without evidence of intraluminal filling. In these cases CT findings may suggest the vascular nature of the lesion more clearly than with angiogram.

The finding of bloody CSF that appears xanthochromic in centrifuged supernatant establishes the diagnosis of SAH. It is possible for blood to obstruct CSF pathways or become entrapped within cisterns or sulcal spaces and not to communicate with CSF circulation. This offers a theoretical explanation for the instances of patients with aneurysmal SAH who have clear nonbloody CSF; however, we have never seen this occur with initial SAH hemorrhage. If lumbar puncture is delayed for several days following aneurysmal SAH, blood has been absorbed and CSF may be clear.

The reliability of CT for detecting subarachnoid blood of ruptured aneurysm is variable. It has ranged from 55 to 95 percent in several reported series.[1-5] This marked variability in positive CT findings in aneurysmal SAH reflects the effects of three factors. First is timing. CT is more likely to be negative following a warning or prodromal hemorrhage. Second is source. Referral aneurysm treatment centers are more likely to evaluate sicker patients in whom CT is more likely to be positive. Third is what we call LP bias. Neurologists are more likely than neurosurgeons to establish the diagnosis of SAH by LP.

Detection of a diffuse thin layer of subarachnoid blood is also dependent on three factors, the first of which is again timing. Delay of CT for longer than 72 hours may result in failure to detect subarachnoid blood. A second factor is improved spatial resolution of new scanners. Third is failure to perform plain scan as contrast-enhanced pattern may mask subarachnoid blood in the initial 72 hours. The most severely neurologically impaired patients have extensive diffuse and localized subarachnoid blood on CT scan and also high red blood cell (RBC) CSF contents. However, there is no correlation of high RBC count with CT findings or for development of vasospasm.[6] CT is most likely to show subarachnoid blood if performed within 48 hours after clinical ictus. Four to 14 days after SAH, cisternal blood may appear isodense; however, there may be diffuse or focal cisternal enhancement to indicate the presence and location of SAH.[7] If dense subarachnoid blood is seen 7 days after the initial hemorrhage, this is evidence of rebleeding. Slight degrees of subarachnoid and tentorial hyperdense blood have been reported to persist into the second week.[3]

In patients with aneurysmal SAH who have CT evidence of dense subarachnoid blood, early angiography and surgery may be indicated even if the patient is in poor clinical condition. This is because these patients are most likely later to develop vasospasm, which may be avoided by early surgery.

LOCATION OF ANEURYSM BY CT ABNORMALITIES

Anterior Cerebral–Anterior Communicating Artery Aneurysm (ACA-ACoA). These patients frequently develop severe headache and have generalized seizures. There may be no neurologically abnormal findings. Bleeding aneurysms may result in these six CT findings: (1) caval-septal hematoma (Fig. 6–55), (2) blood visualized in the pericallosal cistern or anterior interhemispheric fissure, (3) blood within the anterior interhemispheric fissure extending into the bifrontal regions, (4) unilateral frontal hematoma pointing or tracking toward the anterior communicating artery (Fig. 6–56), (5) symmetrical intraventricular hemorrhage extending through the lamina terminalis cistern and (6) hypodense lesions in the frontal or parasagittal regions representing ischemia or infarction in the distribution of the anterior cerebral arterial territory. These may be directly visualized by the finding of a round or ovoid hyperdense anterior paramedian lesion on plain scan; this shows homogeneous dense intraluminal enhancement (Fig. 6–57). In patients with these ruptured aneurysms, at least one of these six CT findings is present in 80 to 90 percent of cases. If CT does not demonstrate blood in the anterior interhemispheric fissure, SAH is unlikely to

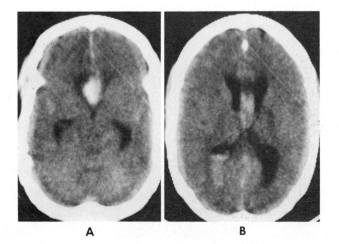

Figure 6–55. A 40-year-old woman complained of severe headache and had generalized seizure. Findings included nuchal rigidity and confusion. CSF was bloody. *CT findings:* blood can be visualized in the caval-septal region and anterior interhemispheric fissure (*A*) and lateral ventricles (*B*). Angiogram showed ACA-ACoA aneurysm.

A   B

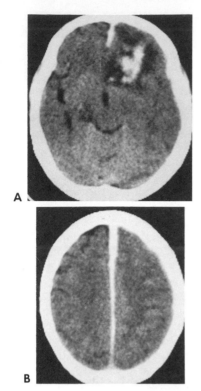

Figure 6–56. This 42-year-old man had generalized seizure. Findings were nuchal rigidity and left hemiparesis. *CT findings*: right frontal hematoma pointing toward the paramedian frontal region (A) with thick blood in the anterior interhemispheric fissure (B). Angiogram showed ACA-ACoA aneurysm.

be related to ACA-ACoA aneurysm. The finding of caval septal hematoma is diagnostic of this aneurysm; however, this is seen in only 50 percent of cases.[8]

Middle Cerebral Artery (MCA) Aneurysm. Focal neurological deficit (hemiparesis, aphasia) is most common with ruptured MCA aneurysms. Characteristic CT findings include: (1) unilateral sylvian cistern and middle cerebral artery cistern blood, (2) temporal lobe hematoma extending across the sylvian fissure

(Fig. 6–58), (3) a round or ovoid hyperdense lesion in the sylvian or MCA cistern with intraluminal enhancement that directly represents the aneurysm (Fig. 6–59), (4) ischemic

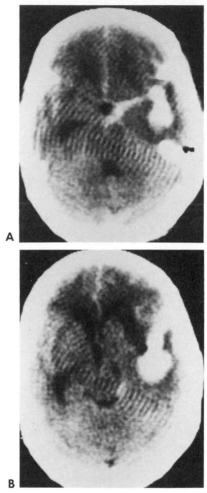

Figure 6–58. A 48-year-old man developed headache and lethargy; findings included nonfluent motor aphasia and right hemiparesis. *CT findings*: left (reader's right) sylvian and MCA cistern blood extending into the suprasellar cistern (A) and temporal lobe (B). Angiogram showed MCA aneurysm.

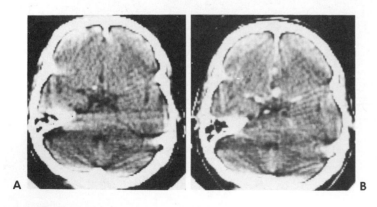

Figure 6–57. A 70-year-old man with bronchogenic carcinoma developed headache and dizziness; neurological examination, EEG and isotope scan were negative. *CT findings*: noncontrast scan shows no abnormality (A); postcontrast scan showed round, densely enhancing masses consistent with anterior cerebral and pericallosal artery aneurysms (B). These were confined by angiography.

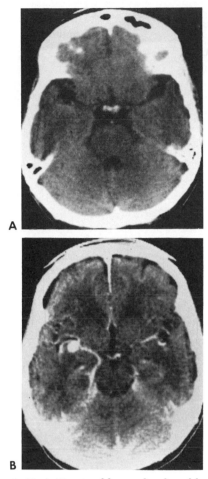

lesions in the lateral frontal, temporal or parietal region. The coronal sections may be of help in determining if the hematoma is located in the temporal lobe or the sylvian cistern. Ventricular extension, that is, temporal horn blood, resulting from ruptured MCA aneurysms usually occurs only if there is a temporal lobe hematoma. Sylvian cistern bleeding is usually caused by MCA aneurysm (Fig. 6–60); however, temporal hematomas are more likely caused by other conditions such as hypertension, angioma, or neoplasm, although they may also be caused by carotid aneurysms.

Internal Carotid–Posterior Communicating Artery Aneurysm. Clinically, these patients frequently develop headache and diplopia. Examination shows complete unilateral oculomotor nerve paresis. When these aneurysms rupture, CT evidence of subarachnoid blood may be seen in several locations, including the suprasellar-interpeduncular cistern, the medial temporal lobe, the sylvian cistern-interhemispheric fissure, and the ganglionic region especially contiguous with the head of the caudate nucleus (Fig. 6–61). The finding on plain scan of a hyperdense round or ovoid mass in the caudate or suprasellar cistern that shows homogeneous sharply marginated enhancement is characteristic of internal carotid aneurysm.

Vertebral-Basilar Aneurysm. There are no clinical features that are characteristic of these ruptured posterior fossa aneurysms. CT evidence of blood in the perimesencephalic or interpeduncular cisterns with or without midbrain hematoma is suggestive of ruptured basilar tip aneurysm. The CT finding of blood in the fourth and third ventricles with minimal blood within the lateral ventricles (sometimes

Figure 6–59. A 60-year-old man developed headache and stiff neck. Findings included confusion and right pronator drift. CSF was bloody. *CT findings:* hypodense region at the terminal portion of the MCA cistern (*A*) with dense intraluminal enhancement (*B*) continuous with normal vessels. This is consistent with saccular aneurysm and was confirmed by angiography.

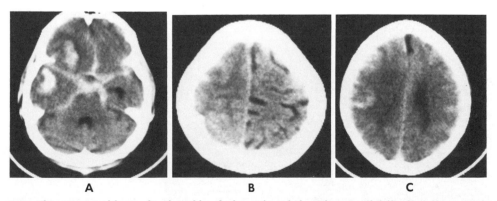

Figure 6–60. This 49-year-old man developed headache, right-sided weakness and difficulty talking. *CT findings:* left sylvian cistern hematoma (*A*) with nonopacification of sulcal spaces (*B*) filled with blood (*C*). Angiogram showed MCA aneurysm.

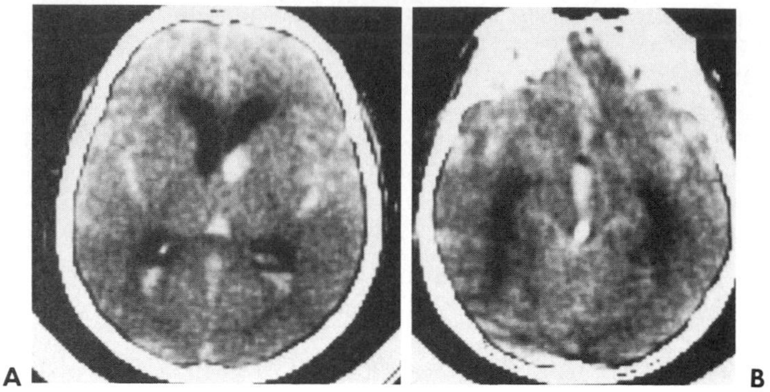

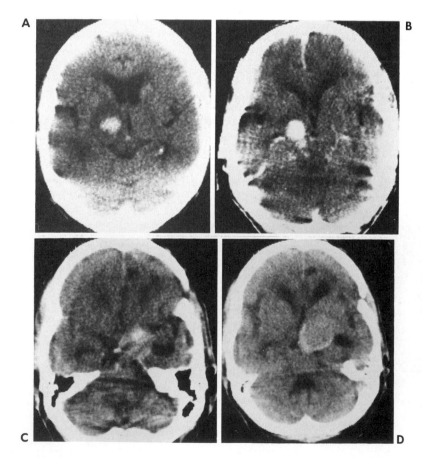

Figure 6–61. A 47-year-old hypertensive man developed headache, lethargy and left hemiparesis. CSF was bloody. *CT findings:* right-sided head of caudate hematoma (*A*) with intraventricular and cisternal blood (*B*). Angiogram showed ICA aneurysm.

blood is seen only in the dependent occipital horns) is usually caused by vertebral–posterior inferior cerebellar artery aneurysm. If there is associated vasospasm, hypodense lesions are seen in the cerebellum, brain stem or occipital region. Large posterior fossa aneurysms may simulate neoplasms.

Direct Visualization of Aneurysms by CT

Thin-walled nonthrombosed patent saccular aneurysms are usually less than 10 mm in diameter. They are not of sufficient size to be directly visualized by CT, although location of subarachnoid blood suggests which aneurysm has ruptured. In rare instances, smaller aneurysms (6 to 9 mm) are visualized by CT, but only when these are located within or directly contiguous with CSF-filled spaces, such as ACA-ACoA aneurysm located within the cistern of the lamina terminalis, and carotid or ACA-ACoA aneurysm projecting into the suprasellar region. On plain scan nonthrombosed aneurysms appear as round or oval

Figure 6–62. A 48-year-old man developed headache and became obtunded. CSF was bloody. *CT findings:* left ganglionic hyperdense lesion and surrounding hypodense rim (*A*) with dense homogeneous enhancement (*B*). Angiography showed ICA aneurysm with broad neck that could not be surgically clipped. The aneurysm size was identical on the basis of CT and angiographical measurements. Two years later, repeat CT showed left (reader's right) suprasellar-ganglionic hyperdense mass (*C*) with a small area of enhancement (*D*). Angiogram showed a large avascular mass with a small area of intraluminal enhancement consistent with partially thrombosed aneurysm. The lesion appeared larger on CT than on angiography.

isodense or hyperdense noncalcified lesions. The cistern in which the aneurysm is located may be enlarged, and this may cause the appearance of hypodense component surrounding the aneurysm. This hypodense region may simulate edema; however, it lacks frond-like projections and mass effect. Following contrast infusion, these aneurysms demonstrate dense homogeneous intraluminal enhancement (Fig. 6–62). CT lacks spatial resolution to demonstrate morphological details of the aneurysm sac, such as size of the neck, multilobulation and bleeding points; therefore, angiography is still essential to define aneurysm morphology. The aneurysm diameter as determined by CT and angiography should be identical. Other lesions with similar CT findings include meningiomas, pituitary adenomas, neuromas (acoustic, trigeminal), metastases, angiomas and gliomas.[9]

Partially thrombosed aneurysms are usually large lesions. The peripheral wall is thickened and frequently calcified. On plain scan this portion appears as a continuous or noncontinuous curvilinear hyperdense rim. The thrombosed portion is usually calcified. The intraluminal patent portion appears isodense on plain scan. Following contrast infusion, enhancement may be seen in the peripheral wall because of contrast extravasation into highly vascularized collagen tissue in the aneurysm wall. The thrombosed portion does not en-

hance; however, the patent central channel shows intraluminal enhancement (Fig. 6–63). CT density and enhancement features create a target or bull's eye appearance. Because the aneurysm has partially thrombosed, the lesion may appear larger on CT than by angiography. Other conditions that may simulate the CT pattern of partially thrombosed aneurysm are ring-enhancing hematomas, tuberculomas, craniopharyngiomas and gliomas.

Completely thrombosed aneurysms have thickened calcified peripheral walls. This wall appears as a curvilinear high-density rim on CT. This rim may be continuous or discontinuous, depending upon the thickness of the calcified portion. The peripheral wall may show peripheral rim enhancement (Fig. 6–64). There may be laminated areas of clot within the thrombosed aneurysm; these appear as multiple hyperdense rings. There is no intraluminal enhancement because the lesion is thrombosed. These aneurysms may be surrounded by a hypodense halo representing enlarged surrounding subarachnoid spaces. There is no surrounding edema and minimal mass effect despite the large size of these aneurysms. CT findings provide a better estimate of size of thrombosed aneurysms than angiography. CT directly visualizes the peripheral wall and central region, while angiography shows the intraluminal component and associated mass effect caused by the aneu-

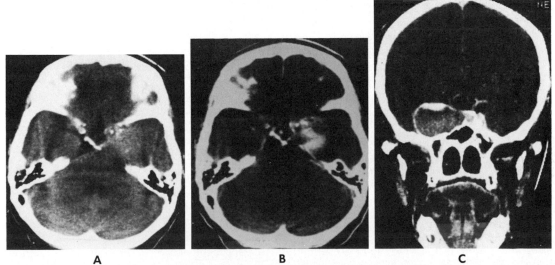

A **B** **C**

Figure 6–63. This 52-year-old woman developed supraorbital numbness and diplopia. Findings were right abducens paresis and dilated pupil. Skull radiogram showed normal-sized sella with erosion of the right anterior clinoid process. *CT findings:* right parasellar hyperdense mass (*A*) with calcification and dense serpiginous enhancement (*B*) that was best seen on coronal sections (*C*). Angiogram showed partially ICA aneurysm.

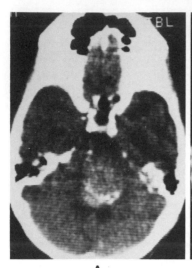 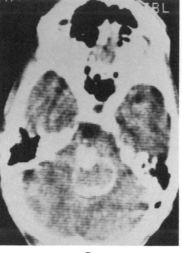

A   B

Figure 6–64. A 66-year-old man developed difficulty walking and dizziness. *CT findings:* midline posterior fossa round mass with posterior curvilinear calcified rim (*A*) with dense ring enhancement and anterior round enhancement (*B*). Angiogram showed partially thrombosed basilar aneurysm.

rysm.[10] On the basis of CT findings, differential considerations include meningioma, craniopharyngioma, glioma and vascular malformation. If a vascular lesion is suspected, angiography and CT are complementary procedures in thrombosed aneurysms.

COMPLICATIONS OF RUPTURED ANEURYSMS

1. Subdural Hematoma (SDH). These occur most commonly in association with ruptured internal carotid and MCA aneurysms.[11] These SDH may cause progressive neurological deterioration and surgical drainage may

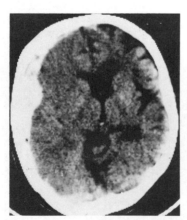

Figure 6–65. A 41-year-old man suddenly became confused and developed right hemiparesis and left dilated pupil. *CT findings:* left convexity semilunar-shaped hyperdense lesion with inward bulge at the pterion. Angiogram showed acute SDH due to ruptured MCA aneurysm.

be necessary. These lesions appear as thin hyperdense semilunar bands contiguous with bone (Fig. 6–65). There are no distinguishing CT features of aneurysmal-related SDH. In patients with aneurysmal SAH, CT findings of edema and mass effect within the initial week after the hemorrhage suggest the possibility of isodense SDH (see Fig. 6–60). Angiography may be necessary in diagnosis of some complicating aneurysmal-related SDH, although the majority are well delineated by CT. In some cases, opacification of cortical subarachnoid spaces by blood may falsely suggest the presence of SDH on the basis of CT findings; however, angiography or surgical or necropsy findings fail to confirm SDH (Fig. 6–66).

2. Intracerebral Hematoma (ICH). Immediately following aneurysmal SAH, some patients are poorly responsive or progress rapidly to poor clinical condition. This deterioration may be related to a large focal ICH contiguous to the ruptured aneurysm. Less commonly, ICH may cause no neurological abnormalities and it is an unexpected CT finding. CT demonstrated ICH in 27 percent of patients with aneurysmal SAH. This is probably higher than its true incidence because patients with poor neurological condition are usually high priority for CT, while patients in good clinical condition may not be scanned. In patients with large ICH who are in poor neurological condition, early angiography is performed. This is sometimes followed by removal of clot *and* clipping of the aneurysm. If the patient with ICH is clinically stable, this is not always removed surgically.

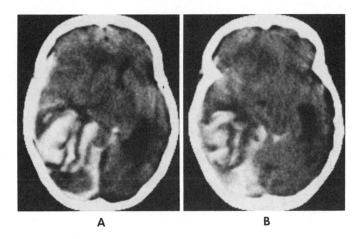

Figure 6–66. This 52-year-old woman developed headache and became obtunded. CSF was bloody. *CT findings*: left occipital hyperdense noncalcified mass with left convexity semilunar (*A*) hyperdense rim with marked mass effect and edema (*B*). Necropsy showed subarachnoid blood but no subdural hematoma. There was hematoma resulting from partially thrombosed posterior cerebral artery aneurysm.

Resolution of density of ICH is usually substantial by 14 to 21 days; however, ring enhancement may develop in the second week and persist for several weeks.

3. Intraventricular Hemorrhage. This occurs with aneurysms in all locations. It is most common with ACA-ACoA aneurysms with blood in the third ventricle and intraventricular foramen region or basilar or posterior inferior cerebellar–vertebral aneurysms with blood best seen in the fourth and third ventricles and minimal lateral ventricular blood. If there is CT evidence or intraventricular hemorrhage, the ventricles are enlarged but periventricular lucencies are not usually initially seen. CT evidence of intraventricular blood usually disappears within two to three weeks and ventricular size is usually normal within four to six weeks after the hemorrhage, although in some cases ventricles remain dilated. Intraventricular hemorrhage is the most complicating factor that predisposes for development of hydrocephalus. This is usually of extraventricular obstructive type.

4. Rebleeding. The peak time interval for rebleeding is 7 to 12 days following the initial episode.[12] The mortality for rebleeding is 50 percent. Symptoms include exacerbation of headache, deterioration in consciousness, bilateral Babinski signs and apnea. CSF analysis shows change in the appearance of the fluid from yellow to pink or red. There is an increased number of red blood cells; however, there may be no reflection of rebleeding in CSF if bleeding is directed into brain parenchyma (Fig. 6–67) or if CSF pathway obstruction has developed. In patients who show subsequent or delayed neurological deterioration, CT is reliable to differentiate rebleeding from edema, ischemia, infarction or hydrocephalus. In assessing the presence of rebleeding with CT, the most reliable CT criterion is demonstration of increased extent or density of hemorrhage in the subarachnoid

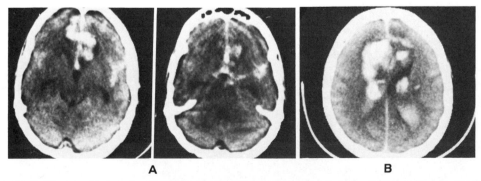

Figure 6–67. A 53-year-old man developed severe headache and nuchal rigidity. CSF was bloody. *CT findings*: frontal hematoma with anterior interhemispheric blood (*A*). Angiogram showed ACA-ACoA aneurysm. Six days later he became comatose with irregular respirations. *CT findings*: massive bifrontal (*B*) and intraventricular blood consistent with rebleeding.

spaces, ventricles and brain parenchyma as compared with initial study. Other causes of delayed neurological deterioration include systemic complications such as gastric bleeding, infection (sepsis, pneumonia, urinary infection), pulmonary embolism and myocardial infarction, and in these cases CT would be expected to be normal. CT has been extremely reliable in defining the occurrence of rebleeding (Fig. 6–68). In some cases, episodes of initial SAH or rebleeding may not be clinically apparent. The CT finding of a ring-enhancing hematoma may help in determining that hemorrhage occurred at least two weeks previously (Fig. 6–69).

5. Cerebral Ischemia and Infarction. Cerebral vasospasm due to aneurysmal SAH initially develops four to six days after initial hemorrhage, although it may begin earlier. Neurological disturbances that develop within five days of initial SAH are rarely caused by vasospasm. This process usually progresses to maximal severity within 7 to 10 days. After this time it usually decreases unless other factors such as rebleeding and edema complicate the patient's condition. Vasospasm causes brain ischemia and increases the potential for rebleeding. The vasospasm usually resolves within two weeks but neurological abnormalities resolve more slowly. There are conflicting data concerning the effect of treatment modalities such as surgery and antifibrinolytic drugs and of systemic arterial hypertension on the incidence and severity of vasospasm. Vasospasm may be diffuse; however, more commonly it occurs in the distribution of a ruptured aneurysm. Neurological symptoms and abnormal CT findings are usually present if the intracranial vessel is narrowed by more than 40 percent.[13, 14] As vasospasm and neurological deficit resolve, the hypodense wedge-shaped lesion decreases in size, mass effect resolves and enhancement may develop. It is quite unusual for CT to show a hypodense lesion caused by vasospasm in the absence of neurological deficit; however, angiogram fre-

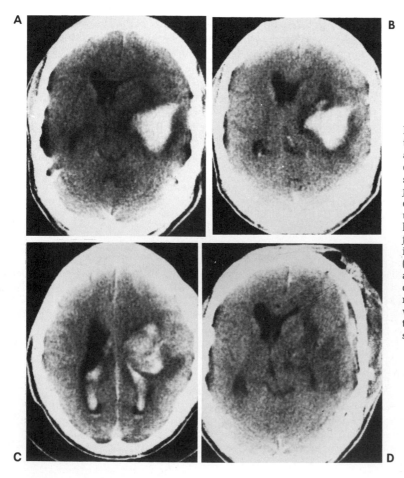

Figure 6–68. A 44-year-old hypertensive man developed headache and became lethargic. Findings included left hemiparesis with sensory deficit. CST was bloody. *CT findings*: right ganglionic and parietal hematoma without intraventricular extension (A). Eight days later he was clinically improved. *CT findings*: hematoma appeared larger in size with ventricular extension (B, C). Angiogram showed ICA aneurysm, which was surgically clipped. Six days after surgery, he remained lethargic. *CT finding*: wedge-shaped hypodense lesion in the MCA territory (D). Angiogram showed marked right MCA spasm.

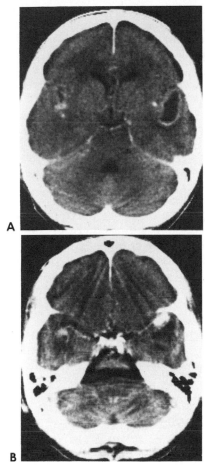

Figure 6–69. This 53-year-old woman had severe headache and was confused for several hours but this rapidly cleared. One month later she had psychomotor seizure. EEG showed right temporal spike focus; CSF was slightly xanthrochromic. CT findings: right temporal hypodense lesion with peripheral rim enhancement (A) and MCA intraluminal enhancement (B). This was consistent with ring-enhancing hematoma due to ruptured MCA aneurysm (surgically confirmed).

in only 8 to 10 percent of patients. Since CT evidence of subarachnoid blood is detected only for the initial several days, reliability of this correlation between CT evidence of subarachnoid blood and vasospasm depends upon early performance of CT.

6. Hydrocephalus. Owing to the presence of blood in the ventricles and subarachnoid spaces, CSF-filled spaces may dilate. Ventricular dilatation may develop immediately after the bleeding episode or it may develop one to six months later. In one study, 33 to 66 percent of patients with SAH developed ventricular enlargement within 48 hours of ictus, whereas others have reported this in only 12 percent. We have found that 33 percent of our patients had CT evidence of ventricular enlargement within five days of SAH, even if there were no complicating lesions. Early CT scan is important to establish baseline ventricular size. When ventricular dilatation is identified in the absence of clinical deterioration, serial scans may provide an alternative to shunting. The development of delayed ventricular dilatation occurs in 7 to 12 percent of patients; 5 to 7 percent are clinically symptomatic and require shunting.[15] CT findings in aneurysmal SAH hydrocephalus include (1) ventricular enlargement with rounding of the frontal horns, (2) periventricular hypodensities, (3) temporal horn dilatation and (4) nonvisualization of cerebral sulcal spaces. CT evidence of thickened subarachnoid clots or intracerebral hematoma does not correlate with development of hydrocephalus; however, there is a definite correlation of subsequent hydrocephalus with intraventricular blood.

POSTSURGICAL CT EVALUATION

Following intracranial surgical clipping of the aneurysm, sensitivity of CT may be decreased because of artifact emanating from metallic surgical clips. Despite this limitation, CT is the initial study if neurological worsening occurs postoperatively or if recovery from surgery is delayed. Immediate postoperative angiogram is frequently performed to determine patency of the carotid artery. If this vessel is patent and the patient develops symptoms several days later with CT evidence of hypodense lesion with mass effect, this is caused by postoperative vasospasm with infarction and is not an effect of surgery on the carotid artery. Negative postoperative CT ex-

quently shows a lesser degree of vasospasm without CT evidence of ischemia or infarction or clinical neurological deficit.

It would be extremely helpful if a reliable method existed to predict development of vasospasm. The finding of thick subarachnoid blood clots in basal cisterns and fissures on initial CT usually correlates with subsequent development of significant vasospasm and delayed neurological deterioration. The presence of intracerebral or intraventricular hematoma does not predispose to vasospasm. If CT shows no blood or only minimal diffuse subarachnoid blood, clinially significant vasospasm develops

cludes intracranial hemorrhage and hydrocephalus as causes of neurological deterioration. This is strong presumptive evidence of vasospasm, and subsequent CT scans usually show evolution of ischemic lesions. If the aneurysm has been visualized by CT before the operation, postoperative CT may be utilized to determine if the lumen is completely occluded, in which case intraluminal enhancement should no longer be seen.

FUSIFORM ANEURYSMS

Atherosclerotic change may result in loss of elasticity of intracranial blood vessel walls with elongation, tortuosity, displacement and widening (ectasia). This most commonly develops in the internal carotid and basilar arteries. Fusiform aneurysms involve the entire thickness of the vessel wall. Ectatic vessels may compress or displace contiguous structures. Despite increase in external diameter, the lumen is narrowed by atherosclerotic change. These patients frequently develop symptoms of cerebrovascular insufficiency. Patients with

basilar artery ectasia do not develop subarachnoid hemorrhage; however, fusiform aneurysms are associated with increased incidence of saccular aneurysms. If SAH occurs in patients with CT and angiographical evidence of fusiform aneurysm, associated saccular aneurysm should be suspected as the cause of the bleeding episode.

Clinical symptomatology caused by basilar artery ectasia results from compression of such contiguous structures as cranial nerves and CSF pathways. These abnormalities include: (1) lower cranial nerve dysfunction (trigeminal neuralgia, hemifacial spasm, vertigo); (2) vertebral basilar ischemic episodes; (3) dementia and gait disturbance caused by hydrocephalus as the tortuous vertebral-basilar aneurysm obstructs the ventricular system (the floor of the third ventricle, the aqueduct of sylvius, the fourth ventricle). In some patients with fusiform aneurysm there is no associated neurological symptomatology.

Vertebral angiography is the appropriate method to demonstrate vertebral-basilar artery ectasia. Utilizing CT, it is possible to establish reliably this diagnosis without an-

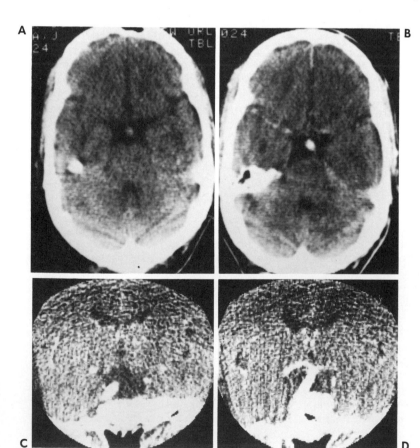

Figure 6–70. A 52-year-old man developed left-sided trigeminal neuralgia but had no neurological abnormalities. *CT findings:* hyperdense suprasellar and interpeduncular eccentric round lesion (*A*), which densely enhanced (*B*). Dynamic CT with coronal section shows marked dilatation and tortuosity of the basilar artery consistent with ectatic fusiform aneurysm (*C, D*).

giography.[16, 17] In normal persons, the basilar artery appears as a round midline hyperdense area located within the interpeduncular cistern. If there is fusiform aneurysm, the artery is tortuous and displaced laterally. More severe degrees of basilar artery ectasia appear as calcified curvilinear lesions coursing through the interpeduncular fossa and extending into the cerebellopontine cisterns. When CT shows a serpiginous hyperdense posterior fossa structure that traverses the pons and extends upward into the interpeduncular cistern to appear as an oval-shaped hyperdense enhancing lesion, this appearance leaves little room for differential considerations. In other cases, scanning angulation and size of tissue sections may result in visualization of only one portion of the ectatic vessel, and this may lead to a false impression of neoplasm. However, utilizing axial and coronal sections, multiple shapes are appreciated and the diagnosis of arterial ectasia is established. Other fusiform aneurysms are visualized as hyperdense round densely enhancing lesions that simulate meningioma, neurinoma or saccular aneurysm in the posterior fossa or pituitary tumor if seen in the interpeduncular-suprasellar region. With dynamic scanning the vascular nature of this lesion is usually apparent (Fig. 6–70).

MYCOTIC ANEURYSMS

Mycotic or septic aneurysms occur in patients with systemic septic conditions such as bacterial endocarditis and meningitis.[18] The blood vessel wall is damaged by inflammatory arteritis caused by infected embolus. These aneurysms are frequently multiple and are located on *distal* arterial branches. Most commonly they are located along the middle cerebral artery in the posterior limb of the lateral fissure. During the course of bacterial endocarditis, aneurysms may change in size and new lesions may form. Following antibiotic therapy, serial angiography may show enlargement, shrinkage or disappearance. These aneurysms may rupture to cause SAH, and there may be multiple bleeding episodes. Other patients undergo spontaneous thrombosis of aneurysm and a normal portion of the artery that causes cerebral infarction.

The diagnosis of mycotic aneurysm is established by angiography. Serial studies are necessary to follow their evolution during antibiotic therapy. Characteristic angiographic findings are multiple small aneurysms located at distal sites and with associated evidence of arteritis. CT may demonstrate location of the bleeding or the presence of infarction. However, the small size of these aneurysms precludes direct visualization by CT.

REFERENCES

1. Weisberg LA: Computed tomography in aneurysmal subarachnoid hemorrhage. Neurology 29:802–808, 1979
2. Davis KR, Kistler JP, Heros RC: Neuroradiologic approach to the patient with diagnosis of subarachnoid hemorrhage. Radiol Clin North Am 20:87, 1982
3. van Gijn J, van Dongen KJ: The time course of aneurysmal hemorrhage on computed tomograms. Neuroradiology 23:153, 1982
4. Kendall BE, Lee BCP, Clavaria E: Computerized tomography and angiography in subarachnoid hemorrhage. Br J Radiol 49:483–501, 1976
5. Silver AJ, Pederson ME, Ganti SM: CT of subarachnoid hemorrhage due to ruptured aneurysm. Am J Neuroradiol 2:13–22, 1981
6. Davis JM, Ploetz J, Davis KR: Cranial computed tomography in subarachnoid hemorrhage. J Comput Assist Tomogr 4:794–796, 1980
7. Inoue Y, Saiwai S, Miyamoto T: Postcontrast CT in SAH from ruptured aneurysms. J Comput Assist Tomogr 5:341, 1980
8. Yock DH, Larson DA: Computed tomography of hemorrhage from anterior communicating artery aneurysms with angiographic correlation. Radiology 134:399–407, 1980
9. Pinto RS, Kricheff II, Butler AR: Correlation of computed tomographic, angiographic and neuropathological changes in giant intracranial aneurysms. J Neurosurg 132:85–92, 1979.
10. Sundt TM, Piepgras DG: Surgical approach to giant intracranial aneurysms. J. Neurosurg 51:731–742, 1979.
11. Handel SF, Perpetus FOL, Handel CH: Subdural hematomas due to ruptured cerebral aneurysms. Am J Roentgenol 130:507–509, 1978
12. Van Crevol H: Pitfalls in the diagnosis of rebleeding from intracranial aneurysm. Clin Neurol Neurosurg 82:1–9, 1980
13. Fischer CM, Kistler JP, Davis JM: Relation of cerebral vasospasm to subarachnoid hemorrhage visualized by computed tomographic scanning. Neurosurgery 6:1–9, 1980
14. Saito I, Shigeno T, Aritake K: Vasospasm assessed by angiography and computerized tomography. J Neurosurg 51:466–475, 1979
15. Vassilouthis J, Richardson AE: Ventricular dilatation and communicating hydrocephalus following spontaneous subarachnoid hemorrhage. J Neurosurg 51:341–351, 1979
16. Weisberg LA: Atherosclerotic deformation of the basilar artery as visualized by computed tomography. Comput Tomogr 5:247, 1981
17. Deeb ZL, Janetta PJ, Rosenbaum AE: Tortuous vertebrobasilar arteries causing cranial nerve syndromes: screening by computed tomography. J Comput Assist Tomogr 3:774–778, 1979
18. Bingham WF: Treatment of mycotic intracranial aneurysms. J Neurosurg 46:428–437, 1977

Cerebrovascular Malformations (Angiomas)

Vascular malformations are the result of incomplete embryonic vascular development. Seven conditions are classified in this category: (1) *Arteriovenous malformations* (AVM), consisting of abnormal tortuous dilated arteries directly connecting to "arterialized veins" without an intervening capillary network. The intervening cortex may undergo atrophic, fibrous, cystic or calcified change. (2) *Venous angiomas*, having normal feeding arteries with enlarged, tortuous (single or multiple) venous drainage and normal intervening neural tissue. (3) *Vein of Galen malformation*, consisting of aneurysmal dilatation of the normal venous structure. (4) *Cavernous angioma*, consisting of multiple dilated sinusoidal vascular spaces without intervening neural parenchyma. (5) *Capillary-venous angioma (Sturge-Weber syndrome)*, which involves meningeal vessels with atrophy and calcification of the underlying cortex. (6) *Telangiectasis*, which consists of multiple dilated capillary vessels separated by normal parenchyma. (7) *Occult (cryptic) cerebrovascular malformations* that are angiomas, such as AVM, venous angioma and cavernous angioma, and cause neurological symptoms, e.g., hemorrhage, seizures and focal deficit. However, angiography and pathological findings show no or minimal evidence of abnormal vessels.

Because abnormal vessels comprising vascular malformations have thickened malformed walls (devoid of elastic and muscle fibers), pathological characterization of these arteries, veins and capillaries is difficult.[1]

ARTERIOVENOUS MALFORMATION (AVM)

These are not neoplasms, but lesion size may increase as contiguous vessels are incorporated or recruited into the angioma's flow pattern. Ninety percent are supratentorial. The majority are located in the frontal-central-parietal distribution of the middle cerebral artery. Ten percent are infratentorial or involve dural vessels.

The angiomas are usually located superficially but may extend into ventricles and the subcortical region. They consist of large dilated tortuous feeding vessels that are drained by single or multiple enlarged veins. Neurological symptoms result from rupture (hemorrhage), altered CSF flow pattern or hemodynamic vascular disturbances (ischemia, infarction). Pathological tissue changes include hemorrhage, infarction, atrophy, cyst formation, calcification and gliosis.

The clinical symptomatology attributed to AVM is highly biased by source of data. In neurosurgical series 40 to 78 percent of patients presented with subarachnoid or intracerebral hemorrhage;[2] in necropsy studies 10 to 40 percent had pathological evidence of hemorrhage.[1, 3] The next most common symptom was seizures. Other symptoms are headache, transient ischemic episodes, and progressive deterioration. The pathogenesis of the nonhemorrhagic symptomatology is not established. Three postulated mechanisms are: (1) increase in lesion size, (2) progressive ischemia as blood is shunted away from underlying normal brain parenchyma and (3) impairment of CSF circulation. Certain patients present with sudden onset of transient or permanent focal neurological deficit caused by ischemia or infarction. In rare cases dementia may develop, possibly related to cerebral blood flow "steal phenomenon" or hydrocephalus. Intracranial hypertension may result from increased cerebral blood volume within the angioma.

Subarachnoid and intracerebral hemorrhage are the most life-threatening complications. Because bleeding occurs at venous pressure, mortality from ruptured angioma is lower than with aneurysmal bleeding. Repeated bleeding episodes are characteristic of the natural history of AVM. There is no correlation between size of AVM and risk of bleeding. Small cryptic or occult angiomas may cause recurrent intracranial bleeding episodes.[4]

In 15 to 20 percent of patients with AVM, plain skull x-ray shows evidence of curvilinear or punctate calcification or enlargement of meningeal arterial grooves if dural vessels are involved.[5] EEG may show lateralized slow-wave focus. The location of EEG abnormality is not always reliable in defining the full extent

TABLE 6–5. CT Findings in 50 Patients with AVM

Characteristics	Percentage of Cases
Noncontrast density pattern	
hyperdense	22
isodense	8
hypodense	16
mixed density	54
Mass effect	36
Hydrocephalus	22
Cerebral atrophy	8
unilateral	6
bilateral	2
Postcontrast enhancement	
nonvisualized	4
present	96
evidence of abnormal vessels	50
homogeneous wedge or ovoid pattern	28
homogeneous with irregular shape	18

curs with increased incidence in these patients. The characteristic angiographical pattern is a tangle of abnormal dilated irregular blood vessels. Mass effect may not be present unless there is acute hematoma.[7] In rare cases of occult or thrombosed AVM, angiography does not demonstrate abnormal vessels; in these cases angiogram may be normal or show an avascular mass.

CT has become an important complementary procedure to isotope scan and angiography in the diagnosis of AVM.[8–12] The findings in 50 cases (angiographically confirmed) of AVM are listed in Table 6–5. The noncontrast density findings may reflect these pathological features: hematoma, calcification, abnormal blood pool, atrophic change, infarction, and unilocular or multilocular cysts.[8, 12] In 18 to 25 percent of patients, the lesion appears iso-

of the angioma or in predicting the type of underlying pathological changes caused by the angioma. In 90 to 95 percent of patients who harbor symptomatic supratentorial AVM, isotope scan is positive. If hemorrhage has not occurred, this uptake is caused by increased blood volume or isotope leak through the angiomas' immature blood-brain barrier. There is usually rapid circulation time through the AVM. The presence of accelerated flow is determined by the dynamic portion of the scan, and by early uptake with rapid washout on later images. One study reported high accuracy with isotope study if early static scan and dynamic imaging were obtained and lower accuracy with delayed scan without dynamic imaging.[6] Positive isotope scan may also occur when hemorrhage occurs; however, blood flow is decreased because of compression of vessels, vasospasm or thrombosis. The finding of normalcy on isotope and CT scan is quite reliable in excluding symptomatic supratentorial AVM.

Angiography is most reliable in detecting an AVM and in delineating supplying and draining vessels. Because circulation time through the AVM is accelerated, rapid-sequence filming is necessary to demonstrate the entire arterial and venous pattern. Four-vessel angiography is usually performed. This is necessary to visualize all abnormal feeding and draining vessels and to exclude the presence of associated berry aneurysm, which oc-

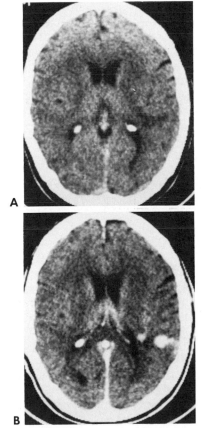

Figure 6–71. A 36-year-old man developed intermittent episodes of left face and arm numbness. EEG and isotope scan were negative. *CT findings:* no abnormality is seen on noncontrast scan (*A*). Postcontrast scan shows right parietal gyral and tubular enhancement with no mass effect (*B*). Angiogram showed AVM supplied by middle cerebral artery.

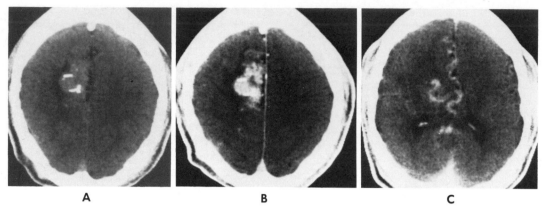

Figure 6–72. This 33-year-old man developed right focal motor seizures. Isotope scan was negative; EEG showed bifrontal spikes. *CT findings:* hyperdense and calcified left parasagittal lesion (A) with dense tubular (B) and serpiginous enhancement (C). Angiogram showed AVM supplied by both anterior cerebral arteries.

dense on noncontrast scan (Fig. 6–71). Sixty percent of AVM have mixed-density pattern (Fig. 6–72). Calcification may be intracerebral and have several patterns (punctate, globular) or located in the blood vessel wall (curvilinear). The hematoma is usually lobar and superficial in location. The hypodense regions may be ovoid or wedge-shaped, and these are believed to result from ischemia or infarction. Others are nonuniform in shape with irregular margination and associated ventricular and sulcal space enlargement. These are believed to represent cystic and atrophic change (Fig. 6–73).

On the basis of the findings of early studies, it was believed that abnormal blood vessels could not be detected by CT. With improved resolution, tortuous and dilated vessels are sometimes large enough to be detected as hyperdense tubular or serpiginous structures on noncontrast scan (Fig. 6–74). The shape of these vessels depends on their orientation to the scanning plane. If the abnormal vessels are parallel to the x-ray beam they may appear round or oval, whereas if they are perpendicular they may appear tubular or curvilinear on CT. Coronal sections are sometimes of value because vessels that may not be imaged in the axial plane are sometimes visualized in the coronal plane in which their orientation to the scanning angulation is different. On the basis of spatial (shape, size, location) features of these abnormal vessels visualized by CT, it is not possible to distinguish arterial from venous structures.

Following contrast injection, 96 percent of patients with AVM showed visual evidence of

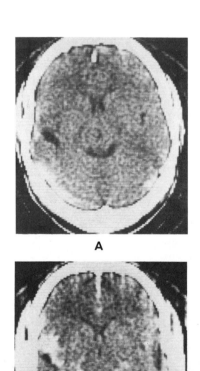

Figure 6–73. A 34-year-old woman developed right-sided clumsiness and numbness that progressively worsened over a 12-month interval. EEG and isotope scan were negative. *CT findings:* noncontrast scan showed a hypodense temporal region (A) with dense diffuse enhancement (B). Angiogram showed AVM supplied by the middle cerebral artery.

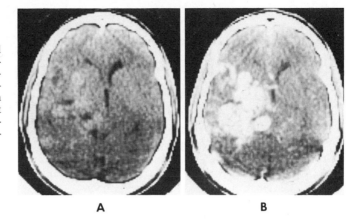

Figure 6–74. A 40-year-old man developed right focal motor seizures. Findings included mild right hemiparesis. *CT findings:* irregular curvilinear hyperdense lesion in the left hemisphere (*A*), which showed dense intraluminal enhancement (*B*). There are multiple interspersed hypodense regions within the angioma. Angiography showed extensive AVM.

A   B

enhancement. There may be either an intravascular or extravascular component. Two thirds of the enhancing lesions showed structures believed to represent abnormal vessels, and one third showed nodular or diffuse enhancement without evidence of vascular structures. The abnormal vessels show dense sharply marginated homogeneous enhancement. They are either tubular, vermian or nodular in shape. It is sometimes possible to visualize a connection of the angioma to the normal vascular structures or to demonstrate that the normal vessels on the involved side appear larger and more prominent (Fig. 6–75). There may be an extravascular enhancement component; in these cases the lesion enhances diffusely and may have wedge or ovoid shape. If the venous drainage occurs through transependymal veins, the apex of the wedge extends toward the ventricular surface.

CT scan that includes both noncontrast and postcontrast study is the most reliable screening procedure for detecting AVM. This should be supplemented by isotope scan. If isotope and CT are negative, angiography is unlikely to demonstrate an AVM.[13] Five to seven percent of these malformations demonstrated by angiography have negative CT study. These patients should have an additional CT scan that utilizes double-dose contrast medium injection and one hour delayed postcontrast scan.

CT evidence of mass effect is seen in only 10 to 20 percent of angiomas unless bleeding has occurred. In these latter cases mass effect is believed caused by hematoma or edema. This paucity of mass effect in AVM is a significant finding that differentiates AVM from

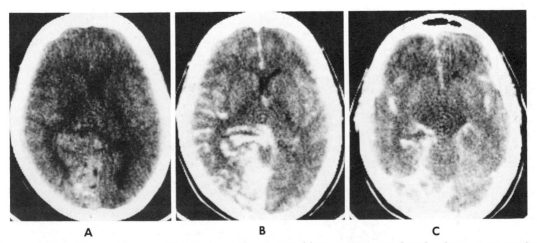

A   B   C

Figure 6–75. A 40-year-old man with symptoms of intracranial hypertension was found to have AVM supplied by the left, middle and posterior cerebral arteries. *CT findings:* hyperdense noncalcified left occipital lesion (*A*) is seen on plain scan. There is ovoid and curvilinear enhancement (*B*). The posterior cerebral artery and tentorial enhancement is more prominent on the left side (*C*).

neoplasms. In patients with angioma, hydrocephalus may result from intraventricular or subarachnoid hemorrhage. Less common causes of hydrocephalus in patients with AVM are mass effect caused by lesion size, increased cerebral blood volume, and ventricular obstruction caused by the presence of enlarged draining veins within the ventricular walls.

In patients who present with apoplectic onset, noncontrast CT detects the location of intracerebral hematoma. This is usually lobar and superficial; however, other locations have been thalamic, brain stem and intraventricular. There may be no evidence of blood on CT if the AVM has caused subarachnoid bleeding, cerebral ischemia or infarction. In young patients who have evidence of lobar or intraventricular hematomas, postcontrast scan is necessary to exclude an AVM. In these cases cerebral angiography is usually also indicated even if postcontrast CT shows no enhancement evidence of angioma. It has been our experience that hematoma formation does not reduce the likelihood of postcontrast enhancement in patients with AVM.

The CT findings of AVM may be quite similar to other pathological processes: enhancing cerebral infarction, ring-enhancing hematoma, glioma and meningioma. Cerebral infarction may appear isodense with serpiginous gyral enhancement to simulate abnormal vessels of AVM; however, enhancement usually decreases markedly within two weeks. On the basis of sequential CT findings and isotope scan results in cerebral infarction (decreased blood flow on dynamic study and positive uptake on static image 7 to 21 days following the ictal episode), it is usually possible to avoid angiography. Ring enhancement is detected in 20 percent of hematomas that have

been studied between 10 and 28 days after the hemorrhage; however, this enhancement characteristic does not suggest the presence of an underlying AVM. Gliomas may simulate AVM and angiography is necessary; however, certain diagnostic criteria make possible differentiation. These include: (1) Gliomas cause significant mass effect and angiomas usually do not. (2) Nonenhancing cysts may be seen with both angiomas and gliomas but cysts with nodular enhancement are seen only with gliomas. (3) Abnormal vessels of gliomas are not seen on CT. In certain cases dense homogeneous enhancement of meningiomas occurred contiguous to normal vascularized structures, e.g., choroid plexus. In these cases, the lesion was initially diagnosed as an angioma because these structures were believed to represent abnormal vessels; however, angiographical findings were diagnostic of meningioma.

VENOUS ANGIOMAS

These are located in the distribution of the middle cerebral artery, cerebellum or vein of Galen (see next section). The angioma is conical or wedge-shaped with its base at the cortex and apex directed toward the ventricular surface. The characteristic feature is a series of abnormal veins that converge on a central vein.[14, 15] There are no abnormal feeding arteries to this angioma. The walls of abnormal vein(s) undergo hyperplasia, fibrinoid change, calcification, loss of muscle fibers and elastic tissue. There is normal intervening brain parenchyma, usually without atrophy, gliosis or calcification.

Clinical findings include seizures (50 per-

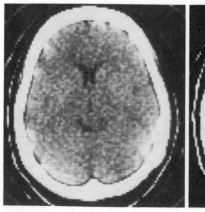
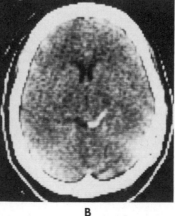

A   B

Figure 6–76. A 21-year-old woman had eight months of intermittent headache. She suddenly developed severe headache and had nuchal rigidity. CSF showed one thousand red blood cells and elevated protein content. *CT findings:* No abnormality is seen on plain scan (A). An abnormal enhancing vascular structure in the quadrigeminal cistern and third ventricle were seen on postcontrast scan (B). Angiography demonstrated venous angioma involving the right thalamus.

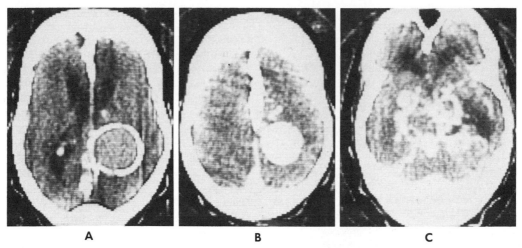

Figure 6–77. This 42-year-old woman was neurologically asymptomatic; skull x-ray showed right parietal calcification. Findings were minimal organic dementia and left pronator drift. *CT findings:* dense parietal calcification (*A*) with dense rim (*B*) and midline tubular and serpentine enhancement representing dilated vessels (*C*). Angiogram showed a venous angioma.

cent) or subarachnoid hemorrhage (17 percent). In one third of patients with venous angioma, there are no neurological symptoms. In these cases diagnostic evaluation has been initiated because skull x-ray defined intracranial calcification usually for a symptom unrelated to the angioma. Isotope scan is usually negative. The CT findings are variable and include: (1) round or curvilinear hyperdense regions that enhance on postcontrast scan; (2) isodense lesion with enhancement of single deep venous structure (Fig. 6–76) and (3) peripheral calcification with evidence of deeply situated enhancing venous structures (Fig. 6–77). The abnormal CT findings in venous angiomas are believed to represent an increased blood pool of the draining central vein.[14] The diagnosis of venous angioma is established by angiography, which shows normal circulation time and normal arterial network with an umbrella radial pattern of abnormal veins that are directed toward the central draining vein. These lesions also cause minimal mass effect.

VEIN OF GALEN MALFORMATION

This venous angioma consists of two types: First, aneurysmal dilatation of the vein of Galen supplied by dilated feeding vessels that originate from both the carotid and vertebral-basilar systems and drain into the dilated straight sinus and torcula and second, vein of Galen aneurysmal dilatation resulting from thalamic or midbrain angioma.[16] Pathological

tissue changes include ischemia, anoxia, calcification and hematoma. These vascular lesions may cause symptoms by compressing adjacent structures, including the midbrain (Perinaud syndrome with impaired upward gaze and pupillary abnormalities) or the posterior third ventricle–proximal aqueductal region (hydrocephalus).

The clinical findings are dependent upon the age at which the patient becomes symptomatic: Congestive heart failure caused by arteriovenous shunts occurs in the neonatal period. Hydrocephalus due to ventricular obstruction occurs in infants. Ocular and cerebellar symptoms due to midbrain compression occur in children and young adults. These angiomas usually cause mass effect and rarely bleed.

Prior to development of CT, the presence of midline posterior third ventricular mass that was causing obstructive hydrocephalus was established by air study; however, angiography was also necessary to define its vascular nature. It is important to perform four-vessel angiography because angioma may be supplied by both the carotid and vertebral-basilar systems. CT scan provides valuable diagnostic information about the presence of the mass and provides important diagnostic clues as to its vascular nature as well as defining the occurrence of pathological tissue change. CT findings include: (1) hyperdense midline posterior third ventricle mass with homogeneous intraluminal enhancement; (2) lesion connects to dilated straight sinus and torcula; (3) tubular and curvilinear enhancing structures in the

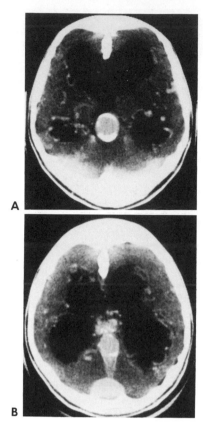

Figure 6–78. A child developed episodic vomiting. Findings included increased head circumference, impaired upward gaze and bilateral Babinski signs. *CT findings:* calcified rim of a midline posterior third ventricular mass (*A*). There is dense intraluminal enhancement and straight sinus and torcular area are dilated (*B*). The lateral and anterior third ventricles are markedly dilated. Angiogram showed vein of Galen malformation.

basal ganglion and thalamus are directed toward the mass and these represent feeding vessels; (4) peripheral curvilinear calcification outlining the wall of the lesion and (5) ventricular dilatation with compression of posterior third ventricle (Fig. 6–78). Associated pathological changes visualized by CT are ischemic and anoxic tissue damage due to shunting, cerebral atrophic change, and hematoma formation.

CAVERNOUS ANGIOMA

These consist of multiple dilated sinusoidal spaces that contain no intervening normal parenchymal tissue. They are usually located in the cerebrum (including the middle fossa and parasellar region) and less commonly in the brain stem.[17] The sinusoidal spaces are large enough to be seen by gross visual inspection. Their size is variable, ranging from several millimeters to four centimeters. The caliber of vessels comprising cavernous angioma is quite small and the walls of these vessels have poorly defined elastic tissue and smooth muscle. These vessels may become hyalinized, fibrosed, thrombosed or calcified. These patients usually present with either bleeding episodes or seizures. Skull x-ray may show evidence of calcification; isotope scan sometimes shows abnormal uptake with normal dynamic flow pattern if the lesion is larger than 2.5 cm in size. Angiography has been reported to show the patterns of capillary

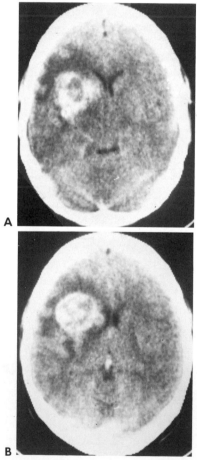

Figure 6–79. A 32-year-old woman developed partial complex seizures. Findings included right pronator drift and hemisensory deficit. EEG showed bitemporal spikes; isotope scan was negative. *CT findings:* hyperdense left hemispheric nonhomogeneous (*A*) mass with enhancement in the peripheral rim and several portions of the central region (*B*). Angiogram showed avascular mass. Surgical finding was cavernous angioma.

blush, avascular mass, or no abnormality. The failure to demonstrate abnormal vessels may be related to slow circulation time, small caliber of vessels, intravascular thrombosis, vascular compression caused by hematoma or vascular spasm.

Noncontrast CT findings that have been reported include: (1) calcification that is nonhomogeneous, mottled or lamellated; (2) hypodense lesion that represents a thrombosed portion or a slowly circulating blood pool; (3) mass effect. Postcontrast scan abnormalities may be variable. The enhancement may be minimal or intense in a diffuse or nonhomogeneous pattern (Fig. 6–79). No abnormal vessels have been detected by CT in cavernous angiomas. In certain cases, the finding of dense homogeneous enhancement has simulated CT findings of meningioma.

CAPILLARY-VENOUS ANGIOMA (STURGE-WEBER SYNDROME)

The primary lesion is a capillary-venous angioma involving the meninges without involvement of the intracranial vessels of the underlying posterior parietal and occipital region. The clinical features include facial angioma seen in the ophthalmic division of the trigeminal nerve, seizures that are usually focal in nature, and radiographical evidence of calcification. Less common findings are mental retardation, hemiparesis and glaucoma. Plain skull x-ray shows gyriform, tram-like calcification. This finding may be absent if the

patient is studied before the age of two. CT is more reliable to detect a calcified lesion than is skull roentgenogram. Isotope scan sometimes shows abnormal uptake caused by a nonspecific defect in the blood-brain barrier. Angiography demonstrates abnormal venous pattern with diversion of flow from the superficial cortical veins and superior sagittal sinus into the deep venous system. The cortical arterial and capillary flow to the involved hemisphere may be decreased and this probably results from cerebral atrophy. Other reported abnormalities include the presence of venous angioma, telangiectasis, arterial thrombosis, anomalous veins and venous sinuses.[18]

The CT findings reflect the underlying capillary-venous angiomatous lesion and resultant pathological cortical abnormalities. CT shows cortical gyriform or tram-like calcifications over the involved cerebral hemisphere (Fig. 6–80). There is frequently ipsilateral ventricular and sulcal enlargement caused by cortical atrophy. This may involve the entire cerebral hemisphere, although angioma usually involves only the parietal-occipital region. CT may show dense calcification in the occipital region with diffuse enhancement pattern. Postcontrast scan sometimes shows a diffuse homogeneous haze over the involved hemisphere or tortuous dilated vessels that may represent the dilated deep venous system and not the angioma. The long-standing cortical atrophy may be associated with reduced size of the hemicranium (Davidoff-Dyke-Masson syndrome). One variant of the Sturge-Weber disorder is Kleppel-Trenaunay-Weber syn

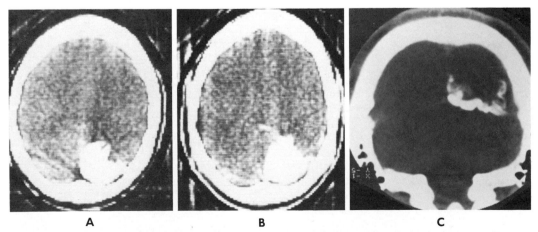

A   B   C

Figure 6–80. A 12-year-old had generalized seizures but no clinical evidence of facial angioma. Skull x-ray showed tram-like calcification. *CT findings:* occipital gyriform calcification (*A*) with minimal diffuse gyral enhancement (*B*). Coronal section shows gyral calcification (*C*) consistent with Sturge-Weber syndrome.

drome, which consists of venous and arteriovenous abnormalities and associated hemihypertrophy of the cranium.

TELANGIECTASIS

These consist of abnormal thin-walled enlarged capillaries that are separated by normal intervening brain parenchyma. These vessels have poorly developed elastic and muscle fibers and this may result in intracranial hemorrhage. These frequently occur in the brain stem (see Fig. 6–51). Clinical symptomatology may develop suddenly because of intracranial bleeding. Less commonly there is progressive neurological worsening, and this mode of presentation may suggest brain stem glioma.[19] Angiography may show an avascular mass caused by parenchymal hematoma, and in certain cases diffuse capillary blush without abnormal arteries or veins is demonstrated. Air studies may show enlarged brain stem that simulates brain stem neoplasm. In patients with brain stem telangiectasis, CT detects brain stem hematoma and intraventricular extension; however, no enhancement has been reported in these cases to indicate a possible source of the hemorrhage.

OCCULT CEREBROVASCULAR MALFORMATIONS

In most cerebrovascular malformations, diagnosis is established by characteristic angiographical findings. In rare instances the lesion is cryptic or occult; this implies that the vascular nature of the lesion is not apparent (clinically, angiographically or pathologically). Necropsy studies have demonstrated unsuspected AVM in clinically asymptomatic patients.[20] In certain young patients who suffer spontaneous ICH, angiography shows no evidence of abnormal feeding or draining vessels; pathological findings show minimal evidence of an abnormal vascular lesion.[21, 22] It is postulated that hematoma may have destroyed or compressed the cryptic vascular lesion, which may be angioma or aneurysm. Postulated explanations for nonvisualization by angiography include: (1) Hemorrhage occurs that destroys the lesion and causes vascular spasm, thrombosis or compression of abnormal vessels. (2) Spontaneous thrombosis occurs, caused by degenerative vascular change (atheroscler-

otic). (3) Supplying vessels are of a caliber that may not be detected by angiography. (4) Technical factors are present such as failure to perform prolonged venous phase to detect venous angiomas or film sequencing that is not rapid enough to detect the early arterial filling phase of AVM.[23]

The CT findings of occult vascular malformations are nonspecific and diagnosis is established by surgical biopsy. Noncontrast scan can show hyperdense (calcification, hematoma) pattern, hypodense (cystic) pattern or isodense pattern. Following contrast infusion, enhancement with tubular, serpiginous, nodular or diffuse pattern may be seen (Fig. 6–81); however, certain lesions do not enhance.

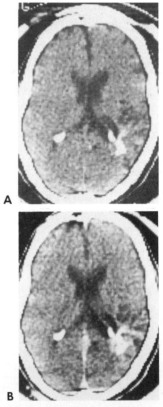

Figure 6–81. A 40-year-old man had a bleeding episode and angiogram showed AVM. No surgery was performed. He developed focal motor seizures that were controlled with anticonvulsants. Fifteen years later he was reassessed because of increasing seizure frequency. EEG showed right parietal-temporal slow wave focus; isotope scan was negative. *CT findings:* right parietal linear calcified lesion with surrounding hypodense portion (*A*). There was ipsilateral ventricular dilation and diffuse and intraluminal enhancement (*B*). Angiography and surgical findings showed thrombosed angioma.

Since this pattern may simulate glioma, irradiation without initial surgical biopsy should not be performed. Biopsy is important because irradiation of vascular malformation may cause further tissue damage; irradiation of occult vascular malformations may explain reports of radiation-cured gliomas. Meningiomas and enhancing infarcts should also be considered.

REFERENCES

1. McCormick WF, Schochet SS: Atlas of Cerebrovascular Disease. W B Saunders Company, Philadelphia, 1976, pp 72–87
2. Paterson JH, McKissock W: Clinical survey of intracranial angioma with special reference to mode of progression and surgical treatment. Brain 79:233, 1956
3. Crawford JV, Russell DS: Cryptic arteriovenous and venous hemartomas of the brain. J Neurol Neurosurg Psychiatr 19:1, 1956
4. McCormick WF, Nofzinger JD: "Cryptic" vascular malformations on CNS. J Neurosurg 24:865, 1966
5. Rumbaugh CL, Potts DG: Skull changes associated with intracranial AVM. Am J Roentgenol 98:525, 1966
6. Handa J, Handa H, Torizuka K, et al: Radioisotopic study of arteriovenous anomalies. Am J Roentgenol 115:751, 1971
7. Ramsey R: Neuroradiology with Computed Tomography. W B Saunders Company, Philadelphia, 1981, pp 536–539
8. Kendall BE, Clavaria LE: The use of CAT for diagnosis and management of intracranial angioma. Neuroradiology 12:141, 1976
9. Hayward RD: Intracranial arteriovenous malformation; experience with CT. J Neurol Neurosurg Psychiatr 39:1027, 1976
10. Terbrugge K, Scotti G, Ethier R, et al: CT in intracranial AVM. Radiology 122:703, 1977
11. Weisberg LA: Computed tomography in the diagnosis of intracranial vascular malformations. Comput Tomogr 3:125, 1979
12. Leblanc R, Ethier R, Little JR: Computerized tomography findings in arteriovenous malformations of the brain. J Neurosurg 51:765, 1979
13. Hayman LA, Fox AJ, Evans RA: Effectiveness of contrast regimens in CT detection of vascular malformations of the brain. Am J Neuroradiol 2:421–425, 1981
14. Michels LG, Bentson JR, Winter J: CT of cerebral venous angiomas. J Comput Assist Tomogr 1:149, 1977
15. Fierstien SB, Pribham HW, Hieshima G: Angiography and computed tomography in the evaluation of cerebral venous malformations. Neuroradiology 17:137, 1979
16. Martelli A, Scotti G, Harwood-Nash DC: Aneurysms of the vein of Galen in children; CT and angiographic correlations. Neuroradiology 20:123, 1980
17. Savoiardo M, Passerine A: Computed tomography, angiography and radionuclide scan in intracranial cavernous hemangiomas. Neuroradiology 16:256, 1978
18. Enzman DR, Hayward RW, Norman D: CT scan appearance of Sturge-Weber disease. Radiology 122:721, 1977
19. Zeller RS, Chutorian AM: Vascular malformations of the pons in children. Neurology 25:776–80, 1975.
20. Noran HH: Intracranial vascular tumors and malformations. Arch Pathol 39:393, 1945
21. Becker DH, Townsend JJ, Kramer RA: Occult cerebrovascular malformations. Brain 102:249, 1979
22. Kramer RA, Wing SD: CT of angiographically occult cerebral vascular malformations. Radiology 123:649, 1977
23. Kamrin RB, Buchsbaum HW: Large vascular malformations of the brain not visualized by serial angiography. Arch Neurol 12:413, 1965

Chapter 7

METASTATIC DISEASE

Intracranial metastases occur in 20 to 30 percent of patients who die with carcinoma.[1] Malignant melanoma causes the highest incidence of brain involvement. Hypernephroma, choriocarcinoma and testicular carcinoma, when fatal, frequently show pathological evidence of brain metastases. Lung and breast cancer represent the largest number of cases of brain metastases; whereas other carcinomas, such as those of the colon, stomach, pancreas, ovary, endometrium and prostate, cause parenchymal lesions less commonly but may involve the calvarium.[1, 2] The reported incidence of brain metastases is quite different according to the source of clinical material; that is, whether it is from surgical, radiation or necropsy studies. Patients with brain metastases comprise only 2 to 10 percent of cases in several neurosurgical series because they represent patients with solitary parenchymal lesions who are good operative risks without other manifestations of metastatic carcinoma.[3–5] Some of these patients present with signs of progressive neurological deterioration without evidence of systemic carcinoma.

There are four types of metastatic intracranial deposits: parenchymal, skull lesions, epidural tumors and leptomeningeal. Intracerebral metastatic tumors may be discrete and sharply marginated nodular lesions. They are commonly located at a gray–white matter junction or superficial cortex. Tumor nodules may be small with extensive peritumoral edema. Metastatic neoplasms usually spread by hematogeneous dissemination, following cerebral blood flow distribution. Eighty percent of metastatic lesions are supratentorial; they are most common in the posterior Rolandic, anterior temporal and frontal regions. Twenty percent occur in posterior fossa—cerebellum (18 percent) and brain stem (2 percent). Metastases may be solitary (35 percent) or multiple (65 percent). Most intracranial metastases usually occur in patients with other signs of systemic carcinoma; however,

CNS involvement is the initial manifestation in 10 to 14 percent.

Neurological symptoms develop rapidly (47 percent) or insidiously (53 percent). There may be generalized dysfunction (confusion, seizures) or focal deficit (hemiparesis, aphasia). The triphasic course may be seen with cerebral metastases.[5] This is characterized by initial sudden neurological deterioration caused by neoplastic arterial embolism or peritumoral hemorrhage. There is subsequent transient improvement. Gradual clinical worsening occurs later with further tumor growth and peritumoral edema. This temporal pattern has been reported in patients with other intracranial lesions such as glioma, abscess and subdural hematoma.

In patients with suspected metastatic lesions, plain skull x-rays may show calvarial lesions, sella erosion or pineal shift. Since the clinical course is usually short, Posner reported that only 11 percent of patients had calvarial lesions; 6.2 percent had sella erosion or pineal shift.[1] In patients with clinically symptomatic supratentorial lesion, focal slow wave (80 percent) and bilateral or diffuse abnormalities (16 percent) are the EEG findings that have been reported. Six percent had no EEG abnormality.[6] EEG does not usually show focal abnormality in asymptomatic patients or in those with lesions smaller than 2 cm. Multiple noncontiguous lesions usually do not cause discrete slow wave patterns but may cause generalized slowing.

Isotope scan detects symptomatic metastatic lesions in 70 to 90 percent.[7, 8] There is 95 percent accuracy with lesions equivalent in size to a sphere 2.67 cm in diameter.[9] False-negative results occur most commonly with lesions of the temporal fossa and juxtaseller and posterior fossa. Maximal tracer uptake occurs at 24 hours with metastases; however, routine isotope scan is usually performed at three hours.

The delayed scan is quite useful. This is

**TABLE 7–1. CT Findings in 400 Patients
with Intracranial Metastases**

	Incidence (Percentage)
Number of lesions	
Single	29
Multiple	71
contiguous	12
noncontiguous	59
Location	
Supratentorial	78
Infratentorial	22
cerebellar	20
brain stem	2
Mass effect	78
Edema	83
Density and enhancement	
hypodense-enhancing	40
hypodense-nonenhancing	6
hyperdense-enhancing	43
hyperdense-nonenhancing	1
isodense-enhancing	10
Multiple lesions detected by postcontrast scan only	26

because 29 percent of metastatic lesions were detected only at 24 hours, multiple lesions were detected in 20 percent of delayed scans, and 24 percent of lesions were more clearly demonstrated on delayed scan when 3-hour scan was only suspicious.[8] Delayed scan defines temporal fossa and cerebellar lesions more effectively because uptake caused by overlying temporal muscle and vascular structures of posterior fossa is no longer present at 24 hours. The finding of multiple lesions makes diagnosis of metastases most likely; however, this occurs with abscesses, granulomas, cerebral embolism and multiple sclerosis. If single homogeneous uptake is seen, differentiation from other pathological processes is not possible. A peripheral rim of uptake is suggestive of central necrosis (doughnut pattern); however, this is seen with abscesses and intracerebral hematomas.[10] Isotope scan is rarely positive in patients with clinically asymptomatic lesions.

If isotope scan detects a single lesion, angiography is indicated to exclude a primary intracranial lesion such as meningioma, aneurysm or angioma; however, differentiation from glioma is not usually possible. In patients with solitary metastases angiography may

show an avascular mass or a mass with abnormal tumor circulation. Neovascularity of metastatic tumor may have four patterns: (1) nodular stain with homogeneous opacification in arterial and capillary phase, (2) pseudoglioblastomous with early draining vein and irregular nonhomogeneous stain, (3) irregular and poorly marginated stain in capillary and venous phase and (4) avascular nonopacified central portion with peripheral stain. If angiography shows avascular mass, differentiation of metastatic lesion from other intracerebral lesions is usually not possible.[11]

Intracranial metastatic lesions are reliably detected by CT. Early studies reported few false-negative results. CT was more effective than angiography or isotope scan.[12–14] Early scanners missed some high-convexity and pos-

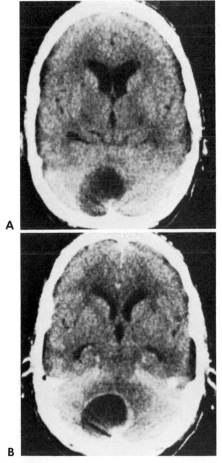

Figure 7–1. A 52-year-old woman developed headache and vomiting. Findings were gait ataxia and papilledema. *CT findings:* paramedian cerebellar hypodense lesion effacing the fourth ventricle (A) with peripheral ring enhancement (B). *Operative findings:* cystic bronchogenic epidermoid carcinoma.

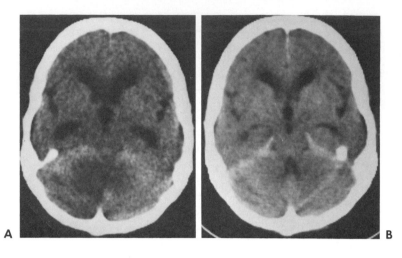

Figure 7–2. A 58-year-old woman with lung carcinoma developed headache and gait instability. Findings were gait and left-limb ataxia. *CT findings*: left cerebellar hemisphere and vermian hypodense lesion. There is nonvisualization of the fourth ventricle and no enhancement is seen (*A*). There is biventricular enlargement. Following irradiation marked decrease was seen in the hypodense region; the midline fourth ventricle is visualized and appears normal (*B*).

terior fossa lesions owing to obscuring artifact from bone. Some isodense lesions were not detected because contrast study was not performed. With the improved resolution and routine use of contrast enhancement in modern scanners, almost all metastatic lesions larger than 5 mm are visualized. CT findings in cerebral metastases are summarized in Table 7–1.[15] Noncontrast scan may show a hypodense component; this represents edema, necrosis or cysts. Hypodense component with irregular margination and frond-like projections is consistent with peritumoral edema.

Cysts appear as round or ovoid sharply marginated hypodense lesions. They sometimes are surrounded by a hyperdense peripheral enhancing rim (Fig. 7–1). This central hypodense lesion with peripheral enhancement is seen in solid tumors and those with central necrosis (Fig. 7–2). This represents hemorrhage (Fig. 7–3) or very rarely calcification (Fig. 7–4). In other cases, the hyperdense component represents high cellular density. Five percent of lesions were isodense. Ninety-five percent of solitary lesions showed mass effect; however, one half of the multiple le-

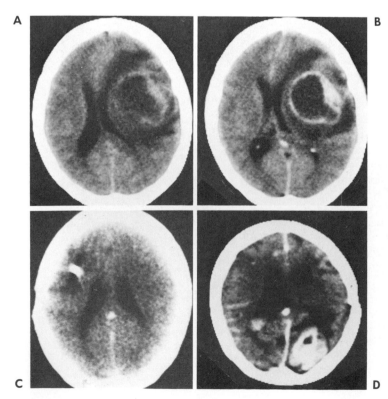

Figure 7–3. A 23-year-old woman with malignant melanoma had been treated with surgical excision and chemotherapy four years previously. She suddenly became unable to express herself and had right-sided weakness immediately after cesarean section. *CT findings*: plain scan shows a left-sided hypodense round lesion (reader's right) with surrounding hyperdense rim (*A*). There is dense ring enhancement of variable thickness (*B*). Following surgical excision and irradiation, no abnormal enhancement or mass effect is seen (*C*). Three years later, she became obtunded. *CT findings*: multiple enhancing hemorrhagic neoplasms with intraventricular extension (*D*).

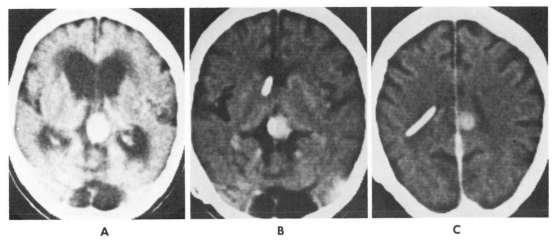

Figure 7–4. A 60-year-old woman had enucleation for orbital melanoma and developed headache; examination was normal. *CT findings*: massive pineal calcification (*A*) with biventricular enlargement. Following insertion of a diversionary shunt, ventricles were normal in size and enhancing lesion was seen contiguous to the pineal (*B*) and falx (*C*).

sions showed only minimal mass effect. Ninety-three percent of metastatic lesions showed contrast enhancement. These patterns included: (1) dense homogeneous nodular (Fig. 7–5), (2) thin peripheral rim, (3) complex irregular-thickness rim, (4) linear gyral and (5) periventricular. Two CT patterns were relatively specific for metastases: first, extensive peritumoral edema with small superficial enhancing tumor nodule and second, multiple noncontiguous mixed-density enhancing lesions. The differential diagnoses for varied CT pattern of metastases are listed in Table 7–2.

The smallest tumor nodule visualized was 4 mm. We have seen CT change from normal to evidence of small metastatic lesion in two weeks. Detection of these small lesions depends on lesion location and the presence of surrounding edema. If a small high-density nodule is surrounded by hypodense component, it is more likely to be visualized than if surrounded by normal brain parenchyma. Sources of false-positive findings are hyperdense superficial artifact emanating from bone in high convexity (vertex) region to simulate small metastases and small cortical vessels that may simulate a small isodense enhancing lesion. Although systemic carcinomas do not have specific CT patterns, certain unique features exist for different neoplasms.

Bronchogenic Carcinoma. Intracranial metastases from adenocarcinoma and small cell undifferentiated carcinoma usually appear as hyperdense nodular or ring lesions (Fig. 7–6).

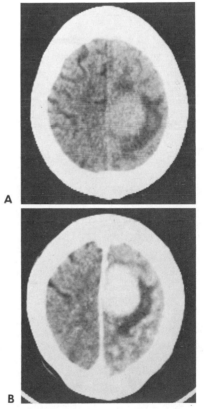

Figure 7–5. This 60-year-old man with bronchogenic carcinoma developed left-sided weakness and confusion. Isotope scan showed right parasagittal uptake; angiogram showed avascular mass. *CT findings*: right parasagittal hyperdense noncalcified lesion with surrounding hypodense region (*A*). There is dense homogeneous enhancement with dural thickening (*B*). *Operative findings*: solid metastatic carcinoma.

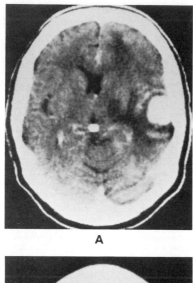

A

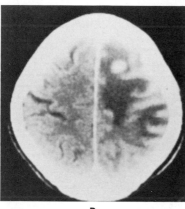

B

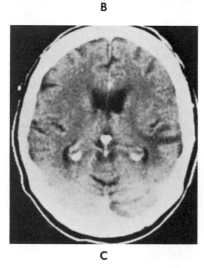

C

Figure 7–6. A 51-year-old woman had partial complex seizures; examination was normal. Isotope scan showed right frontal uptake. *CT findings:* right hemispheric mixed-density lesion with nodular (*A*) and gyral enhancement (*B*). Bronchoscopy showed adenocarcinoma. Following corticosteroids and irradiation, there is marked decrease in size and enhancement of lesions (*C*).

There is extensive surrounding edema and dense enhancement. Metastases may be hemorrhagic or necrotic. These neoplasms appear as mixed density with heterogeneous and variable-thickness ring enhancement. Squamous cell (epidermoid) carcinoma usually appears as round or ovoid hypodense lesions with thin peripheral enhancing rims. This pattern may represent cystic lesions. Cerebral metastases caused by squamous cell carcinoma were solitary in 50 percent; however, 95 percent of patients with other lung carcinoma showed multiple lesions.

In patients with bronchogenic carcinoma who are neurologically asymptomatic, isotope scan was positive in only 1 to 3 percent, but at autopsy 15 to 32 percent have microscopic evidence of intracranial metastases. CT is positive in 8 to 12 percent of neurologically asymptomatic patients; 75 percent were solitary and 25 percent were multiple. CT is an effective screening procedure in patients with lung cancer and should be performed prior to thoracotomy.[16] The finding of clinically silent intracranial metastases may modify plans for surgical resection of lung tumor.

Breast Carcinoma. This is the second most frequent source of intracerebral metastases. It is the most common solid neoplasm to cause epidural deposits and leptomeningeal involvement.[17] Ten to 15 percent of patients with breast carcinoma develop intracranial metastases. This may occur many years after treatment of breast tumor. If a patient develops neurological symptoms after successful treatment of a breast lesion, the possibility of unrelated primary intracranial lesion should be considered. For example, the incidence of meningioma in patients with breast carcinoma is quite high. In neurologically asymptomatic patients with breast cancer, isotope scan and CT are unlikely to demonstrate intracranial lesion; therefore, we do not recommend CT as a routine screening procedure.

Of patients with breast carcinoma with CT evidence of intracranial metastases, locations were intracerebral (87 percent), extradural (8 percent) and leptomeningeal (5 percent). Intracranial lesions are not usually the initial manifestation of breast cancer. Seventy-five percent of patients with intracranial lesions had metastases to bone, lung or liver. The time interval from detection of primary breast lesion to diagnosis of cerebral metastases was quite variable—six months to eight years. Seventy percent of metastatic lesions were

TABLE 7–2. Differential Diagnostic Considerations for the Varied CT Patterns of Cerebral Metastases

Pattern	Other Diagnoses
hyperdense nonenhancing	hemorrhagic infarct intracerebral hematoma
hyperdense enhancing	meningioma glioma lymphoma abscess ring-enhancing hematoma aneurysm
hypodense nonenhancing	cerebral infarct cerebritis contusional injury demyelination radiation necrosis gliosis glioma leukoencephalopathy cystic angioma
hypodense enhancing	infarct cerebritis abscess contusional injury demyelination radiation necrosis gliosis glioma meningioma angioma granuloma

solitary; 30 percent were multiple. CT findings were similar to other brain metastases. Of solitary lesions, three CT patterns were common: (1) hypodense sharply marginated round or oval-shaped lesion with peripheral enhancement (Fig. 7–7); (2) hypodense sharply marginated nonenhancing lesions and (3) hypodense lesions with central or peripheral nodular enhancing region. Breast metastatic lesions were nonenhancing in 25 percent; this was more common than other metastases. Twenty percent of breast metastases had pathological evidence of cystic component; this was anticipated by CT findings. Neurological outcome was poor if the solitary lesion was larger than 4 cm; however, there was no prognostic correlation with number of metastatic lesions or with CT pattern. Extradural deposits appear as hyperdense lens-shaped or semilunar lesions. These were usually associated with bone lesions. Leptomeningeal involvement was usually not diagnosed by CT.

Melanoma. Forty-six percent of patients have clinical neurological dysfunction; however, 75 percent have necropsy evidence of intracranial metastases. The majority of melanomas metastasizing to CNS are located in upper extremities, face, head and neck. The location of melanoma cannot be determined in 10 percent of patients with cerebral metastases. CNS was the only site of metastases in 25 percent of patients; 70 percent of these lesions were solitary. Forty percent of metastatic melanomas were solitary and 60 percent were multiple noncontiguous lesions. Frontal and parietal lobes were most common sites; posterior fossa (18 percent), intraventricular

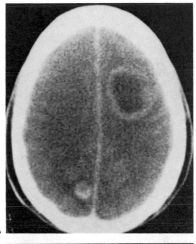

A

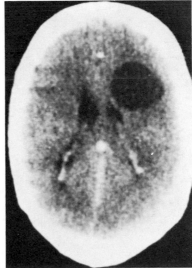

B

Figure 7–7. A 52-year-old woman with breast carcinoma developed left arm weakness. *CT findings:* right frontal-parietal sharply marginated hypodense lesion with ring enhancement and left occipital enhancing lesion (*A*). Following surgical drainage of cystic lesion and irradiation, CT showed a hypodense nonenhancing round lesion (*B*).

(four percent) and orbital (two percent) were less frequent.

All our patients with CT evidence of intracranial melanoma were symptomatic. Several studies have reported 10 percent of neurologically asymptomatic patients had CT findings of cerebral metastases; however, not all patients were examined by neurologists. The exact incidence of asymptomatic lesions is important to ascertain, because this will determine whether or not CT should be part of the routine staging procedure in melanoma.[18, 19] The onset of neurological symptomatology was apoplectic in 12 percent, usually but not always caused by peritumoral hemorrhage. All hemorrhagic lesions were larger than 2.5 cm. Some patients with CT evidence of hemorrhage did not have apoplectic onset.

CT findings of intracerebral melanoma reflect a high incidence of peritumoral hemorrhage (Fig. 7–8). Seventy percent of solitary lesions appear hyperdense; 25 percent are hypodense and 5 percent are isodense. At least 60 percent of multiple lesions were isodense, but only 5 percent of solitary lesions were isodense. Sixty percent of hyperdense lesions had pathological evidence of hemorrhage. All lesions larger than 1.2 cm had peritumoral edema and mass effect. Features of hyperdense lesions indicating hemorrhage were: intraventricular or cisternal blood, fluid level within the lesion and irregular margination and heterogeneity of hyperdense component. Metastatic melanoma lesions usually show contrast enhancement. This enhancement also occurred in hemorrhagic lesions.

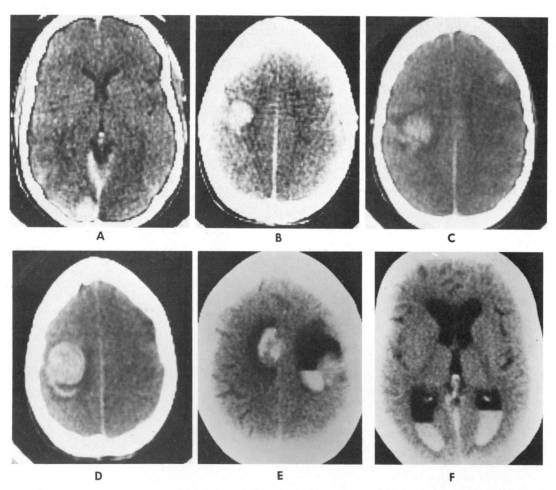

Figure 7–8. A 39-year-old man had metastatic melanoma but was neurologically asymptomatic. Isotope scan was negative. *CT findings*: left occipital (*A*) and parietal (*B*) enhancing lesion. He received corticosteroids and irradiation. Three weeks later he developed right focal motor seizures and became aphasic. *CT findings*: left parietal hyperdense lesion (*C*) with enhancement (*D*). Six weeks later he became obtunded. *CT findings*: left parietal hyperdense lesion with fluid level (*E*) with right parasagittal enhancing lesion with intraventricular blood (*F*).

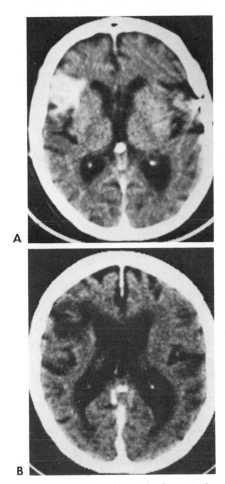

Figure 7–9. A 60-year-old man had surgical excision of melanoma and three years previously had surgical drainage of subdural hematoma. He developed confusional episodes; finding was slight right pronator drift. CT findings: left parietal isodense gyral gray matter enhancing lesion (A). Three months later he was neurologically asymptomatic. CT showed left parietal sharply marginated hypodense nonenhancing lesion (B).

In patients with melanoma, it is especially important to perform both plain and enhanced scan. This is because if hyperdense lesion is seen on enhanced study, the hemorrhagic component within the presumed enhancing component may not be recognized without plain scan for comparison. Five percent of patients with melanoma developed neurological symptomatology (Fig. 7–9) that was not caused by metastatic neoplasms, e.g., cerebral infarction, intracerebral hemorrhage, subdural hematoma and meningioma. In questionable cases isotope scan and repeat CT (two weeks later) were usually sufficient to establish the diagnosis.

Patients with melanoma who have solitary CNS metastases are usually initially treated with corticosteroids and surgical resection. The remission rate is highest in patients who subsequently have radiation therapy, notwithstanding the belief that melanomas are radioresistant. Patients with multiple hemorrhagic metastatic lesions from melanoma were treated with corticosteroids. All our patients died before surgery or irradiation. The outcome of irradiating metastatic lesions with hemorrhagic component lesions is not known.

Hemorrhagic Metastatic Neoplasms.[20] Tumors most likely to cause hemorrhage are metastatic choriocarcinoma, melanoma, bronchogenic carcinoma and hypernephroma. Hemorrhage may occur in any intracranial location. They may rupture into ventricles. Bleeding usually occurs in well-developed tumor nodules. This is frequently seen in the rapidly growing peripheral portion. Factors increasing risk of tumor hemorrhage include rapid growth, vascular erosion, hypervascularity, and hemorrhagic infarction or necrosis. Other contributing factors predisposing to peritumoral hemorrhage are coagulation disorders and head trauma. Onset of symptoms is usually sudden; however, in 25 percent, onset and progression were insidious. CT shows hyperdense lesion sometimes with fluid level and intraventricular extension. There may be postcontrast enhancement within hemorrhagic lesions or in peripheral region. If multiple metastatic lesions are present, hemorrhage is sometimes seen within all lesions. CT findings in patients with solitary lesion with peritumoral hemorrhage may be difficult to differentiate from those of intracerebral hematomas.

Leptomeningeal Metastasis. This is defined as diffuse or multifocal involvement of subarachnoid space by metastatic tumor.[21] It is most commonly caused by breast or lung carcinoma, lymphoma and malignant melanoma. Neurological abnormalities are cerebral (seizures, motor weakness, altered mentation); cranial nerve (extraocular and facial nerve dysfunction) and spinal root (headache, radicular pain, nuchal rigidity, decreased reflexes). Diagnosis is established by the CSF findings of lymphocytic pleocytosis, positive cytology for neoplastic cells, negative cultures and decreased sugar and elevated protein content. Myelography may show multiple nodular filling defects. CT is usually normal, but rarely diffuse cisternal and gyral enhancement with hydrocephalus are seen. CT findings reflect

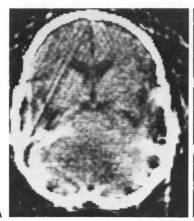
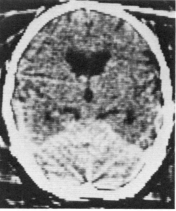

A   B

Figure 7–10. A 52-year-old man became confused and unable to walk. CSF showed anaplastic cells with decreased sugar content. *CT findings:* hypodense midline cerebellar lesion with nonvisualization of the fourth ventricle (A) and diffuse posterior fossa enhancement (B). Necropsy showed carcinomatosis meningitis.

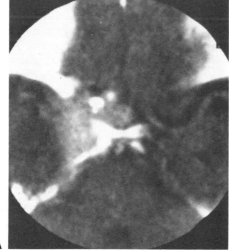

A

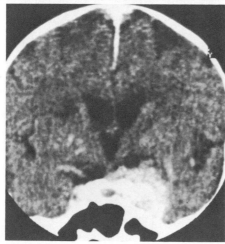

B

Figure 7–11. A 52-year-old with widely disseminated breast carcinoma developed diplopia; findings were ophthalmoparesis with decreased sensation in upper face. *CT findings:* left medial sphenoid and sella bone erosion (A) with dense parasellar cavernous sinus enhancement. This is well seen on coronal sections (B).

the pathological findings of thickening and opacification of leptomeninges by tumor infiltration (Fig. 7–10). Obstruction of CSF pathways by tumor results in hydrocephalus.

Metastatic Intracranial Bone Lesions. Metastatic lesions of the skull base may be divided into five patterns.[22]

Orbital Syndrome. This involves pain and paresthesias in the ophthalmic branch of the trigeminal nerve, ophthalmoparesis, proptosis and normal visual acuity. Skull x-ray shows erosion in the orbital region (superior orbital fissure). CT shows orbital bone destruction and evidence of a hyperdense homogeneous sharply marginated retroglobal mass.

Parasellar Syndrome. Unilateral frontal headache, ophthalmoparesis with no proptosis and normal visual acuity are seen. Skull x-ray shows sella and petrous apex bone erosion; CT shows hyperdense enhancing parasellar and cavernous sinus mass (Fig. 7–11).

Middle Fossa Syndrome. Pain and paresthesias are present in one or multiple branches of trigeminal nerve; skull radiogram is usually normal. CT shows a soft tissue mass in the temporal fossa.

Jugular Foramen Syndrome. Hoarseness and dysphagia with dysfunction of glossopharyngeal, vagus and spinal accessory nerve are symptoms. Skull x-ray or tomograms show bone erosion in the jugular foramen; CT indicates bone erosion or soft tissue mass.

Occipital Condyle Syndrome. Present are unilateral neck pain, palpable soft tissue neck mass, hypoglossal and spinal accessory nerve dysfunction. Skull base tomograms indicate erosion of occipital condyle; CT shows bone erosion but no soft tissue mass.

Metastatic calvarial lesions are most reliably

detected by skull roentgenograms or isotope bone scan. Skull x-ray shows abnormality if there is 50 percent decrease in mineral content of the bone and if the lesion is larger than 15 mm. Isotope bone scan is more sensitive than skull x-ray in detecting bone metastases; however, positive bone scan is seen in nonneoplastic conditions causing increased bone turnover. Early CT studies failed to demonstrate metastatic bone lesions because of technical factors that failed to highlight bone detail. With wide window settings, calvarial metastatic lesions are more frequently detected; but isotope bone scan remains a very sensitive study. If CT shows a solitary calvarial lesion, isotope bone scan usually detects other bone lesions. Fifty percent of patients with CT evidence of calvarial lesions have parenchymal lesions; therefore, it is important to utilize both narrow (brain) and wide (bone) window settings. Metastatic bone abnormalities defined by CT include: (1) osteolytic-hypodense lesions that thin the calvarium and erode through the inner or outer tables of skull, sometimes associated with soft-tissue mass (Fig. 7–12); (2) osteoblastic-hyperdense lesion causing bone expansion and (3) mixed osteolytic-osteoblastic lesions.[23]

Solitary Intracranial Metastasis

In patients with systemic carcinoma who have CT evidence of a solitary intracerebral lesion, surgical biopsy is sometimes necessary to confirm the diagnosis pathologically. CT findings are not always specific enough to exclude nonmetastatic lesion. If solitary lesions are surgically accessible (superficial supratentorial, cerebellar), complete tumor removal is sometimes attempted.

Patients should receive irradiation even after surgical removal.[24] The rationale for irradiation of solitary metastasis is based upon two assumptions: first, microscopic tumor foci remain in peripheral margins of tumor despite complete gross total tumor removal and second, small undetected microscopic metastatic lesions are present in contiguous or distant intracranial regions despite negative CT. With the sensitivity of CT, which may detect lesions as small as 3 to 6 mm in size, the validity of the latter assumption may be challenged. We have studied patients who had negative CT immediately postoperatively but who developed CT evidence of metastases within one month if irradiation was not utilized. No patient with solitary CT lesion who received irradiation showed evidence of recurrent or

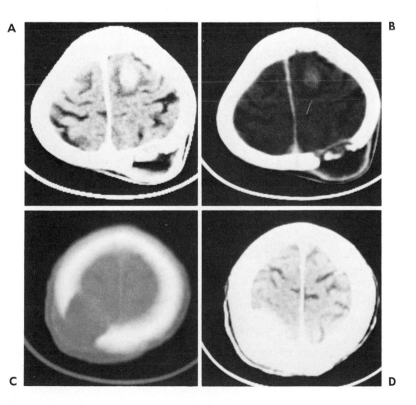

Figure 7–12 *A,* A 40-year-old man developed a lump on his scalp with left leg weakness. Skull x-ray showed lytic skull lesion; isotope scan was negative. *CT findings:* right frontal enhancing nodular lesion (*A*) with scalp lesion. With bone settings, bone destruction is well visualized (*B*). *B,* A 52-year-old man with prostate carcinoma developed a mass with swelling in the left parietal region. *CT findings:* left-sided calvarial lytic lesion with soft-tissue density (*C*) and epidural enhancing lesion (*D*).

additional metastatic lesions within nine months of irradiation.

The factors that influence survival in patients with solitary cerebral metastases include extent and progression of carcinoma outside CNS, severity of neurological deficit and time of onset of cerebral metastasis. Because cerebral metastases are associated with significant peritumoral edema, the neurological condition may improve rapidly following initiation of corticosteroid treatment. This improvement is most marked in patients with symptoms of recent onset and if CT shows extensive edema. Clinical improvement is frequently seen within 24 hours; however, CT findings reflecting decreased edema and mass effect are sometimes not detected for five to eight days. Patients with solitary superficial cerebral metastases had the best outcome.

Solitary brain metastases were the initial manifestation of systemic neoplasm in 10 percent (Fig. 7–13). If clinical course and neurological findings are consistent with expanding intracranial mass, CT characteristics of solitary intracranial lesion must be analyzed carefully because CT alone is not usually reliable in delineating the lesion as metastasis. In patients with solitary intracranial lesion, we suggest the following approach: (1) careful physical examination with special attention directed to skin, oral mucosa, abdomen and complete breast examination in women; (2) rectal ex-

amination and sigmoidoscopy; (3) chest radiogram and (4) intravenous pyelogram. If patients have no clinical findings to suggest the presence of a primary lesion, "blind" testing is unlikely to have significant yield[25] and this workup may delay surgery. Angiography should be performed to exclude the possibility of a primary intracranial neoplasm (meningioma, angioma, aneurysm). If the pathological nature of the lesion remains in doubt and the patient remains clinically stable, repeat CT scan is sometimes helpful if performed 7 to 10 days later. It may demonstrate increase in lesion size and exclude the occurrence of other lesions, e.g., infarction or hematoma (Fig. 7–14). It may also detect the possible occurrence of additional lesions (Fig. 7–15). The finding of a small superficial hyperdense homogeneously enhancing nodule with a large frond-like hypodense region has been found to represent metastases in 80 percent of cases; however, we have observed an identical pattern in gliomas, lymphomas and meningiomas. We do not believe that double-dose contrast administration utilizing both immediate and delayed (3-hour) scan provides additional information. Use of high-dose contrast material may cause increased neurotoxicity; some patients have developed neurological deterioration such as seizures and encephalopathy.

Reticuloendothelial Tumors

Primary Reticulum Cell Sarcoma. This is a rare CNS tumor. It is seen in immunologically deficient patients, including transplant recipients and patients receiving high-dose immunosuppressive medication. Patients with this neoplasm present with two clinical patterns: (1) basal-meningeal syndrome (headache, nuchal rigidity, cranial nerve dysfunction, hydrocephalus), with CSF showing neoplastic cells; (2) symptoms of intracranial expanding mass such as seizures, confusion, dementia, weakness, ataxia, with diagnosis established by neurodiagnostic studies. If primary reticulum cell sarcoma causes mass effect, it may be detected by isotope scan and angiography; however, if it is infiltrating tumor, these studies may be negative and CSF cytological studies may be needed.[26] Reticulum cell sarcoma tumors may be multiple (Fig. 7–16) or solitary (Fig. 7–17).

Multiple sarcomas are frequently located in the basal ganglia, thalamus, corpus callosum and cerebellar vermis and extend into the

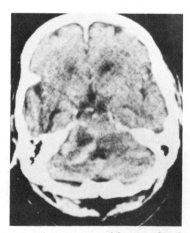

Figure 7–13. This 48-year-old man developed left facial weakness and gait instability. Findings were gait and left-limb ataxia, left-sided decreased hearing and abducens paresis. Petrous bone x-ray and isotope scan were negative. *CT findings:* left cerebellopontine angle hypodense lesion with ring enhancement. The fourth ventricle is displaced to the right. *Operative findings:* metastatic adenocarcinoma. The primary source of carcinoma was never determined.

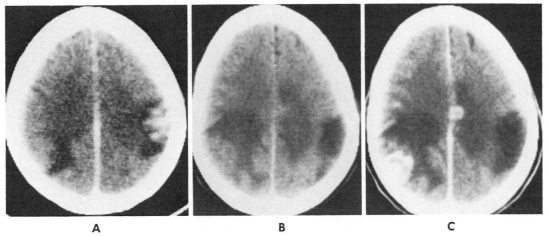

A   **B**   **C**

Figure 7–14. A 52-year-old man who had prior irradiation for bronchogenic carcinoma developed atrial fibrillation. He suddenly developed left hemiplegia. *CT findings:* right parietal hypodense lesion with interspersed gyral blood (*A*) consistent with hemorrhagic infarct. Left parieto-occipital nonenhancing triangular-shaped hypodense lesion is also seen, and this was believed to be an infarct. He improved clinically but two months later had a right focal motor seizure. *CT findings:* left hypodense and right parasagittal hypodense (*B*) lesions with small ring and nodular enhancement (*C*). Necropsy findings confirmed the diagnosis of multiple metastases and two old areas of cerebral infarction.

periventricular white matter. Solitary sarcoma usually appears in the cerebral hemispheres.

CT finding of reticulum cell sarcoma is that of an isodense or hyperdense lesion. Larger lesions are surrounded by edema and there is associated mass effect; however, mass effect may be minimal with smaller lesions. If smaller lesions appear isodense and do not cause mass effect, they are not detected on plain scan. Following contrast infusion, sarcomas show homogeneous nodular enhance-

ment with a central hypodense region. Despite clinical evidence of meningeal syndrome, CT evidence of cisternal enhancement was not always seen. CT findings in multiple primary reticulum cell sarcoma are quite characteristic; however, differentiation from systemic lymphoma, leukemia, metastases, abscesses or granulomas is not possible without biopsy.[27]

Secondary Intracranial Lymphoma. In Hodgkin's and other lymphomas, intracranial involvement is uncommon. This usually occurs

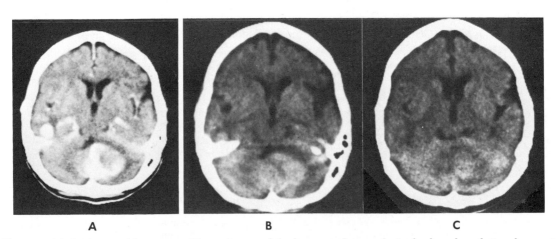

A   **B**   **C**

Figure 7–15. A 70-year-old woman with carcinoma of the larynx and supraclavicular lymph node involvement developed left arm clumsiness. She showed clinical improvement and was believed to have "lacunar infarct." Isotope scan was negative. *CT findings:* right cerebellar and multiple supratentorial hyperdense (*A*) and enhancing lesion. The fourth ventricle is effaced (*B*) and the shape of quadrigeminal cistern is distorted consistent with ascending tentorial herniation (*C*).

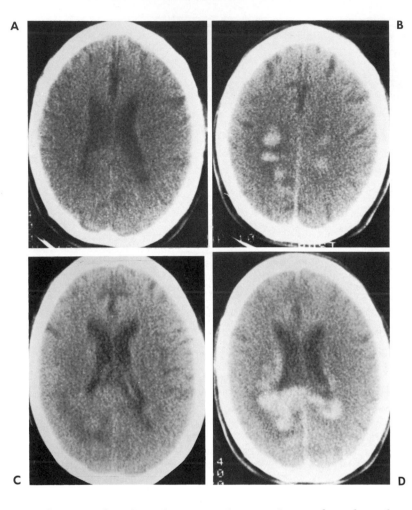

Figure 7–16. A 68-year-old developed fever and confusion. He was demented and had no focal neurological findings. CSF showed malignant cells consistent with reticulum cell sarcoma. *CT findings*: isodense (*A*) periventricular lesions (*B*). Two weeks later, he became obtunded. *CT findings*: hyperdense left occipital lesions (*C*) with dense periventricular enhancement (*D*).

with certain histological types such as Hodgkin's disease and diffuse histiocytic and undifferentiated lymphoma. Neurological dysfunction usually occurs in patients with widespread systemic manifestations. Leptomeningeal infiltration is most common; dural and parenchymal involvement is less frequent. The CT finding of intracerebral lesions is that of multifocal isodense regions that show nodular or ring enhancement. In patients with dural involvement, CT may show a hyperdense semilunar-shaped lesion contiguous to bone. If

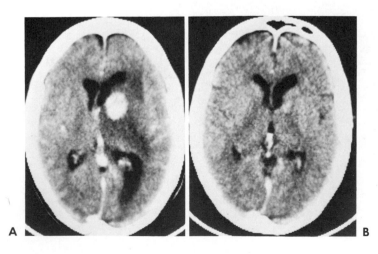

Figure 7–17. A 40-year-old man with histiocytic lymphoma developed left-sided weakness. EEG and isotope scan were negative. *CT findings*: right ganglionic sharply marginated densely enhancing lesion with surrounding hypodense component (*A*). Following cranial irradiation he was neurologically asymptomatic. CT showed minimal enhancement and mass effect (*B*).

lymphoma involves the orbit, CT shows hyperdense nonenhancing sharply marginated inferior retroglobal mass. In patients with lymphomatous meningitis, CT is usually negative. In patients with lymphoma who are neurologically asymptomatic, orbital and cranial CT scans are invariably negative; therefore, CT does not appear indicated in lymphoma staging. All patients with lymphoma who develop neurological symptoms should be carefully investigated to exclude nonlymphomatous disorders, such as subdural hematoma, intracerebral hemorrhage, abscess and infarct.[28]

Plasmacytoma. Neurological symptomatology caused by plasma cell dyscrasias (multiple myeloma, Waldenström's macroglobulinemia) usually is associated with skull and vertebral body involvement. Parenchymal and dural involvement is uncommon without evidence of direct extension from adjacent bone; however, extraosseous intracranial involvement has rarely been reported. Intracranial lesions have usually been solitary. CT findings have included isodense or hyperdense lesion with dense and homogeneous enhancement. If there is no evidence of bone involvement on CT or skull x-ray, pathological diagnosis must be established by surgical biopsy (Fig. 7–18). In patients with plasma cell dyscrasias, cerebral infarction may result from hyperviscosity, and intracranial hemorrhage may result from thrombocytopenia or coagulation disorders.

Leukemia. Ten to 15 percent of patients with acute lymphocytic or myelogenous leukemia develop CNS involvement. This is manifested by meningeal leukemic infiltration. These patients clinically present with meningeal signs or cranial nerve dysfunction. Patients with acute leukemia may present with meningeal signs and have papilledema; this suggests intracranial lesion. CT should be performed before lumbar puncture is done. In patients with CSF evidence of leukemic meningitis, CT rarely shows diffuse meningeal enhancement. This CT finding should suggest the possibility of complicating infectious-inflammatory meningitis (fungal, tuberculous) in leukemic patients. Some patients with acute leukemia show CT evidence of localized intracerebral (Fig. 7–19) or dural tumor. This most frequently occurs in acute myelogenous leukemia (chloroma). This develops in some patients in hematological remission. The CT finding of parenchymal leukemic lesion is an isodense enhancing lesion; this pattern is similar to other reticuloendothelial tumors.[29]

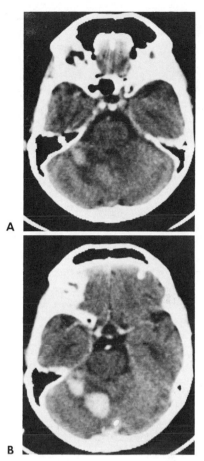

Figure 7–18. A 57-year-old man with multiple myeloma was in hematological remission. He developed headache and gait ataxia. *CT findings:* bilobulated hyperdense left cerebellar lesion (*A*) with dense sharply marginated enhancement (*B*). The fourth ventricle is effaced and there is biventricular enlargement. *Operation findings:* cerebellar plasmacytoma without calvarial involvement.

Other neurological abnormalities are not caused by leukemic infiltration. These complications include: (1) intracranial hemorrhage resulting from platelet or coagulation disorders, (2) cerebral infarcts relating to hyperviscosity, (3) intracranial infections caused by impaired immune response, (4) central pontine myelinolysis, (5) therapy related complication such as basal ganglia calcification, cerebral atrophy and leukoencephalopathy. Progressive necrotic leukoencephalopathy is characterized by focal necrosis of white matter and dystrophic intracerebral calcification. Clinical findings include altered mentation, gait ataxia, seizures, spasticity and dementia. In the active stage of this disorder, CT findings include low-density white matter lesions, ven-

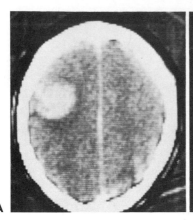
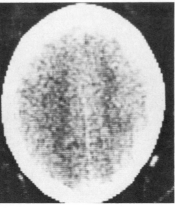

A

B

Figure 7–19. A 23-year-old woman with acute myelocytic leukemia was in hematological remission. She developed left-sided headache. *CT findings:* round homogeneous hyperdense parietal lesion with dense enhancement (A). Following cranial radiation, CT shows complete lesion resolution (B).

tricular compression and diffuse or focal enhancement. The enhancing lesions that represent leukoencephalopathy may simulate a leukemic mass; differentiation may be established only by pathological findings (see page 214). In the chronic form of leukoencephalopathy, the findings are somewhat different. The periventricular lucencies are most localized and there is minimal enhancement and mass effect. Periventricular and basal ganglia calcification and ventricular dilatation may also be seen. Leukoencephalopathy developing in patients with leukemia is related to treatment with methotrexate. The risk of this complication is increased in patients who receive both intrathecal methotrexate and CNS irradiation.[30, 31]

Hematological Conditions

Hemophilia. Intracranial bleeding occurs in 4 to 10 percent of these patients. Two thirds of episodes occur when patients are less than 18 years old and one third occur in patients younger than 3 years old. History of recent head trauma is obtained in one half of cases. Certain patients have an interval-free period of up to seven days following trauma before developing neurological symptoms. Bleeding may occur in any location of the CNS; those patients with intracerebral hemorrhage have a worse prognosis than those with subarachnoid or subdural hemorrhage. Mortality of hemophiliac patients with intracranial bleeding is 30 to 40 percent; one quarter of survivors have episodes of recurrent bleeding at other intracranial locations. When intracranial bleeding is suspected, CT is utilized and lumbar puncture and angiography may be avoided. Treatment includes component (fac-

tor) replacement therapy, usually with corticosteroids or other agents such as mannitol and glycerol to reduce cerebral edema. If the patient's clinical condition remains stable, nonsurgical management may be effective and the patient is followed with serial CT scans. There is a high incidence of neurological sequelae such as seizures and dementia in patients who have survived an episode of intracranial hemorrhage.[32, 33]

REFERENCES

1. Posner JB: Diagnosis and treatment of metastases to the brain. Clin Bull Sloan Kett Cancer Ctr 4:47, 1974
2. Lesse S, Netsky MG: Metastasis of neoplasm to CNS and meninges. Arch Neurol Psychiatr 72:133, 1954
3. Richards P, McKissock W: Intracranial metastases. Br Med J 1:15, 1963
4. Vieth RG, Odom GL: Intracranial metastases and their neurosurgical treatment. J Neurosurg 23:375, 1965
5. Paillais JE, Pellet W: Brain metastases. *In* Handbook of Clinical Neurology, vol 18, Vinken PJ, Bruyn GW (eds). North Holland Publishing Company, Amsterdam, 1975, pp 201–252
6. Strang R, Almonc Mason C: Brain metastases. Arch Neurol 4:20, 1961
7. McCormack KR: Scanning of liver and brain in evaluation of patients with bronchogenic carcinoma. J Nucl Med 9:222, 1968
8. Schlesinger EG, Michelsen WJ, Antunes JL: Value of sequential scanning in detection of metastatic tumors. Surg Neurol 6:239, 1976
9. Boller F, Patten DH, Howes D: Correlation of brain scan results with neuropathological findings. Lancet 1:1143, 1973.
10. Tarcon YA, Fajman W, Marc J: "Doughnut" sign in brain scanning. Am Roentgenol 126:842, 1976
11. Zachrisson L: Angiography of cerebral metastases. Acta Radiol (Diagn) 1:521, 1963
12. New PFJ, Scott WR, Schnur JA: Computed tomog-

raphy in diagnosis of primary and metastatic intra-cranial neoplasms. Radiology 114:75, 1975

13. Deck MDF, Messina AV, Sackett JR: Computed tomography in metastatic disease of the brain. Radiology 119:115, 1976

14. Potts GD, Abbott GF, von Sneidern JV: National cancer institute study: evaluation of computed tomography in the diagnosis of intracranial neoplasms. III. Metastatic tumors. Radiology 136:657–664, 1980

15. Weisberg LA: Computed tomography in the evaluation of CNS metastases. Arch Neurology 36:630–634, 1979

16. Jacobs L, Kinkel WR, Vincent RG: Silent brain metastases from lung carcinoma determined by computerized tomography. Arch Neurology 34:690, 1977

17. Dearnaley DP, Kingsley DPE, Husband JE: The role of CT of the brain in the investigation of breast cancer patients with suspected intracranial metastases. Clin Radiol 32:375–382, 1981

18. Holtas S, Cronquist S: Cranial computed tomography of patients with malignant melanoma. Neuroradiology 22:123 – 127, 1981

19. Ginaldi S, Wallace S, Shalen P: Cranial computed tomography of malignant melanoma. Am J Neurol 1:531–535, 1980

20. Mandybur TI: Intracranial hemorrhage caused by metastatic tumors. Neurology 27:650–655, 1977

21. Glass JP, Shapiro WR, Posner JB: Treatment of leptomeningeal metastases. Neurology 28:351, 1978

22. Greenberg HS, Deck MDF, Vikram B: Metastasis to the base of the skull: clinical findings in 43 patients. Neurology 31:530, 1980

23. Kido DK, Gould R, Taati F: Comparative sensitivity of CT scans, radiographs and radionuclide bone scans in detecting metastatic calvarial lesions. Radiology 128:371–375, 1978

24. Galicich JH, Sundaresan N, Thaler HT: Surgical treatment of single brain metastasis. J Neurosurg 53:63–67, 1980

25. Voorhies RM, Sundaresan N, Thaler HT: The single supratentorial lesion: an evaluation of preoperative diagnostic tests. J Neurosurg 53:364–368, 1980

26. Schaumberg HN, Plank CR, Adams RD: Reticulum cell sarcoma–microglioma group of brain tumors. Brain 95:199, 1972

27. Enzmann DR, Krikorian J, Norman D: Computed tomography in primary reticulum cell sarcoma of the brain. Radiology 130:165–170, 1979

28. Brent-Zawadzki M, Enzmann DR: Computed tomographic brain scanning in patients with lymphoma. Radiology 129:67–71, 1978

29. Kingsley DPE, Kendall BE: Cranial computed tomography in leukemia. Neuroradiology 16:543–546, 1978

30. Peylan-Ramu N, Poplack DG, Pizzo PA: Abnormal CT scans of the brain in asymptomatic children with acute leukemia after prophylactic treatment of the CNS with radiation and intrathecal chemotherapy. N Engl J Med 298:815–818, 1978

31. Pederson H, Clausen N: Development of cerebral CT changes during treatment of acute lymphocytic leukemia in childhood. Neuroradiology 22:79-84, 1981

32. Gastaut JA, Gastaut JL, Carcassonne Y: Computerized axial tomography in the study of intracranial complications in hematology. Cancer 41:487–501, 1978

33. Eyster ME, Gill FM, Blatt PM: Central nervous system bleeding in hemophiliacs. Blood 51:1179–1188, 1978.

Chapter 8

JUXTASELLAR REGION ABNORMALITIES

Patients with juxtasellar pathological conditions present with endocrine, visual or neurological abnormalities. Endocrine manifestations of disturbed hypothalamic-pituitary function are (1) anterior pituitary failure (amenorrhea, infertility, cold intolerance, short stature, loss of body and pubic hair, orthostatic hypotension, hypoglycemia); (2) neurohypophyseal hypofunction (diabetes insipidus); (3) hypersecretion syndromes (acromegaly [growth hormone], amenorrhea-galactorrhea [prolactin], Cushing's syndrome [adrenocorticotrophic hormone]). Laboratory tests such as basal hormone levels, provocative stimulation and suppression studies are necessary to confirm the clinical impression of hypothalamic-pituitary endocrine dysfunction.[1, 2] Visual and neurological disturbances are dependent upon the vector of tumor expansion rather than tumor pathological characteristics. Neurodiagnostic studies delineate the presence and location of lesions. They are less reliable in determining the precise nature of a juxtasellar lesion (Table 8–1).

Visual impairment is the most common symptom of juxtasellar lesions and this represents the most significant morbidity. Visual loss results from tumor compression of the optic nerve and chiasm. Reduced visual acuity and dimming of perception of color brightness have been reported in 58 to 88 percent of patients. Careful tangent screen or perimetry visual field examination is essential to detect early signs of anterior visual pathway (optic nerve, chiasm) dysfunction. The characteristic visual field defect is bitemporal hemianopsia. This is caused by impingement upon central crossed chiasmal fibers. Because the optic chiasm is located 10 mm above the diaphragma sella, visual field defect indicates occurrence of significant suprasellar extension. Fifteen to 20 percent of patients with visual field defects have no visual symptoms; therefore, careful visual examination is essential in all patients with radiographic evidence of abnormal sella or endocrine symptoms of hypothalamic-pituitary dysfunction.[3]

Primary intrasellar tumors such as pituitary adenoma grow upward to compress the undersurface of the optic chiasm. The initial finding is superior bitemporal quadrantanopsia. Paracentral and inferior temporal quadrant involvement may be later detected to cause bitemporal hemianopsia. Suprasellar lesions such as craniopharyngioma initially compress the superior chiasmal fibers (representing the inferior temporal fields) to result in inferior bitemporal quadrantanopsia. If the optic chiasm is located anterior to the sella turcica (prefixed chiasm), the initial visual defect may be bitemporal scotomas. This results from compression of macular fibers located in the posterior part of the optic chiasm. This defect is sometimes missed unless careful tangent screen examination utilizing small (1 to 6 mm) colored, i.e., red, test objects is performed and the examiner directs specific attention to the central visual region.

Anterior extension of juxtasellar lesions compresses the prechiasmal optic nerve. This results in reduced visual acuity, impaired pupillary reactivity (Marcus-Gunn pupil response) and optic atrophy. Lateral growth into the cavernous sinus results in diplopia, ophthalmoparesis and supraorbital facial sensory disturbances (pain, paresthesias). Inferior extension through the sellar floor into the sphenoid sinus may result in rhinorrhea or a nasopharynx mass. Psychomotor seizures and memory loss result from middle fossa extension. Anterodorsal extension to the undersurface of the frontal lobes may cause behavioral

174

TABLE 8–1. **Pathological Processes Involving the Juxtasellar Region**

Common Lesions
pituitary adenoma
craniopharyngioma
meningioma
anterior (optic nerve and chiasm) visual pathway glioma

Less Common Lesions
aneurysm (internal carotid, anterior communicating artery)
atypical teratoma
sella metastases
chordoma
carcinoma (sphenoid sinus, nasopharynx)
mucocele
granuloma, (sarcoid, tuberculous of the pituitary and hypothalamus pituitary abscess)
cyst (epidermoid, dermoid, subarachnoid)
arachnoiditis involving the optic chiasm
demyelination of the optic chiasm
intracranial hypertension
empty sella
third ventricular tumor
    colloid cyst
    pineal region tumor
    glioma

aberrations or dementia. Suprasellar extension may result in intraventricular foraminal obstruction or third ventricular compression; this causes intracranial hypertension or hypothalamic involvement (diabetes insipidus, galactorrhea). Posterior extension causes brain stem compression; this results in cranial nerve, cerebellar and pyramidal tract signs.

Previous clinical studies of patients with suspected juxtasellar lesions utilized conventional radiography, sella tomography, air studies and angiography. DuBoulay reported sella turcica radiographic abnormalities in 67 to 77 percent of juxtasellar lesions. Ninety percent of pituitary adenomas have abnormal sella turcica.[4] If the sella appears normal in size and shape and without erosive changes, pluridirectional thin-section conventional tomography is performed. This is especially important in patients with symptoms of hypersecreting pituitary tumors because these may result from microadenomas that do not necessarily enlarge the pituitary fossa. In patients with pituitary microadenoma, hypocycloidal tomography may show evidence of localized bulging of the anterolateral sella wall or a "blistering" pattern of the sella floor.[5, 6] Sella tomography permits precise intrasellar volume measurements and accurate delineation of normal anatomical variants. Certain of these normal but inconsistently seen structures may be incorrectly interpreted as effects of expanding intrasellar masses. These anatomical variants are (1) differences in sellar floor density underlying aerated or nonaerated sphenoid sinus, (2) double sella floor when attachment of sphenoid sinus is lateral rather than midline, (3) extensive thinning of the sellar cortex and (4) sloping of the sellar floor.[7]

If the sella appears enlarged, the presence of accompanying findings are sometimes helpful in distinguishing intrasellar tumors from nontumorous sella enlargement, e.g., empty sella syndrome. Symmetrical sella enlargement with normal position and contour of clinoid processes and no evidence of bone erosion are most suggestive of nontumorous etiology; however, exclusion of an intrasellar mass usually requires complementary studies.[8] In patients with suspected juxtasellar lesions, supplemental radiographic projections are sometimes needed to visualize the optic foramina and the superior orbital fissure if optic glioma or carotid aneurysm is suspected. The characteristic finding of juxtasellar aneurysms is unilateral sella enlargement with erosion of the clinoid process and widening of the superior orbital fissure.[9] Optic nerve gliomas and meningiomas may enlarge the optic foramina.

The most compelling reason to perform angiography in patients with suspected juxtasellar lesions is to exclude the presence of juxtasellar aneurysm. Features of this lesion may simulate clinical and radiographic features of pituitary adenoma. Certain patients with intrasellar neoplasms have accompanying juxtasellar aneurysms. Failure to identify aneurysms by preoperative angiography may cause operative mortality. In patients with juxtasellar tumors, angiography may show evidence of extrasellar extension. Lateral displacement of the posterior portion of the cavernous segment of the carotid artery is an early sign of extrasellar lateral extension. If tumor extends into the middle fossa, there is lateral displacement and elevation of the anterior portion of the basal vein of Rosenthal. Posterior displacement of the basilar artery and elevation of the posterior cerebral arteries indicates retrosellar extension. Elevation of the horizontal portion of the middle and anterior cerebral arteries is evidence of suprasellar extension.

Conventional angiography has shown that pituitary adenomas are avascular. The finding of abnormal supplying vessels and vascular stain pattern is consistent with malignant invasive tumors. These tumors are usually large and grow rapidly. They frequently infiltrate into contiguous structures and encase major arteries. These pituitary adenomas frequently develop hemorrhagic necrosis. With magnification and subtraction techniques, the presence of extensive arterial feeding vessels derived from the dilated and hypertrophied meningohypophyseal trunk have been identified in pituitary adenomas. Solid adenomas may show feeding capsular vessels and homogeneous stain, whereas cystic tumors show less intense homogeneous stain or mottled heterogeneous stain pattern. The latter pattern is suggestive of degenerative tumor change.[10]

Plain skull radiographic and angiographic findings are sometimes characteristic for certain juxtasellar lesions: (1) Meningiomas show hyperostosis and blistering of the planum sphenoidale or tuberculum sella with supplying vessels derived from the external carotid artery. (2) Craniopharyngiomas show suprasellar calcification with angiographic findings of avascular mass. (3) Gliomas of the optic nerve or chiasm are associated with J-shaped sella deformity. Angiogram may show suprasellar and anterior third ventricular mass with abnormal feeding vessels derived from the superior and premamillary branches of the posterior cerbral arteries. (4) Malignant neoplasms such as metastases, rhabdomyosarcoma, paranasal sinus carcinoma and chordomas cause radiographic evidence of destructive skull base changes. Angiography may show encasement of internal carotid artery with persistent diffuse stain. Pathological characterization of the majority of juxtasellar lesions requires surgical exploration.

In CT evaluation of suspected intra- and juxtasellar lesions, the suprasellar (chiasmatic) cistern is an important anatomical landmark.[11] The suprasellar cistern appears hypodense; its shape is hexagonal, pentagonal or tetragonal. Anatomical and technical factors may cause variations in configuration. Anterior clinoid processes and dorsum sella project into the suprasellar cistern; this may simulate abnormal calcification. Optic nerves may appear as paired round hyperdense masses located anterior to a V-shaped hyperdense optic chiasm within the suprasellar cistern. Anterior recesses (supraoptic and infundibular) of the third ventricle are located superior to the suprasellar cistern. They may appear as slit-like hypodense structures projecting into the suprasellar cistern. This cistern has the following perimeters: frontal lobes form the anterior border, the medial temporal lobe (uncus) forms the lateral border and the brain stem forms the posterior border.[12]

Utilizing thin-section high-resolution axial and coronal projections, pituitary fossa contents (pituitary gland, infundibulum) and contiguous structures (cavernous sinus, carotid arteries, sphenoid sinus) may be visualized.[13] On coronal sections the pituitary gland appears isodense or hyperdense. The size and configuration of the pituitary gland is best appreciated on postcontrast scan in which the gland normally shows diffuse enhancement. The top of the pituitary is flat or concave downward with CSF spaces located directly superior to the pituitary, which rests on the sellar floor. The infundibulum is a linear-shaped hyperdense enhancing structure. It extends from the top of the pituitary to the infundibular recess of the third ventricle. The sphenoid sinus is located inferior to the sella floor. The relationship of the sphenoid sinus to the sellar floor is best visualized on coronal sections. Supraclinoid carotid arteries appear as paired enhancing structures located in the anterolateral portion of the suprasellar cistern. Cavernous sinuses appear as densely enhancing vertically oriented symmetrical bands located lateral to the sella.

The presence of an intrasellar mass is defined by these four findings: (1) the pituitary fossa is enlarged, (2) the height of the pituitary

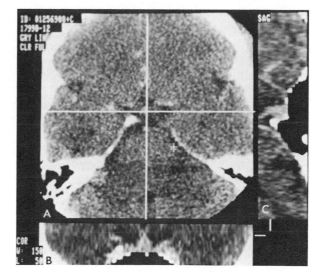

Figure 8–1. A 26-year-old man was evaluated for impotence. He had increased prolactin level. Skull x-ray, other endocrine studies and visual fields were normal. *CT findings:* intrasellar enhancing mass (*A*) extending upward into the infundibulum. This is seen with coronal (*B*) and sagittal (*C*) reformated views. *Operative finding:* pituitary microadenoma.

gland is greater than 9 mm and bulges convex upward, (3) abnormal intrasellar enhancement is present and (4) there is elevation of the infundibulum (Fig. 8–1). Suprasellar extension is manifested by mass effect and abnormal density within the suprasellar cistern (Fig. 8–2). With extensive suprasellar extension there is compression of the intraventricular foramina. Anterior extension of sellar lesions is manifested by abnormal enhancing lesions projecting into the frontal lobes and frontal hypodensities. Lateral extension is manifested by asymmetrical enhancement of the cavernous sinus, lateral displacement of the supraclinoid carotid arteries, and enhancing lesions extending into the middle fossa.[14] Posterior extension is manifested by abnormal densities and enhancement extending into the interpenduncular and ambient cisterns. With inferior extension there is a soft-tissue mass projecting into the sphenoid sinus and erosion of the sellar floor. Inferior extension into the sphenoid sinus and relationship of the juxtasellar mass to the third ventricle is most clearly delineated by coronal views.

Pituitary Adenoma

This is the most common intra- and juxtasellar lesion. These tumors may be an incidental necropsy finding in 30 percent of asymptomatic patients. Pituitary adenomas originate within the pituitary fossa. They cause ballooning and enlargement of the sella turcica with bone erosion. However, certain symptomatic hypersecreting microadenomas originate as small (less than 10 mm) discrete nodules; they may not cause sella enlargement. Macroad-

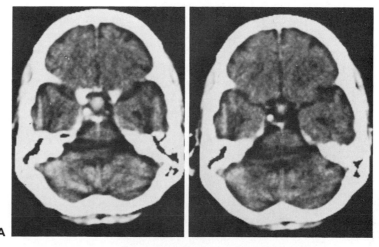

Figure 8–2. A 37-year-old woman had amenorrhea. Skull radiogram showed enlarged sella turcica. Visual fields were normal. *CT findings:* small enhancing intrasellar mass (*A*) with extension into the suprasellar region (*B*). *Operative finding:* solid pituitary adenoma.

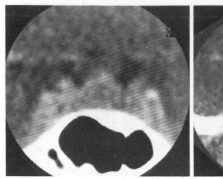

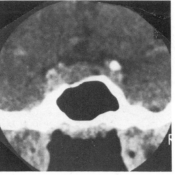

Figure 8–3. A 17-year-old girl had amenorrhea and galactorrhea. She had elevated serum prolactin but normal sella tomograms. *CT finding:* coronal views show enlarged pituitary gland (*A*). This has a convex upward shape and a hypodense region in the lateral portion of the gland (*B*). *Operative finding:* pituitary adenoma.

enomas may expand upward into the suprasellar cistern to compress the undersurface of the optic chiasm or grow inferiorly into sphenoid sinus. The majority of pituitary adenomas are benign slow-growing tumors; they are usually encapsulated and solid. Degenerative change (cysts, hemorrhage, necrosis and calcification) occurs in one quarter of adenomas.[15]

In patients with symptoms of pituitary hypersecretion syndromes, the responsible lesion is either microadenoma or macroadenoma.[16–18] Hypocycloidal tomography may

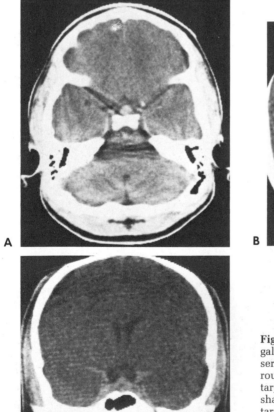

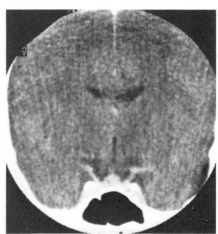

Figure 8–4. This 15-year-old girl had amenorrhea and galactorrhea. Skull radiogram showed enlarged sella; serum prolactin was elevated. *CT finding:* intrasellar round homogeneous enhancing mass (*A*). The pituitary gland appears enlarged with convex upward shape (*B*) on coronal views. *Operative finding:* pituitary macroadenoma.

detect microadenomas even if plain skull radiography is negative. However, in some cases tomography may be negative, or an abnormal finding may represent false-positive. CT scan may show no abnormalities in some pituitary microadenomas; nevertheless, with high resolution technology some lesions have been detected. Several types of CT findings have been reported in pituitary microadenoma: First is focal hypodensity within hyperdense pituitary gland. This finding is visualized on coronal views (Fig. 8–3). Second is increased height of the pituitary gland with upward bulging and convexity (Fig. 8–4). Third is upward deviation of the infundibulum. A focal hypodense area is believed to represent the microadenoma and is frequently located laterally and inferiorly. This hypodense lesion does not always correlate with cyst formation. Other normal and pathological conditions such as pars intermedia cysts, metastases, infarcts, abscesses and epidermoid cysts may cause a hypodense region within the pituitary gland and may simulate microadenoma.[19] The height of the pituitary gland is most reliably assessed on enhanced coronal projection. Microadenoma has been reported in association with "empty sella" in one quarter of cases.[20] If CT shows a small hyperdense enhancing intrasellar mass located in the posterior-inferior portion of the enlarged pituitary fossa that contains CSF density, this suggests the occurrence of microadenoma within empty sella; however, this may also represent a normal compressed pituitary gland.

For diagnosis of pituitary macroadenoma, CT has been quite sensitive in detecting abnormalities of the pituitary fossa and suprasellar cistern.[21] These adenomas are usually located centrally and symmetrically within the anterior portion of the suprasellar cistern. They are usually round in shape; less commonly, they are multilobulated or have irregular margination. There is usually no surrounding hypodense rim. Solid pituitary adenomas appear isodense or slightly hyperdense on plain scan and demonstrate dense homogeneous sharply marginated contrast enhancement (Fig. 8–5). Cystic adenomas appear hypodense. They usually have density values consistent with CSF; cyst fluid may be more proteinaceous and appear denser than CSF. Cysts are sometimes surrounded by a thin and regularly shaped hyperdense rim (Fig. 8–6). There is a thin rim of peripheral enhancement with minimal intracystic en-

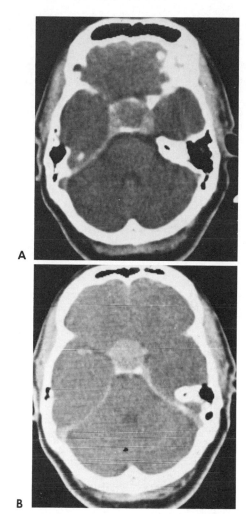

Figure 8–5. A 38-year-old man developed visual blurring. He had superior bitemporal quadrantanopsia. CT findings: enlarged sella turcica (A) with round homogeneously enhancing mass extending to the suprasellar region (B).

hancement. Hemorrhagic adenomas appear as hyperdense round or irregularly marginated suprasellar lesions. These are frequently surrounded by a hypodense peripheral collar. This lesion may appear heterogeneous because of the combined presence of hemorrhagic necrosis and viable tumor tissue (Fig. 8–7). In the acute stage of pituitary hemorrhage, enhancement may be seen in the portion of the lesion that represents viable residual pituitary neoplasm. As the hematoma degenerates, it appears isodense or hypodense with peripheral rim enhancement. In certain patients with suspected pituitary apoplexy, differentiation of hemorrhagic from cystic pituitary adenomas cannot always be established as both lesions

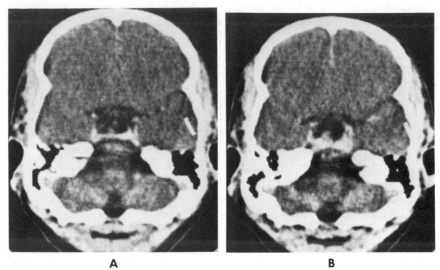

Figure 8–6. A 42-year-old woman developed increased fatigue and visual blurring. Visual fields demonstrated superior bitemporal quadrantanopsia. Skull x-ray showed enlarged eroded sella turcica. *CT findings:* hypodense intrasellar lesion (*A*) with variable-thickness enhancing rim (*B*). *Operative finding:* cystic pituitary adenoma.

show ring enhancement, and densities of degenerating hematomas may be variable.[22]

The finding on CT and at surgery of hemorrhage within a pituitary neoplasm is more common than the clinical syndrome of pituitary apoplexy. Not all patients with hemorrhagic pituitary neoplasm present with sudden neurological deterioration (Fig. 8–8). Conversely, not all patients with rapid worsening of chiasmal or parasellar symptoms have hemorrhagic lesions.

Pituitary adenomas may be invasive and infiltrative into contiguous regions. The CT finding of this neoplasm is a heterogeneous mixed-density lesion with irregular margination and dense irregular complex ring enhancement. These tumors are usually large; they frequently extend laterally through the cavernous sinus into the middle fossa (Fig. 8–9).

Pituitary adenomas may rarely show peritumoral calcification. This may outline the periphery of the adenoma with a lamellar ring pattern or show diffuse or globular configura-

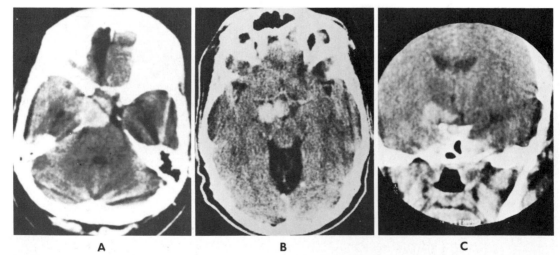

Figure 8–7. A 52-year-old man developed headache and confusion. He had nuchal rigidity and left abducens paresis. CSF was bloody. *CT findings:* hyperdense and enhancing intrasellar (*A*) mass extending into the suprasellar (*B*) and left parasellar region (*C*). *Operative finding:* hemorrhagic pituitary adenoma.

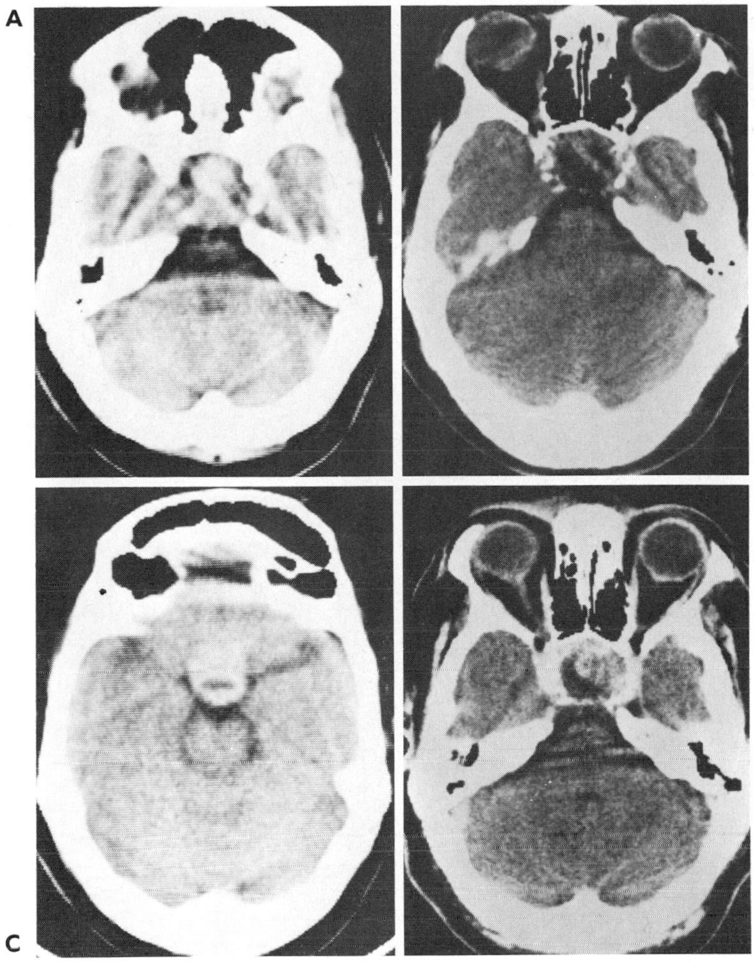

Figure 8–8. A 44-year-old man developed headache and visual blurring that progressively worsened over 8 months. Skull x-ray showed enlarged eroded sella. *CT findings:* hyperdense intrasellar and suprasellar mass (*A*) with slight heterogeneous enhancement (*B*). *Operative findings:* hemorrhagic necrotic pituitary adenoma. Two years later he developed facial paresthesias. *CT findings:* enlarged sella (*C*) with enhancing mass (*D*) extending inferiorly.

tion. Peripheral capsular rim calcification is also seen with craniopharyngioma carotid aneurysm; globular calcification also develops in craniopharyngioma, meningioma or chordoma. In rare cases, patients with no endocrine or visual symptoms are found to have skull radiographic and CT evidence of intrasellar calcification with normal-sized sella turcica. This has been defined as *pituitary stones.*[23] CT may show intrasellar calcification without abnormal soft-tissue densities or enhancement.

Following surgical decompression and postoperative irradiation of pituitary adenomas, CT shows an enhancing mass; however, it is not possible to differeniate complications of surgery (abscess or hematoma) or radiotherapy (radionecrosis) from recurrent tumor. In some cases, CT shows the pituitary fossa filled with CSF-density fluid. This represents secondary empty sella. Some patients with prolactin-secreting pituitary adenomas are treated with bromocriptine, and serial CT may demonstrate normalization in size and appearance of the pituitary fossa. Reduction in tumor size usually correlates with decreased serum prolactin content.[24] There has been no CT documentation of pituitary hemorrhage following medical treatment with bromocriptine.

Craniopharyngioma

This tumor usually occurs in childhood, but 30 percent occur in adults.[25, 26] Radiographic evidence of juxtasellar calcification is demonstrated in 90 percent. These tumors have varied pathological features—cystic, solid, calcified. The majority of craniopharyngiomas originate in the suprasellar region; however, 20 percent arise in the pituitary fossa (intrasellar). They may rarely originate in the thalamic, third ventricular or posterior fossa region.

The initial visual field abnormality usually detected in patients with craniopharyngioma

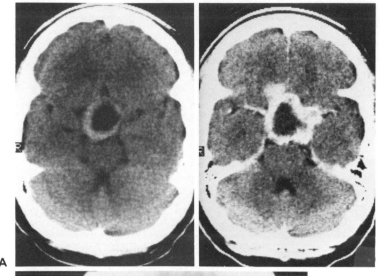

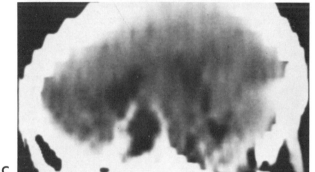

Figure 8–9. A 34-year-old man developed visual blurring and headache. He had bitemporal hemianopsia and left optic atrophy. *CT findings:* hypodense intrasellar and suprasellar core with peripheral hyperdense rim (A). There is dense variable-thickness ring enhancement (B) extending into the left frontal and right middle fossa. The extent of the mass is seen on sagittal views (C). *Operative finding:* invasive pituitary adenoma.

is inferior bitemporal quadrantanopsia. This results from compression of the superior surface of the optic chiasm. Endocrine symptoms reflect disturbed hypothalamic-pituitary function. Children develop diabetes insipidus, growth retardation and pubescence dysfunction (delayed or precocious); adults may initially develop diabetes insipidus and symptoms of hyperprolactinemia (galactorrhea,

infertility, amenorrhea). Intracranial hypertension may develop early because of intraventricular foramina obstruction. Retrosellar extension may cause brain stem and cerebellar dysfunction. Dementia may result from bifrontal extension or obstructive hydrocephalus. In adults, clinical findings of craniopharyngioma may simulate pituitary adenoma.

CT diagnosis of craniopharyngiomas is reli-

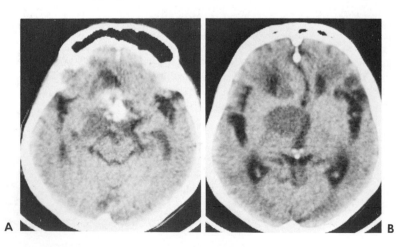

Figure 8–10. A 70-year-old man developed headache and dementia but had no visual field abnormalities. Skull x-ray showed suprasellar calcification. *CT findings:* mixed density calcified with heterogeneous nonenhancing suprasellar mass (A) with a large sharply marginated hypodense component distorting the third ventricle (B). *Operative finding:* cystic craniopharyngioma.

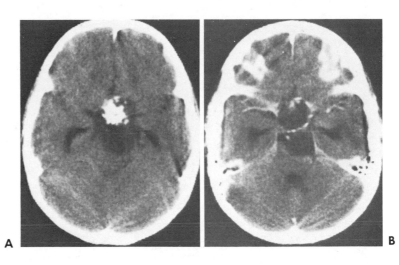

Figure 8–11. An 8-year-old developed visual impairment and hallucinations that consisted of crawling bugs. Findings were bitemporal hemianopsia and optic atrophy. *CT findings:* suprasellar dense globular calcification (*A*) with a hypodense component projecting into the brain stem (*B*). There is no visible evidence of enhancement. *Operative findings:* calcified craniopharyngioma with cystic component.

ably established by axial CT. Intrasellar component and intraventricular extension is best determined by supplemental coronal views. CT is more sensitive than conventional radiography for demonstrating calcification. One half of patients with CT evidence of calcification have none seen with skull x-ray. The pattern on plain and enhanced CT scan is frequently helpful in delineating pathological features of craniopharyngioma. Noncontrast CT findings include: (1) suprasellar soft-tissue mass that may be irregular in shape and contain heterogeneous attenuation values (Fig. 8–10); (2) calcification that is central or peripheral in location (Fig. 8–11); (3) round homogeneous hypodense region representing cyst; (4) effacement of the suprasellar cistern; (5) obstruction of the intraventricular foramen with lateral ventricular dilation and (6) effacement or compression of the anterior third ventricle. The calcified portion of the tumor may appear as multiple round or linear-shaped discrete noncontinuous peripheral hyperdense structures. These may surround hypodense or isodense regions, and this is seen with both cystic and solid tumors. Dense globular juxtasellar calcification is characteristic of craniopharyngioma. Three quarters of craniopharyngiomas contain cystic components. Cysts may appear hypodense. These may have three density appearances: (1) similar to CSF, (2) very low densities caused by fat content (cholesterol) and (3) slightly less dense than brain or surrounding solid tumor. Cysts are sharply marginated and well-delineated; they usually have round or oval shape. In rare instances, cysts are isodense or hyperdense. These unusually high attenuation values for the cystic component are the result of high protein content. The solid tumors usually appear irregularly marginated and heterogeneous in density (Fig. 8–12). Contrast enhancement is demonstrated

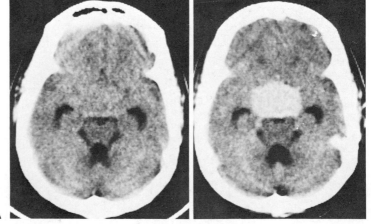

Figure 8–12. This 35-year-old man developed headache and vomiting. Findings were papilledema and bitemporal hemianopsia. *CT findings:* isodense suprasellar mass (*A*) extending to the intraventricular foramina and interpeduncular cistern. There is dense homogeneous enhancement (*B*). *Operative finding:* solid craniopharyngioma.

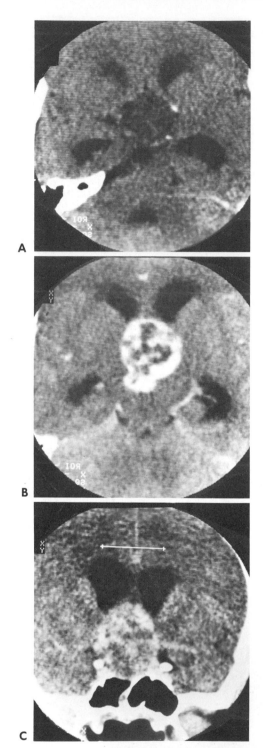

Figure 8–13. A 22-year-old man developed headache and visual obscurations. He had bitemporal hemianopsia. *CT findings:* round sharply marginated hypodense suprasellar lesion with several flecks of peripheral calcification (*A*) and irregular variable-thickness ring enhancement (*B*). Coronal projections show an egg-shaped mass extending to intraventricular foramina (*C*) and obstructive hydrocephalus. *Operative finding:* solid craniopharyngioma.

in 80 percent of craniopharyngiomas. This includes the following patterns: (1) thin peripheral rim, (2) thick complex variable-thickness ring (Fig. 8–13), (3) irregularly shaped and heterogeneous configuration and (4) dense homogeneous and sharply marginated. Craniopharyngiomas frequently appear larger on enhanced scan, especially if the isodense noncystic component enhances.

On the basis of CT findings, a preoperative diagnosis of craniopharyngioma is not always possible. The finding of discrete noncontinuous calcified bands that subsequently show a connecting thin enhancing rim is characteristic of cystic craniopharyngiomas. A similar pattern may be seen in partially thrombosed aneurysms. Solid neoplasms may show dense homogeneous sharply marginated enhancement or dense heterogeneous irregularly shaped enhancement. This is seen with other malignant tumors such as gliomas.

Meningiomas

The majority of juxtasellar meningiomas originate from the tuberculum sella or planum sphenoidale. Less common sites of origin include the clinoid processes, diaphragma sella and the lesser or greater sphenoid wings.[27] The initial symptom is usually unilateral painless visual loss; however, carefully performed tangent screen visual field examination usually shows temporal defect in the *contralateral* eye. Plain skull x-ray shows juxtasellar abnormalities (66 percent). This includes thickening of bony cortex, loss of distinct cortical margins and blistering of the planum sphenoidale. If meningioma expands into the intrasellar region, the radiographic findings may simulate those caused by pituitary adenoma. Meningiomas may extend forward to the orbit to widen the optic foramina or superior orbital fissure and also cause hyperostosis (Fig. 8–14). Isotope brain scan is positive if meningioma extends 1 cm above the diaphragma sella; however, small tumors are usually not detected. Angiographic findings of juxtasellar meningiomas include: (1) elevation and posterior displacement of the anterior cerebral artery, (2) downward and posterior distortion of the supraclinoid portion of the carotid artery, (3) enlargement of the feeding meningeal vessels and (4) tumor stain that appears early in the arterial phase and persists through the venous phase. Selective internal and external carotid angiography may be necessary to dem-

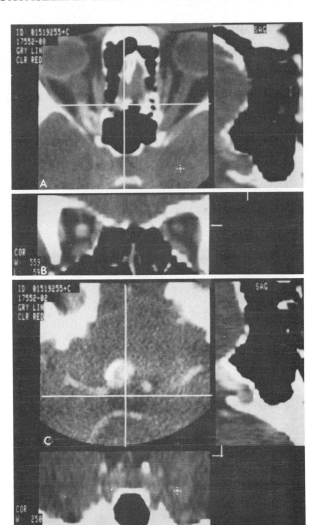

Figure 8–14. A 42-year-old man developed visual blurring in the left eye. Findings were unilateral papilledema and decreased pupillary light reactivity. *CT findings:* enlarged left optic nerve seen on axial (*A*) and coronal projections with apical calcification (*B*). There is an enhancing left anterior parasellar enhancing mass (*C*). *Operative findings:* orbital meningioma with parasellar extension.

onstrate sunburst stain with abnormal vessels derived from the dural meningeal vessels of the external carotid artery or the ophthalmic branch of the internal carotid artery.

CT findings of juxtasellar meningiomas are quite characteristic. Noncontrast scan shows either isodense or speckled hyperdense round mass located laterally and eccentrically within the anterior portion of the suprasellar cistern. They may be multilobulated and surrounded by a thin hypodense rim. Meningiomas show dense homogeneous sharply margined enhancement. Coronal sections are helpful in delineating the full extent of lesion, including intrasellar component and sphenoid bone erosion. With appropriate bone settings, hyperostotic bone reaction may be demonstrated. Juxtasellar meningiomas do not usually contain cystic or hemorrhagic components. The calci-

fied portion is usually speckled and not globular. Meningiomas most commonly simulate solid pituitary adenomas. Meningiomas are more likely to show these CT features: (1) multilobulation, (2) lateral and eccentric location in the suprasellar cistern, (3) extension into the cavernous sinus and orbit (Fig. 8–15), (4) the presence of a surrounding hypodense rim, (5) sphenoid bone erosion and (6) small intrasellar and large extrasellar components.

Gliomas

Juxtasellar involvement may result from primary optic chiasmal glioma, tumor extension from the intraorbital optic nerve glioma or from hypothalamic–third ventricular glioma.[28–30] The initial symptoms of optic glioma include proptosis, visual loss and optic atrophy. Radio-

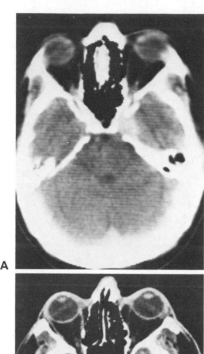

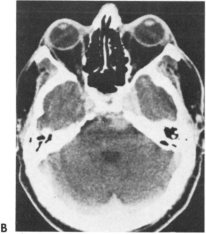

Figure 8–15. A 50-year-old man developed horizontal diplopia. Findings were right partial ophthalmoparesis with normal visual acuity. Skull roentgenogram and carotid angiogram were negative. *CT findings:* right carotid cavernous sinus enhancement (*A*). One year later CT showed parasellar-middle fossa enhancing mass extending posteriorly to the interpeduncular cistern (*B*). *Operative finding:* meningioma.

graphic studies show the optic foramina to be asymmetrically (greater than 1 mm) enlarged in patients with primary orbital optic glioma. Chiasmal gliomas initially cause bitemporal visual field defects. Skull x-ray may show J-shaped sella turcica and normal optic foramina. Initial symptoms of hypothalamic glioma include intracranial hypertension, endocrine dysfunction (diabetes insipidus, growth retardation, diencephalic syndrome, sexual precocity) and visual field defects. Skull x-ray may show sella changes caused by intracranial hypertension rather than direct effect of tumor.

CT diagnosis of optic nerve glioma is established by demonstration of fusiform enlargement of the optic nerve. To delineate the presence of intracranial extension of optic glioma, thin sections through the optic foramen and suprasellar cistern are necessary. If intracranial tumor is present, there is a sharply marginated enhancing soft-tissue lesion extending into the suprasellar cistern. This lesion may extend backward into optic radiations. Primary chiasmal gliomas appear isodense or hyperdense. These are suprasellar masses and extend to the third ventricular region. They may show dense homogeneous enhancement (Fig. 8–16). Large chiasmal gliomas may show irregularly marginated and heterogeneous variable-thickness enhancement. Chiasmal gliomas may extend along the visual pathways. This differentiates these neoplasms from craniopharyngiomas and hypothalamic gliomas. Hypothalamic gliomas are invasive and infiltrative tumors. They frequently have interspersed cystic components. CT shows an irregularly marginated mixed-density suprasellar–third ventricular soft-tissue mass. They may show no enhancement or dense complex variable-thickness enhancement; depending on pathological characteristics. They cause obstruction of the anterior third ventricle and may extend into the thalamic, ganglionic and cortical (frontal, temporal) regions (Fig. 8–17).

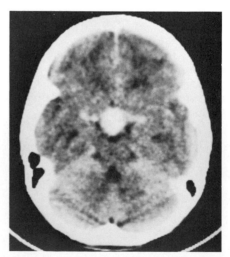

Figure 8–16. An 18-year-old girl developed amenorrhea and visual blurring. Finding was bitemporal hemianopsia. Skull x-ray showed J-shaped sella turcica. *CT findings:* hyperdense intrasellar and suprasellar soft-tissue enhancing mass. *Operative finding:* chiasmal glioma.

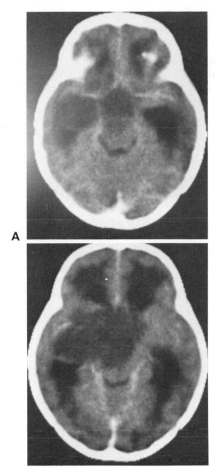

Figure 8–17. A 5-year-old developed headache and vomiting. Findings were papilledema and right hemiparesis. *CT findings:* left hypothalamic and thalamic hypodense nonenhancing (*A*) mass with marked lateral ventricular enlargement (*B*). *Operative finding:* hypothalamic glioma.

Chordomas

These are congenital neoplasms originating from notochord remnants. They are located within the clivus.[31] They may grow anteriorly into the sella, the nasopharynx or the sphenoid sinus. They may also originate within the sella or middle fossa. Early symptoms of clival chordomas include ophthalmoplegias and lower cranial nerve dysfunction. Later symptoms are caused by posterior displacement of the aqueduct, fourth ventricle and brain stem. Parasellar chordomas may cause trigeminal nerve sensory symptoms. Skull x-ray usually shows bone erosion of the clivus and posterior sella region. Angiography is necessary to define the location of the tumor as an extradural

postclival or parasellar mass. This also detects evidence of encasement, irregularity and occlusion of vessels by the chordoma.

CT findings of juxtasellar chordomas reflect their varied pathological characteristics. Chordomas may be highly cellular and infiltrating neoplasms. CT finding in these cases is that of a round multilobulated irregularly shaped soft-tissue density mass located posterior to the dorsum sella. These lesions may show dense heterogeneous complex enhancement (Fig. 8–18). There may be extensive bone erosion at the skull base. Other juxtasellar chordomas consist of gelatinous or mucoid material within the thin capsule. These tumors are calcified and have low cellular density. CT shows hypodense lesions with interspersed hyperdense calcified components, and they do not enhance.

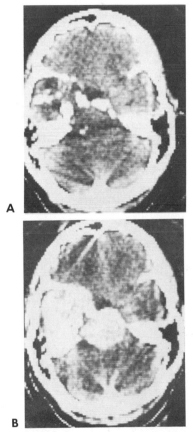

Figure 8–18. A 34-year-old man developed left facial numbness and psychomotor seizures. Skull x-ray showed sella and clivus erosion. *CT findings:* multiple juxtasellar and middle fossa calcifications (*A*) with dense thick irregular enhancement (*B*). *Operative finding:* chordoma.

Metastases

Breast carcinoma is the most frequent cause of juxtasellar metastases. Most commonly these tumors involve the posterior pituitary region. Initial clinical symptomatology may be diabetes insipidus. Skull x-ray usually shows a normal-sized sella turcica with marked erosive changes. CT usually shows an isodense intrasellar lesion with dense nodular homogeneous or ring enhancement. In most cases there are many other intracranial metastases; however, in 10 percent, CT demonstrates a solitary intrasellar lesion. Certain neoplasms secondarily extend to the juxtasellar region from contiguous regions (Fig. 8–19).

Granulomatous Disorders

Granulomas due to intracranial sarcoidosis may involve the suprasellar region. They cause hypothalamic-pituitary and chiasmal dysfunction. These usually develop in patients with systemic illness but may occur rarely as the initial manifestation. Skull x-ray is usually normal; however, CSF may show sterile pleocytosis with decreased glucose content. CT shows isodense homogeneous enhancing suprasellar lesion. This may extend into the frontal region. There may also be diffuse basal cisternal enhancement. Orbital CT may show lacrimal gland enlargement. Following corticosteroid treatment, resolution of an enhancing suprasellar lesion may occur. This response may obviate the need for surgical biopsy. The reticuloendothelioses (eosinophilic granuloma, Schüller-Christian disease) are associated with histiocytic granuloma. Patients may develop diabetes insipidus without other signs of hypopituitarism. Skull x-ray usually shows characteristic bone destruction in the skull. CT may show juxtasellar enhancing nodular lesions. These may simulate sarcoid granulomas.

Pituitary Abscess

This may occur spontaneously or in patients with pituitary tumors that have undergone hemorrhagic necrosis.[32] Initial symptoms include sudden development of headache with accompanying polydipsia and polyuria (diabetes insipidus). Skull x-ray shows abnormalities of an expanding intrasellar mass. Radiographic analysis of the paranasal sinuses is essential as this may delineate the potential source of primary infection. Pituitary abscesses are unusual lesions; CT experience has therefore been limited. Plain scan has shown a heterogeneous hyperdense suprasellar lesion with dense enhancement. None of the reported cases of pituitary abscess have shown ring enhancement that is characteristic of other brain abscesses.

Demyelinating Disorders

Multiple sclerosis may involve the chiasmal region. There have been no CT abnormalities in the suprasellar or orbital region in patients with this disorder; however, demyelinated lesions may appear as hypodense or isodense periventricular lesions in other locations.

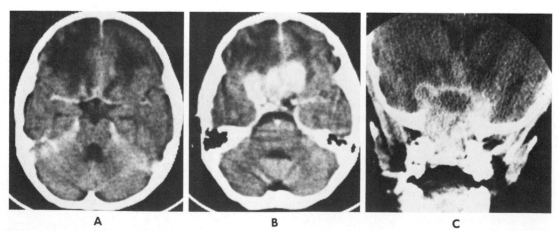

Figure 8–19. A 13-year-old developed visual loss and was found by biopsy to have rhabdomyosarcoma. CT findings: bifrontal hypodense lesion (A) with dense enhancing juxtasellar and bifrontal enhancement (B) with extension anteriorly and inferiorly seen on coronal projection (C).

Aneurysms

Sites of predilection for juxtasellar aneurysms include: (1) the intracavernous internal carotid artery, (2) the internal carotid–ophthalmic artery, (3) the internal carotid–posterior communicating artery and (4) the anterior communicating–anterior cerebral artery. Intracavernous carotid aneurysms cause ophthalmoplegias and trigeminal sensory disturbances. Skull x-ray shows unilateral anterior clinoid erosion, sphenoid wing erosion and widening of the superior orbital fissure. Supraclinoid ophthalmic and anterior communicating artery aneurysms may cause optic nerve and chiasmal compressive syndromes. Skull x-ray usually shows no sella abnormalities. Posterior communicating–carotid artery aneurysms present with subarachnoid hemorrhage, whereas other juxtasellar aneurysms simulate neoplasms in presenting clinically with progressively worsening visual or endocrine disorders.

CT findings of juxtasellar aneurysms are varied, depending on such factors as location, size, the presence of intraluminal calcification, mural thrombus, and intraluminal blood pool. Anterior communicating artery aneurysms appear as isodense or hyperdense calcified round densely enhancing lesions located in the anterior suprasellar cistern and extending into the interhemispheric fissure. Intracavernous carotid artery and ophthalmic aneurysms may show mural thrombus formation; therefore, lesion size is sometimes better assessed by CT than angiography. Partially thrombosed aneurysms have peripheral wall calcification and enhancement within the intraluminal component, whereas completely thrombosed aneurysms are calcified and do not enhance. Nonthrombosed juxtasellar aneurysms may simulate pituitary adenomas or meningiomas (Fig. 8–20). Thrombosed aneurysms may stimulate craniopharyngiomas or pituitary adenomas. CT findings of juxtasellar tumors are not specific enough to exclude the presence of aneurysm without angiography.

Cysts

Arachnoid cysts may be entirely intrasellar or they may be more extensive and extend into the suprasellar region and the middle and posterior fossa.[33] CT shows a hypodense (consistent with CSF) sharply marginated lesion. Failure of subarachnoid juxtasellar cysts to enhance differentiates these lesions from cystic pituitary adenomas or craniopharyngiomas. Communication of cyst with ventricular or subarachnoid spaces may be determined by metrizamide cisterography. Epidermoid cysts may appear as sharply marginated hypodense nonenhancing suprasellar lesions, but they may have calcified components (Fig. 8–21). Dermoid cysts and lipomas (Fig. 8–22) appear as hypodense nonenhancing juxtasellar lesions. These may contain very hypodense regions representing fat and interspersed calcified portions to simulate craniopharyngiomas.

Empty Sella Syndrome

This refers to findings of enlarged sella turcica that is filled by enlarged suprasellar subarachnoid space extending into the intrasellar region. There is bone remodeling of the sella. The pituitary gland is compressed and flattened in the posterior-inferior region of the

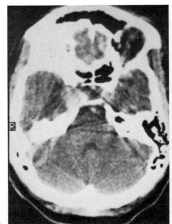 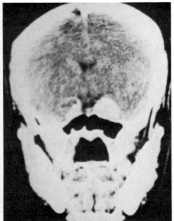

Figure 8–20. A 36-year-old woman developed diplopia and facial parasthesias. Skull x-ray showed erosion of the left anterior clinoid process. CT findings: left parasellar hyperdense mass (A) that shows dense homogeneous sharply marginated enhancement (reader's right) (B). Angiogram showed carotid aneurysm.

A

B

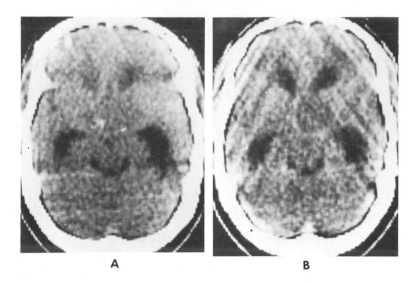

A   B

Figure 8–21. A 48-year-old woman developed headache and vomiting. Findings were bilateral papilledema. *CT findings:* isodense suprasellar mass (*A*) extending to the intraventricular foramina. There is calcification (*B*) and a thin peripheral enhancing rim. *Operative finding:* epidermoid cyst.

Figure 8–22. An elderly man was beaten with a wooden stick. He had no endocrine or visual symptoms. *CT findings:* intrasellar hypodense (consistent with fat) intrasellar nonenhancing mass (*A*) extending into the sphenoid sinus and suprasellar region (*B*). *Operative finding:* lipoma.

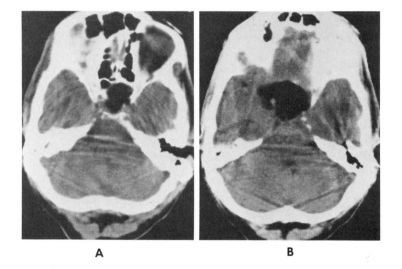

A   B

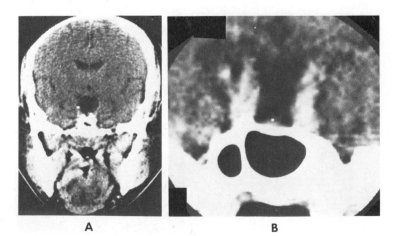

A   B

Figure 8–23. A 42-year-old obese woman was amenorrheic. Skull x-ray showed enlarged sella turcica. Endocrine studies and tangent screen visual fields were normal. *CT findings:* a hypodense intrasellar region is seen (*A*). The hypodense (consistent with CSF) component is seen extending to the sella floor (*B*). The compressed and flattened pituitary gland is seen in the sella floor.

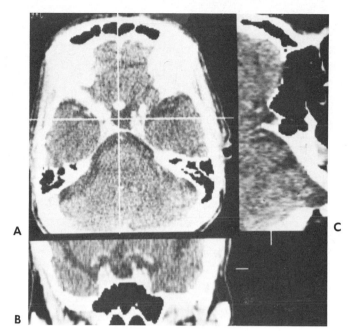

Figure 8–24. A 52-year-old man was asymptomatic but had enlarged sella on routine skull x-ray. *CT findings:* a hypodense intrasellar region (*A*) extending to the sella floor seen on reformated coronal projection (*B*). The small hyperdense pituitary gland is seen on sagittal projections (*C*).

pituitary fossa. Diagnosis of "empty sella syndrome" has been established in 10 percent of routine air studies. Abnormal pituitary function has been described; however, visual and neurological findings are rarely seen in patients with *primary empty sella*.[34] These clinical abnormalities may develop in patients with *secondary empty sella*. This latter condition results from surgery or irradiation of a pituitary tumor.

A typical radiographic abnormality of empty sella is symmetrically ballooned sella turcica; the sella has normal shape and shows no bone erosion. This pattern is frequently different from that seen with an expanding intrasellar neoplasm. This usually shows four characteristics: (1) bone is eroded, (2) there is open configuration of the sella, (3) the clinoid processes appear elevated and (4) the dorsum appears straightened. Plain skull and hypocycloidal tomographic findings are not always specific enough to differentiate empty sella from other conditions such as cystic intrasellar tumor, intrasellar cyst and dilated intrasellar third ventricular recess. Empty sella is diagnosed most reliably by air studies, which demonstrate air entering intrasellar space in sitting or brow-up position.

Figure 8–25. A metrizamide cisternogram shows that contrast material extends to sella floor on axial (*A*) and coronal (*B*) projections. This confirmed the diagnosis of empty sella.

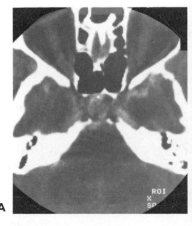
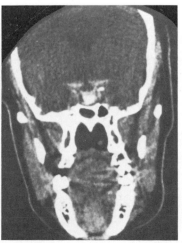

The diagnosis of empty sella syndrome may also be established by CT. This requires coronal projections and thin-section scans (Fig. 8–23). This may be seen on direct or reformated coronal or sagittal projections (Fig. 8–24). The detection of CSF density extending into an enlarged sella turcica with no evidence of abnormal intravenous enhancement rests on characteristic findings; however, cystic lesions or a dilated intrasellar third ventricle recess may show similar findings.[35] Demonstration of a normal pituitary infundibulum extending into the intrasellar region on coronal sections excludes intrasellar mass. The pituitary infundibulum is best visualized with 1.5 or 2.0 mm sections.[36] If the infundibulum position is not demonstrated, diagnosis of empty sella may require metrizamide cisternography (Fig. 8–25). Complete opacification of the intrasellar and suprasellar cistern with metrizamide establishes this diagnosis.[37]

REFERENCES

1. Abboud CF, Laws ER: Clinical endocrinological approach to hypothalamic-pituitary disease. J Neurosurg 51:271–291,1979
2. Zervas NT, Martin JB: Management of hormone-secreting pituitary hormones. N Engl J Med 302:210–214,1980
3. Knight CL, Hoyt WF, Wilson CB: Syndrome of incipient prechiasmal optic nerve compression. Arch Ophthalmol 87:1–12,1972
4. DuBoulay G, Tricky S: The choice of radiological investigation in the management of tumors around the sella. Clin Radiol 18:349,1967
5. Vezina JL, Sutton TJ: Prolactin-secreting pituitary microadenoma. Am J Roentgenol 120:46, 1974
6. Geehr RB, Allen WE, Rothman S: Pluridirectional tomography in the evaluation of pituitary tumors. Am J Roentgenol 130:105–109,1978
7. Tenner MS, Weitzner I: Pitfalls in the diagnosis of erosive changes in expanding lesions of the pituitary fossa. Radiology 137:393–396,1980
8. Weisberg LA, Zimmerman EA, Frantz AG: Diagnosis and evaluation of patients with an enlarged sella turcica. Am J Med 61:590,1976
9. Macpherson P, Anderson DE: Radiological differentiation of intrasellar aneurysms from pituitary tumors. Neuroradiology 21:177–183,1981
10. Powell DF, Baker HL: The primary angiographic findings in pituitary adenomas. Radiology 110:589,1974
11. Kuuliala I: The normal suprasellar subarachnoid space in computed tomography. Clin Radiol 31:155–159,1980
12. Leeds NE, Naidich TP: Computerized tomography in the diagnosis of sellar and parasellar lesions. Semin Roentgenol 12:121, 1977
13. Syvertsen A, Haughton VM, Williams AL: The computed tomographic appearance of the normal pituitary gland and pituitary microadenomas. Radiology 133:385–391, 1979
14. Kline LB, Acker JD, Post MJD: The cavernous sinus: a computed tomographic study. Am J Neuroradiol 2:299–305, 1981
15. Weisberg LA: Pituitary apoplexy. Am J Med 63:109, 1977
16. Faria MA, Tindall GT: Transphenoidal microsurgery for prolactin-secreting pituitary adenomas. J Neurosurg 56:33–43, 1982
17. Bonafe A, Sobel D, Manelfe C: Relative value of CT and hypocycloidal tomography in the diagnosis of pituitary microadenoma. Neuroradiology 22:133–137, 1981
18. Taylor S: High-resolution computed tomography of the sella. Radiol Clin North Am 20:207–236, 1982
19. Chambers EF, Turski PA, LaMasters D: Regions of low density in contrast enhanced pituitary gland: normal and pathologic processes. Radiology 144:109, 1982
20. Domingue JN, Wing SG, Wilson CB: Coexisting pituitary adenomas and partially empty sellas. J Neurosurg 48:23–28, 1978
21. Banna M, Baker HL, Houser OW: Pituitary and parapituitary tumors on computed tomography. Br J Radiol 53:1123–1143, 1980
22. Post MJD, David JN, Glaser JS: Pituitary apoplexy: diagnosis by computed tomography. Radiology 134:665–670, 1980
23. Rilliet B, Mohr G, Robert F: Calcifications in pituitary adenomas. Surg Neurol 15:249, 1981
24. Scotti G, Scialfa G, Chiodini PG: Macroprolactinomas: CT evaluation of reduction of tumor size after medical treatment. Neuroradiology 23:123, 1982
25. Fitz CR, Wortzman G, Harwood-Nash DC: Computed tomography in craniopharyngioma. Radiology 127:687–691, 1978
26. Bartlett JR: Craniopharyngiomas: a summary of 85 cases. J Neurol Neurosurg Psychiatr 34:37–41, 1971
27. Kadis GN, Mount LA, Ganti SR: The importance of early diagnosis and treatment of the meningiomas of the planum sphenoidale and tuberculum sellae. Surg Neurol 12:367, 1979
28. Tenny RT, Laws ER, Younge BR: The neurosurgical management of optic glioma. J Neurosurg 57:452, 1982
29. Byrd SE, Harwood-Nash DC, Fitz CR: CT of the intraorbital optic nerve gliomas in children. Radiology 129:73–78, 1978
30. Savoiardo M, Harwood-Nash DC, Tadmor R: Gliomas of the intracranial anterior optic pathways in children. Radiology 138:601–610, 1981
31. Poppen JL, King AB: Chordoma. J Neurosurg 9:139, 1952
32. Blackett PR, Bailey JD, Hoffman HJ: Pituitary abscess simulating an intrasellar tumor. Surg Neurol 14:129, 1980
33. Spaziante R, Divitis E, Stella L: Benign intrasellar cysts. Surg Neurol 15:274, 1981
34. Neelon FA, Goree JA, Lebovitz HE: The primary empty sella. Medicine 52:73, 1973
35. Sage MR, Chan ES, Reilly PL: The clinical and radiological features of the empty sella syndrome. Clin Radiol 31:513–519, 1980
36. Haughton VM, Rosenbaum AE, Williams AE: Recognizing the empty sella by CT: the infundibulum sign. Am J Neuroradiol 1:527–529, 1980
37. Gross LE, Binet EF, Esguerro JV: Metrizamide cisternography in the evaluation of pituitary adenoma and the empty sella syndrome. J Neurosurg 50:472–476, 1979

Chapter 9

INCREASED INTRACRANIAL PRESSURE

Intracranial hypertension may be caused by diverse pathological conditions, including those of neoplastic, vascular, infectious-inflammatory, toxic, traumatic, metabolic and endocrine origins. Symptoms of intracranial hypertension include headache, vomiting, double vision and visual blurring. Funduscopic examination usually shows papilledema. Absent spontaneous pulsations represents an early sign of elevated intracranial pressure; however, it is possible for the patient to have intracranial hypertension without papilledema.[1] Lumbar puncture should be cautiously performed after neurodiagnostic studies have excluded the presence of hydrocephalus or mass lesions.[2] Neurological signs resulting from intracranial hypertension may be caused by brain parenchyma compression, obstructive hydrocephalus or cerebral edema. Supratentorial mass lesions may cause downward herniation of the uncus and hippocampus (transtentorial) or herniation of the cingulate gyrus underneath the falx (subfalcine). Infratentorial lesions may cause superior vermis upward herniation through the tentorium or downward herniation of the cerebellar tonsils through the foramen magnum.

Nonlocalizing neurological signs may develop in patients with intracranial hypertension. Abducens nerve involvement is manifested by horizontal diplopia caused by lateral rectus paresis. This is usually unilateral; less commonly, it is bilateral. Increased intracranial pressure may cause dilation of the anterior third ventricle with optic chiasm compression to result in visual field defects such as bitemporal or binasal hemianopsia. Distention of the optic nerve sheath by transmitted increased intracranial pressure causes optic nerve compression. Clinical findings are impaired visual acuity, inferior nasal quadrant defect and optic atrophy. Hypopituitarism may result from ballooned anterior third ventricle pulsatile pressure being transmitted to the hypothalamic-pituitary region. Rhinorrhea and "empty sella" may rarely develop in patients with chronic intracranial hypertension.[3]

DIAGNOSTIC ASSESSMENT

Patients with intracranial hypertension without localizing neurological signs represent difficult diagnostic problems. Ophthalmological conditions may simulate papilledema (optic neuritis, central retinal vein thrombosis, diabetic or hypertensive retinopathy, congenital optic disc anomalies). However, exclusion of intracranial lesions in these cases sometimes requires neurodiagnostic investigation. Lumbar puncture is necessary to establish the diagnosis of subarachnoid hemorrhage or meningoencephalitis. If these patients have papilledema, CT should be initially performed because of the risk of neurological deterioration resulting from herniation. Extremely high CSF pressure has been reported in these conditions; however, herniation does not develop following lumbar puncture because pressure gradient does not exist within the brain and CSF spaces unless there is a complicating process—for example, intracranial hematoma, subdural empyema or brain abscess.

Diagnostic evaluation of patients with intracranial hypertension without localizing signs once required invasive contrast diagnostic studies. Many patients had mass lesion or ventricular obstructive process; however, certain patients underwent craniotomy or ventriculography and no mass lesion or ventricular abnormality was detected (pseudotumor cerebri).[4] Kelly reported findings in 21 patients with papilledema only; 10 had midline obstructive lesions of which 7 were colloid cysts, and nine patients had lateralized supratentorial lesions.[5] Berg reviewed the results of ventriculography and craniotomy in patients with nonlocalized increased intracranial pressure: (1) lateralized supra- or infratentorial lesions (50 percent), (2) midline obstructive process (27 percent), (3) subacute or chronic meningitis (13 percent) and (4) no abnormally detected by air studies with normal CSF examination (10 percent). Careful follow-up of patients with initial normal studies showed that occasionally lesions were subsequently demonstrated.[6] In the next decade isotope scan and percutaneous angiography were developed and most lesions were detected on initial evaluation.

Noninvasive studies were used to screen for lateralized supratentorial lesions. EEG may fail to demonstrate one third of supratentorial lesions;[6] however, EEG and isotope scan detected 96 percent.[7] When intracranial hypertension is caused by obstructive hydrocephalus, EEG may demonstrate bilateral frontal or posterior monorhythmic delta pattern. Plain skull x-ray may show sella abnormalities caused by chronic intracranial hypertension. The finding of pineal shift suggests supratentorial mass lesion; however, the pineal is not always visualized because insufficient calcification may exist to make it a midline indicator. Angiography is important to define the shape of the thalamostriate vein, which is a reliable indicator of lateral ventricular size. If this vein appeared normal and no mass effect was seen, pneumoencephalogram was performed; however, if ventricles were enlarged, ventriculography was necessary.

In one study that analyzed 100 patients who presented with nonlocalized intracranial hypertension, 82 had no evidence of mass lesions or hydrocephalus. These patients had normal consciousness; EEG and isotope scan were negative. CSF studies were abnormal only for elevated CSF pressure in 71 patients to confirm the diagnosis of benign intracranial hypertension. Six patients had infectious or neoplastic meningitis; their CSF pressure was markedly elevated. In some cases angiogram and air studies were not performed; the diagnosis of benign intracranial hypertension was established by CSF examination and subsequent clinical course.[8] This approach is associated with certain risks because patients with posterior fossa neoplasms may have increased intracranial pressure with normal-sized ventricles.[9]

The diagnostic assessment of these patients has been modified by CT such that invasive contrast diagnostic studies are rarely necessary. Of 100 patients with nonlocalized intracranial hypertension, CT was the most reliable diagnostic study; no lesion was subsequently detected by angiography or air studies.[10] The accuracy of CT is demonstrated by the following example. Three patients with papilledema and bitemporal hemianopsia had radiographic evidence of enlarged sella turcica to suggest suprasellar mass; however, CT showed evidence of empty sella. This was confirmed by air studies and metrizamide cisternogram.[11]

CAUSES OF THE SYNDROME OF NONLOCALIZED INCREASED INTRACRANIAL PRESSURE

Benign Intracranial Hypertension (BIH). This condition occurs most commonly in young obese but otherwise healthy patients. Symptoms include headache, nausea, vomiting and diplopia; neurological findings are bilateral papilledema. Visual fields examination shows blind spot enlargement caused by optic nerve swelling. One third of patients have visual symptoms; however, only 1 to 8 percent suffer permanent visual sequelae such as impaired acuity, visual field defect (inferior nasal quadrantanopsia) or optic atrophy. The diagnosis of BIH is established by lumbar puncture and radiographic studies; CSF examination is normal except for elevated pressure. Diagnostic studies should exclude enlarged ventricles or a mass lesion.[12-14]

The cause of benign intracranial hypertension is not established. Venous sinus thrombosis elevates venous pressure and impairs CSF resorption; however, angiography rarely shows evidence of this disorder. Metabolic-endocrine factors such as use of corticosteroids, obesity and menstrual disorders have been implicated as casual factors. In BIH, it has been postulated that there is increased CSF volume because of impaired CSF reabsorption; this results from impaired flow across arachnoid granulation microvilli. This causes distention of these spaces with normal or small-sized ventricles.[13]

In BIH, EEG and isotope scan are negative. Skull x-rays may show sella turcica abnormalities; these may be caused by chronic intracranial hypertension or associated empty sella. Angiography has been performed to assess these features: (1) ventricular dilatation, (2) mass effect, (3) patency of venous system to exclude venous sinus thrombosis (lateral, sagittal), (4) caliber of intracranial blood vessels as segmental arterial lesions may develop in vasculitis (systemic lupus erythematosus) and (5) intracranial or dural vascular malformation. Air studies show the ventricles to be normal in size. There are reports of small-sized ventricles, and in one study ventricular volume was small in 24 percent of patients with BIH. Mild ventricular dilatation has been reported in BIH; however, ventricles were never prominently dilated. Because gas artificially distends ventricles and subarachnoid spaces, small-sized ventricles may be obscured by air study.[14] The theory that the ventricles may be small is derived from the hypothesis that benign intracranial hypertension is caused by a form of cerebral edema. This is supported by this evidence: (1) cerebral biopsy specimens showing intra- or extracellular edema, (2) production of cerebral edema in animals by obstruction of the torcular herophili and in humans by lateral sinus occlusion and (3) occurrence of cerebral edema in animals with vitamin A deficiency (etiological factor for BIH in humans). However, normal mental state of patients and normal EEG findings are not consistent with cerebral edema.

It was predicted that plain and enhanced cerebral CT would be normal in patients with BIH, and this assumption has been confirmed.[10, 15, 16] Because air studies had shown that ventricles were sometimes small, nonvisualization of the ventricles by CT was predicted; however, an alternative explanation for nonvisualization is that it is artifactual as a result of partial volume effect.[17] With high-resolution scanners nonvisualization of the lateral and third ventricles and perimesencephalic cisterns is strongly suggestive of cerebral edema. We have observed this pattern in five percent of patients with BIH. Following successful reduction of CSF pressure, ventricles and cisternal spaces were well visualized. This indicated that the intracranial hypertension was responsible for small-sized CSF spaces. Five percent of patients with BIH showed lateral and third ventricular enlargement, usually without supratentorial cortical CSF space enlargement.[18] The temporal horns and fourth ventricle were not enlarged and there were no periventricular hypodensities.

Metrizamide cisternography showed no abnormal CSF circulation. Two percent of patients showed biventricular enlargement with sulcal space enlargement. Following successful reduction of CSF pressure with repeated lumbar puncture or diuretics, CSF spaces decreased in size in these patients.

In several other cases CT showed an enlarged hypodense midline posterior fossa lesion; this was round or triangularly shaped and did not enhance or cause mass effect. This represents an enlarged cisterna magna as confirmed by metrizamide cisternography. It probably represents an *incidental* finding because the appearance did not change when CSF pressure normalized. This was initially believed to be an important finding because when subtemporal decompression had been performed for patients with BIH it had been observed that subarachnoid spaces were distended and ventricles were compressed.

Two patients with BIH had unilateral visual impairment; CT showed bilateral enlargement of the optic nerves. This undoubtedly reflects the effect of distention of subarachnoid spaces surrounding the optic nerves because of papilledema. Following reduction in CSF pressure, visual acuity improved; CT showed reduction in optic nerve size. In two other patients who developed permanent visual loss and optic atrophy, high-resolution CT showed no abnormality of optic nerves. There does not appear to be a correlation of visual impairment with CT findings in BIH.

Supratentorial Lesions. Lateralized supratentorial lesions were diagnosed by CT in 10 percent of patients with intracranial hypertension and no localizing signs. In 40 percent of these cases EEG, skull x-ray and isotope scan were normal. In all cases, plain scan showed abnormal findings and enhanced scan further delineated the lesion; however, pathological characterization required angiography and surgical biopsy. Huckman et al. suggested that patients with nonlocalized increased intracranial pressure should have an enhanced scan despite negative plain scan. Metastatic lesions or angiomas that are isodense and do not cause mass effect may be detected on enhanced scan only.[15] This would be most unusual; in patients with nonlocalized intracranial hypertension there have been no reports of this occurrence. Certain diffusely infiltrating neoplasms (microgliomas, sarcomas) may present with nonlocalized increased intracranial pressure and these lesions show characteristic CT patterns.

Conventional diagnostic tests may show no abnormalities: (1) EEG may be diffusely slow or normal, (2) CSF may show no cytologic abnormalities if the neoplasm does not seed into the subarachnoid spaces and (3) angiogram may be normal and if the tumor is infiltrative without mass effect.

Midline Obstructive Lesions. These lesions represented 10 percent of lesions detected by CT. Colloid cysts were most common; other midline tumors were craniopharyngioma, pinealoma, intraventricular meningioma and choroid plexus papilloma. CT demonstrates abnormal density and enhancement caused by the lesion and hydrocephalus proximal to the site of obstruction. CT obviates the need for air studies in most patients.

Posterior Fossa Lesions. Twenty percent of patients with nonlocalizing intracranial pressure had cerebellar or fourth ventricular tumors diagnosed by CT. Sixty percent were midline in location; 40 percent were located in cerebellar hemispheres. These usually were cerebellar astrocytomas or medulloblastomas. The diagnosis was established by CT; air studies and angiography were not required in any case. In several cases, CT showed evidence of aqueductal stenosis with no contiguous areas of abnormal density, mass effect or enhancement. Ventriculography is frequently performed prior to shunting to exclude occult neoplasm; however, with characteristic CT findings of aqueductal stenosis, this is probably unnecessary.

VENOUS SINUS THROMBOSIS[19, 20]

Thrombosis of the large dural venous sinuses (sagittal, lateral, sigmoid) may result from hypercoagulable states (polycythemia, hyperfibrinogenemia), pregnancy, use of oral contraceptives, infiltration of the venous sinus by neoplasm, or complications of infection (meningitis, mastoiditis, paranasal sinusitis). It may also develop without precipitating factors. Clinical features are influenced by pathological factors: site of occlusion, collateral venous channels, cerebral edema and venous infarction. Thrombosis of the transverse and sigmoid sinus may simulate such symptoms of benign intracranial hypertension as headache and papilledema. Superior sagittal sinus thrombosis may present with papilledema, impaired mentation and alternating hemiparesis. Focal neurological deficit and seizures develop if there is cortical venous infarction or intracerebral hemorrhage. Diagnosis of venous sinus thrombosis is established by angiography. This may show three abnormalities: first, nonfilling of the venous sinus and cortical veins; second, mass effect due to cerebral edema and third, avascular mass caused by intracranial hematoma.

CT findings depend upon pathological changes such as edema, infarction and hemorrhage. Ventricles may be small and perimesencephalic cisterns may be effaced; this pattern reflects cerebral edema. The "cord sign" is seen on plain scan and represents clot in a cerebral cortical vein; it is characteristic of cortical vein thrombosis. Superficial hem-

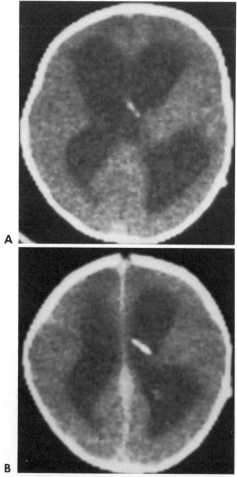

Figure 9–1. A 6-month-old boy with bacterial meningitis developed seizures and increasing lethargy despite antibiotic therapy and diversionary shunt for hydrocephalus. *CT findings:* filling defect in the superior sagittal sinus is consistent with venous occlusion (proved angiographically) seen on both plain (A) and enhanced scan (B). Marked ventricular enlargement and shunt tube are seen. (Courtesy of Dr. T. P. Naidich.)

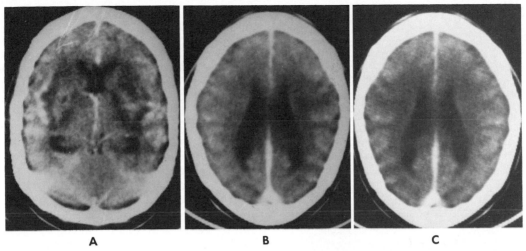

Figure 9–2. A 23-year-old woman in third trimester of pregnancy developed fever and stiff neck and became confused. CSF showed pleocytosis with 70 percent polymorphonuclear cells and decreased sugar content; however, culture was negative. She was treated with intravenous ampicillin. She became increasingly obtunded and developed generalized status epilepticus. CT findings: symmetrical bilateral hypodense lesions with interspersed enhancement (A). The filling defect is seen in the sagittal sinus (B), and is best seen at wide window settings (C).

orrhagic infarcts may be solitary or multiple; they result from venous infarcts. Multiple intracerebral hematomas are seen in 20 percent of cases. On postcontrast scan, abnormal patterns have been reported: (1) gyral-gray matter enhancement, (2) tentorial enhancement and (3) empty delta sign (filling defects in contrast-enhanced sagittal sinus). The filling defect is caused by clot in the sagittal sinus with contrast enhancement in the sinus wall (Fig. 9–1). Filling defects in the superior sagittal sinus may not be detected at routine viewing mode (Fig. 9–2). They may be appreciated best at wider settings (window width, 200; window level, 100). In several cases of angiographically documented sinus thrombosis, CT did not show any filling defect in the superior sagittal sinus. Conversely, we have seen artifacts that are small and adjacent to bone that have simulated venous sinus filling defect[21, 22] Tentorial enhancement represents tentorial collateral channels and this is most frequently seen in sagittal sinus thrombosis. Unilateral visualization of the cavernous sinus may suggest the occurrence of thrombosis of this structure. However, filling defects in the cavernous sinus may be artifactual as a result of head tilt or may represent the presence of cranial nerves located within this structure. With high-resolution thin section axial and coronal sections it may be possible to differentiate cavernous sinus thrombosis from normal-appearing cranial nerves visualized within the cavernous sinus.

Cerebral Edema[23, 24]

This is defined as increased brain volume caused by increased water content. Cerebral edema may be focal or diffuse. If cerebral edema is mild and focal it may cause no clinical neurological dysfunction; however, if it is more severe and diffuse, neurological dysfunction may result. Severe cerebral edema may cause brain herniation. Cerebral edema commonly occurs in association with intracranial hypertension; however, this is not invariable. Focal cerebral edema resulting from middle cerebral artery ischemia may be well-localized and not cause intracranial hypertension. Intra-cranial hypertension may occur without accompanying cerebral edema. This may result from transient brain engorgement caused by increased cerebral blood flow (carbon dioxide intoxication, Reye's syndrome or trauma) or from other mechanisms in benign intracranial hypertension.

On the basis of pathological studies, several different types of cerebral edema have been described.

Vasogenic Edema. This is most common and occurs in association with neoplasm, abscess, intracerebral hematoma and contusional in-

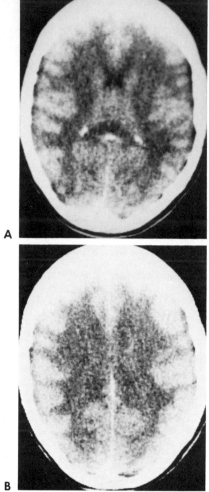

Figure 9–3. A 30-year-old woman developed a prolonged hypoxic episode during induction of anesthesia. She was akinetic and mute with bilateral Babinski signs. *CT findings:* white matter symmetrical hypodensities with scalloped edges *(A)* and bilateral ventricular compression *(B)*. This is consistent with vasogenic edema.

jury. There is increased permeability in brain capillary endothelial cell junctions in vasogenic edema. It usually develops in cerebral white matter (Fig. 9–3). Extracellular fluid volume is increased by edema fluid containing plasma proteins. CT findings include (1) hypodense regions that are slightly more dense than CSF but less dense than brain, (2) location of edema fluid in white matter with sparing of gray matter, (3) frond-like projections that represent indentations in edema fluid in normal gray matter, (4) mass effect manifested by ventricular compression and displacement, (5) enhancement in linear or gyral pattern caused by the effect of impaired blood-brain barrier (Fig. 9–4). The most prom-

inent enhancement is that which occurs within the pathological lesion responsible for the edema. Because normal gray matter density is accentuated by surrounding hypodense edema, this may falsely suggest tumor nodule. Following treatment with corticosteroids, there is usually decreased edema, mass effect and enhancement.

Ischemic Edema. This most commonly results from ischemic stroke but is seen in other conditions in which the brain becomes ischemic (Fig. 9–5). In acute stroke, hypoxia causes neuronal swelling; vasogenic edema results if cerebral infarction subsequently develops. Ischemic edema affects both gray and white matter. There is neuronal swelling and blood-brain barrier impairment. The edema fluid is intra- and extracellular; it consists of both plasma ultrafiltrate and plasma proteins. CT findings include (1) hypodense regions involving both gray and white matter, (2) sharp margination of hypodense fluid, (3) mass effect and (4) enhancement. If there is hypoperfusion, there is no enhancement; the finding of gray matter (linear, gyral) enhancement represents hyperperfusion. In ischemic edema, enhancement occurs at the periphery of hypodense regions. Corticosteroids and hyperosmolar agents do not modify ischemic edema.

Cytotoxic Edema. This most commonly results from generalized hypoxic-ischemic disorders such as respiratory or circulatory arrest. Less commonly, it may be seen in water intoxication, dialysis dysequilibrium syndromes, diabetic ketoacidosis, severe purulent meningitis, hypoglycemia and methanol intoxication. There is swelling of all cellular components (neurons, gilia, ependyma, endothelial cells); therefore, this is a diffuse process involving gray and white matter. The edema fluid is intracellular and consists of plasma ultrafiltrate. CT findings include (1) diffuse mass effect with bilateral ventricular compression, (2) symmetrical hypodense regions throughout both hemispheres, (3) involvement of subcortical nuclear gray matter masses and (4) enhancement absent within hypodense regions or normal cerebral vascular channels (Fig 9–6). The absence of enhancement within normal brain parenchyma reflects decreased cerebral perfusion. If edematous regions are symmetrical and only slightly hypodense, this may cause diagnostic problems. It is difficult to define absolute attenuation values for gray and white matter because of the instability and variability of these measurements.

Following treatment with corticosteroids or

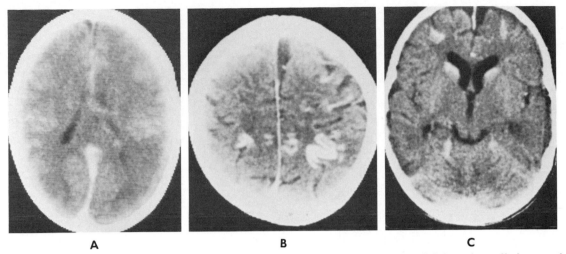

Figure 9–4. A 4-year-old girl was the victim of child abuse. She was comatose with bilateral papilledema and subhyaloid retinal hemorrhages. *CT findings*: symmetrical ventricular compression (*A*) with no abnormal density or enhancement. Following corticosteroid and osmotherapy she clinically improved. *CT findings*: ventricular and subarachnoid space enlargement with gyral (*B*) and subcortical nuclear enhancement (*C*).

osmotic agents, there is no modification in CT findings.

Interstitial (Hydrocephalic) Edema. Interstitial periventricular edema occurs in obstructive (intraventricular) or communicating (extraventricular) hydrocephalus. This is most prominent in the anterolateral portion of the frontal horns. There is disruption of the ependymal cells that comprise the ventricular walls. CSF extravasation occurs across ventricular surfaces into periventricular white matter; however, the endothelial cell blood-brain barrier remains intact. There is increased extracellular fluid volume. Interstitial edema is accompanied by rapid decrease of myelin lipid content because of increased hydrostatic pressure resulting from extravasated CSF. CT findings include (1) the presence of hypodense

symmetrical dome-like structures in the periventricular white matter that are most prominent surrounding the anterolateral portions of the frontal horns; (2) gray matter appears normal and cortical sulcal spaces are not visualized; (3) frontal horns have a rounded configuration; (4) ventricles are dilated, including temporal horns and (5) abnormal enhancement is not seen. In patients with periventricular hypodensities that represent CSF flow impairment, these disappear following successful shunting. We have seen periventricular hypodensities in other patients whose isotope or metrizamide cisternogram did not confirm the diagnosis of impaired CSF ventricular circulation. These include multi-infarct dementia, senile dementia of the Alzheimer type and white matter degenerative processes.

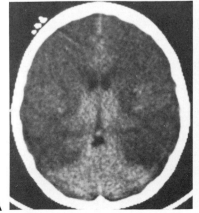
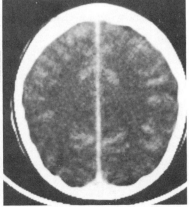

Figure 9–5. A 9-year-old asthmatic girl suddenly collapsed. She was rapidly ventilated but she remained comatose with fixed dilated pupils. *CT findings*: bilateral gray and white matter hypodense nonenhancing symmetrical hemispheric lesions (*A*) with sparing of subcortical nuclear masses and posterior fossa (*B*).

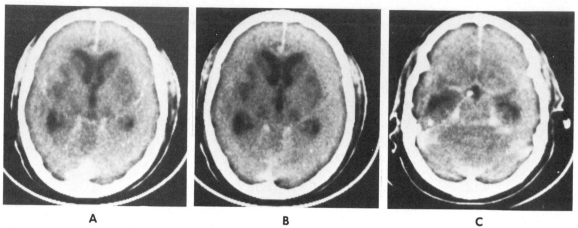

| A | B | C |

Figure 9–6. A 68-year-old man suffered cardiopulmonary arrest. He was comatose with fixed dilated pupils and absent caloric response. *CT findings*: ventricular enlargement with subcortical [ganglionic (A), thalamic (B)] sharply marginated hypodense lesions. Temporal horns are dilated with medial temporal and cerebellar hypodense lesions (C).

Herniation Syndromes

Descending Transtentorial

Certain supratentorial lesions expand rapidly to produce downward dislocation of the medial temporal region (uncus, hippocampus) through the tentorial incisura. Clinical features are (1) fixed and dilated pupil that has limited motion in medial and upward directions due to oculomotor nerve paresis (ipsilateral to lesion) (2) hemiparesis (contralateral to lesion) caused by cerebral peduncle compression against the tentorial notch, (3) altered mentation resulting from diencephalon and upper midbrain reticular activating involvement, (4) homonymous hemianopsia (contralateral to the lesion) caused by posterior cerebral artery compression. Angiographic findings[25] of descending transtentorial herniation include medial displacement and straightening of the anterior choroidal artery, and posterior communicating and proximal posterior cerebral arteries appearing displaced downward (lateral projection) and medially (anteroposterior projection). CT findings of transtentorial herniation include (1) distortion of the lateral aspect of the suprasellar cistern, (2) displacement of the brain stem toward the contralateral side with increase in the width of subarachnoid spaces between the mass and ipsilateral free tentorial edge, (3) medialstretching of the ipsilateral posterior cerebral

artery that is seen on enhanced scan, (4) occipital hypodense lesion representing infarction (Fig. 9–7), (5) brain stem hyperdense lesions representing hemorrhage, (6) distortion of the elongated U-shaped tentorial incisura and (7) contralateral temporal horn widening.[26, 27]

Ascending Transtentorial

Posterior fossa masses—especially those involving the superior cerebellar vermal region such as medulloblastoma, hematoma and metastases—may cause upward (ascending) herniation of the superior vermis and accompanying blood vessels through the tentorial incisura. This may cause midbrain compression. Upward herniation has been reported to occur immediately following ventricular drainage.[28] Clinical features of herniation may be difficult to differentiate from those directly caused by posterior fossa mass; therefore, there is no consistent pattern. This combination of clinical findings suggests the occurrence of upward herniation: (1) sequence of change from equal and briskly reactive pupils to anisocoria and then midposition fixed pupils, (2) the finding of vertical eye movements (pretectal compression) with intact horizontal eye movements, (3) progressively worsening level of consciousness, (4) neurogenic hyper-

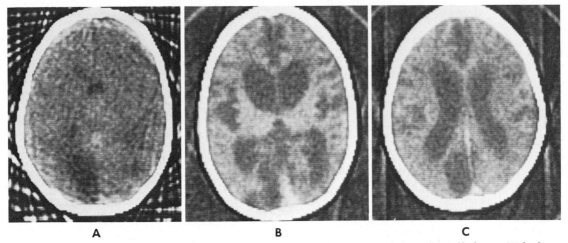

Figure 9–7. A 48-year-old woman suddenly became obtunded. Findings were bilateral papilledema. *CT findings:* ventricles and cisterns spaces are not visualized, with a left occipital sharply marginated hypodense lesion *(A)*. Despite treatment with corticosteroids and osmotherapy she suffered cardiac arrest. She remained in a chronic vegetative state. *CT findings:* marked ventricular and subarachnoid space *(B)* with left occipital hypodense lesion *(C)*.

ventilation and (5) motor dysfunction, e.g., decerebration, decortication, Babinski sign. Angiographic findings of ascending herniation include: (1) superior displacement of proximal segments of the superior cerebellar and posterior cerebral arteries, (2) stretching of these vessels as they course around the midbrain, (3) elevation of the precentral cerebellar, superior vermian and posterior mesencephalic veins.

CT abnormalities consistent with upward herniation vary with severity of the process. Detection of these abnormalities depends on the scanning plane extending fully through the tentorial and quadrigeminal posterior third ventricular region. Initial findings are caused by compression of the quadrigeminal cistern by the superior vermis; this CSF-filled structure appears flattened with posterior indentation. Superior and anterior displacement of the vermis by the lesion causes distortion of the superior cerebellar and quadrigeminal cistern such that the normal triangular-shaped area becomes effaced or square-shaped (see Fig. 7–15). There may be reversal of the shape of the normally posterior-convex quadrigeminal cistern. In the most advanced stage, there are these changes:

(1) effacement of superior cerebellar and quadrigeminal cistern,

(2) flattening or reversal of the curvative of the posterior third ventricle and

(3) severe obstructive hyprocephalus.[29]

Downward Tonsillar Herniation

This is usually caused by infratentorial lesions. The cerebellar tonsils herniate downward through the foramen magnum to compress the medulla. Associated obstructive hydrocephalus is usually present, exerting downward force at the tentorial notch to oppose the upward movement of the cerebellum. There is sudden respiratory and circulatory collapse. One angiographic finding of tonsillar herniation through the foramen magnum is inferior displacement of the tonsillar branch of the posterior inferior cerebellar arteries below the foramen magnum. A second finding is that hemispheric branches of the posterior inferior cerebellar arteries are stretched and pulled down below the foramen magnum as visualized on frontal projection. In the Arnold-Chiari malformation, tonsils may also extend several millimeters below the foramen magnum; however, this condition is better tolerated by the patient and does not invariably cause rapid clinical deterioration. Because of rapid clinical deterioration associated with tonsillar herniation, we have seen no examples of this with CT.

Subfalcine Herniation

Extension of the medial surface of the cerebral hemisphere may occur underneath the falx cerebri. This is most common with frontal and parietal lesions. They cause the anterior cingulate gyrus to be moved underneath the falx with these five abnormalities: (1) the frontal horn is compressed; (2) rotation and shift of the frontal horn occurs contralaterally; (3) the ipsilateral corpus callosum is depressed and the contralateral corpus callosum is elevated; (4) the ipsilateral anterior cerebral artery is stretched and shifted to the opposite side; (5) anterior cerebral artery infarction may result from compression against the free surface of the falx cerebri. Clinical features caused by subfalcine herniation cannot be differentiated from those resulting from the primary lesion. Angiographic findings are caused by displacement of the pericallosal and medial hemispheric arteries across the midline and underneath the falx cerebri. Frontal masses cause round shift of the anterior cerebral artery whereas parietal lesions cause square shift of the pericallosal branch of the anterior cerebral artery. As the cingulate gyrus is displaced under the falx, the callosomarginal branches are contralaterally displaced. CT characteristics of subfalcine herniation include (1) compression and rotation of frontal horns with displacement across the midline, (2) distortion or effacement of the anterior portion of the suprasellar cistern, (3) contralateral shift of the anterior cerebral artery, (4) cingulate gyral hypodensity, (5) marked stretching and bowing of the falx, (6) extension of the medial frontal hypodensity underneath the falx to the contralateral side and (7) frontal hypodensity consistent with anterior cerebral artery infarction.

REFERENCES

1. Levin BE: Spontaneous venous pulsations as an indicator of intracranial pressure. Neurology 27:346, 1977
2. Kahana L, Lebovitz H, Lusk W: Endocrine manifestations of intracranial extrasellar lesion. J Clin Endocrinol 22:304, 1962
3. Weisberg LA, Housepian EM, Saur DP: Empty sella syndrome as complication of benign intracranial hypertension. J Neurosurg 43:177, 1975
4. Zuidema GD, Cohen SJ: Pseudotumor cerebri. J Neurosurg 11:433, 1954
5. Kelly R: Colloid cysts of the third ventricle. Brain 74:23, 1951
6. Berg L, Rosomoff HL, Aronson N: The syndrome of increased intracranial pressure without localizing signs. Arch Neurol Psychiatr 78:498, 1955
7. Murphy JT, Gloor P, Yamamoto YL: Comparison of EEG and brain scan in supratentorial tumors. N Engl J Med 276:309, 1967
8. Weisberg LA: The syndrome of increased intracranial pressure without localizing signs: a reappraisal. Neurology 25:85, 1975
9. Yashon D, White R, Croft TJ: Midline posterior fossa neoplasms without lateral ventricular enlargement. JAMA 215:89, 1971
10. Weisberg LA, Nice CN: CT evaluation of increased intracranial pressure without localizing signs. Radiology 122:133, 1977
11. Buckman MT, Husain M, Carlow TJ: Primary empty sella syndrome with visual field defects. Am J Med 61:124, 1976
12. Weisberg LA: Benign intracranial hypertension. Medicine 54:197, 1975
13. Johnston I, Paterson A: Benign intracranial hypertension. Brain 97:301, 1974
14. Broddie HG, Banna M, Gradley WG: Benign intracranial hypertension: Survey of clinical and radiological features. Brain 97:313, 1974
15. Huckman MS, Fox, JS, Ramsey RG: Computed tomography in the diagnosis of pseudotumor cerebri. Radiology 119:593, 1976
16. Vassilouthis J, Uttley D: Benign intracranial hypertension: clinical features and diagnosis using CT and treatment. Surg Neurol 12:384, 1979
17. Hahn FJY, Schapiro RL: The excessively small ventricle on CAT of the brain. Neuroradiology 12:137, 1976
18. Weisberg LA: Computed tomography in benign intracranial hypertension. Comput Radiol (in press).
19. Rao KCVG, Knipp HC, Wagner EJ: Computed tomographic findings in cerebral sinus and venous thrombosis. Radiology 140:391, 1981
20. Buonanno FS, Moody DM, Ball MR, Lester DW: Computed cranial tomographic findings in cerebral sinovenous occlusion. J Comput Assist Tomogr 2:281, 1978
21. Segall HD, Ahmadi J, McComb JG, Zee CS: Computed tomographic observations pertinent to intracranial venous thrombotic and occlusive disease in childhood. Radiology 143:441, 1982
22. Zilkha A, Stenzler SA, Lin JH: Computed tomography of normal and abnormal superior sagittal sinus. Clin Radiol 33:415, 1982
23. Fishman RA: Brain edema. N Engl J Med 293:706, 1975
24. Drayer BP, Rosenbaum AE: Brain edema defined by cranial computed tomography. J Comput Assist Tomogr 3:317–323, 1979
25. Perrett LV, Margolis MT: Brain herniations. In Newton TH, Potts DG (eds). Angiography in Radiology of the Skull and Brain. CV Mosby, St. Louis, 1971, pp. 2671–2699
26. Osborn AG: Diagnosis of descending transtentorial herniation by cranial computed tomography. Radiology 123:93, 1977
27. Stovring J: Contralateral temporal horn widening in unilateral supratentorial mass lesions. J Comput Assist Tomogr 1:3, 1977
28. Cuneo RA, Caronna JJ, Pitts L: Upward transtentorial herniation. Arch Neurol 36:618, 1979
29. Osborn AG, Heaston DK, Wing SD: Diagnosis of ascending transtentorial herniation by cranial computed tomography. Am J Roentgenol 130:755, 1978

Chapter 10

NEUROBEHAVIORAL SYNDROMES

Patients with the clinical diagnosis of dementia may represent as many as 30 percent of admissions to psychiatric facilities.[1] These patients comprise 10 to 15 percent of neurological admissions; dementia is the second most common neurological discharge diagnosis. Patients who become demented demonstrate diffuse intellectual impairment, including defects in memory, orientation (they forget the time and where they are), adaptive capability, judgment, reasoning, and abstractive ability. Because of these intellectual deficits patients become incapable of handling financial responsibilities and are no longer able to live independently. Personality and behavioral disturbances (anxiety, agitation, depression, apathy, hypochondriasis and perplexity) may be early symptoms; acute psychoses and hallucinations may be later clinical abnormalities. In one study, one quarter of patients with organic dementia were initially diagnosed as having functional psychiatric disorders.[2]

Dementia has multiple etiologies.[3-5] Common etiologies include degenerative brain diseases such as Alzheimer's disease (50 to 60 percent), multi-infarct dementia (8 percent), normal pressure hydrocephalus (6 percent), intracranial masses (5 percent), alcoholic dementia (6 percent) and Huntington's disease (5 percent). Dementias occurring as part of diseases caused by transmissible agents (syphilis, fungal and viral diseases) are uncommon (2 percent) but important etiologies. Potentially treatable factors include drug intoxication and systemic disorders such as thyroid disease, pernicious anemia and liver and renal disease. In several studies 14 percent of patients with the initial diagnosis of dementia had a clinical course with response to antidepressant therapy and no subsequent intellectual deterioration; this is consistent with "depressive pseudodementia."[3,6] Twenty to 30 percent have potentially treatable disorders causing dementia.[7] This is more common in younger patients. Senile dementia of the Alzheimer type is most common in older patients.

In patients with suspected dementia, assessment of intellectual function is based upon clinical history and mental status examination. Formal psychometric evaluation may be necessary to confirm the diagnosis of dementia in some complicated cases. Metabolic studies to look for potentially treatable conditions are also necessary; however, positive results are obtained in less than 2 percent. EEG is utilized as a screening study. Focal slowing suggests intracranial mass lesion, and diffuse slowing with periodic burst of spikes is characteristic of Creutzfeldt-Jakob disease. EEG has limited value in the early stages of Alzheimer's dementia. It may be normal or mildly slow. The significance of mild diffuse slowing is not established because this may be seen in normal subjects, especially geriatric patients. However, demonstration on serial studies of change from a normal to a slow pattern is significant in the absence of drugs that may slow the EEG. Isotope scan has been utilized as a screen for focal lesions; however, this rarely shows abnormal uptake unless focal deficit is also present. Lumbar puncture is occasionally performed if an infectious-inflammatory disorder such as neurosyphilis or fungal meningitis is suspected. CT has replaced air studies, angiography and even EEG as routine study in the evaluation of patients with suspected dementia.

CONDITIONS ASSOCIATED WITH DEMENTIA

Alzheimer's Disease. This may develop in the presenium or senium (person older than

65 years). Memory loss and impaired reasoning and constructional ability are prominent features; seizures and focal neurological deficit are uncommon. Prior to the development of CT, diagnosis was established by air study findings of "walnut-like" brain with dilatation of ventricular and subarachnoid space (SAS).[8] There is an approximate correlation of severity of clinical dementia with degree of cerebral atrophy.[9, 10] However, there are normal patients who have air study evidence of enlarged ventricles, and many normal elderly subjects have widened sulcal space.[11, 12] In some patients with clinical and proved Alzheimer disease, air study shows no evidence of cerebral atrophy. Discrepancies between clinical and air study findings may result from two possible mechanisms: First, early brain damage may occur before pathological changes develop and second, technical factors. Ventricular and subarachnoid space size may be artificially dilated by air injection (pseudocortical atrophy). CSF space size may also be modified by dehydration or cerebral edema. Because patient discomfort and chemical meningitis were associated with air study, serial studies were usually not performed. This limited our air study results to those patients who showed definite evidence of dementia; therefore, some patients in early stages were probably not studied. With CT, it is now possible to obtain an initial early baseline study and subsequently compare *change* that develops in ventricular and sulcal space size.

With CT, several techniques are utilized to assess CSF space size.[13] These were linear measurements, planimetry measurements, CSF space volume determinations, and gray and white matter attenuation value determinations. The numerical gradient exists at the ventricular edge between pixels containing CSF and those representing brain tissue; however, edges may be obscured and ventricular size appear artificially small if pixels contain more brain parenchyma than CSF. Conversely, if pixels contain more CSF compared with brain tissue to lower average attenuation values, ventricles appear larger. Despite partial volume averaging, which may over- or underestimate CSF space size, and the potential problem of overestimation of ventricular size by air study, correlation between air study and CT measurements has been high.

Huckman analyzed ventricular and subarachnoid space size by linear measurements of the distance between the lateral portions of the frontal horns, the maximum lateral ventricular bicaudate width, and the width of the four largest cortical sulcal spaces. The results were classified: (1) normal, maximum ventricular span less than 15 mm with sulci less than 5 mm; (2) borderline atrophy, maximum ventricular size being 16 to 20 mm with sulci less than 5 mm; (3) mild atrophy, ventricles being 16 to 20 mm with sulci 6 to 9 mm; (4) moderate atrophy, ventricles greater than 20 mm with sulci 6 to 9 mm, or maximum ventricular size 16 to 20 mm and sulci larger than 9 mm and (5) severe atrophy, ventricles larger than 20 mm and sulci larger than 9 mm (Fig. 10–1). Patients with senile atrophy of the Alzheimer type showed more cerebral atrophy than nondemented subjects of the same age; how-

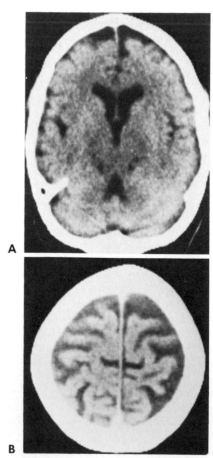

Figure 10–1. A 52-year-old man developed memory lapses and grandiose paranoid ideation. Examination showed evidence of organic dementia. Blood serology for syphilis was positive. CSF showed markedly elevated VDRL titer and protein content of 150 mg percent. *CT findings:* mild enlargement of the ventricles *(A)* with marked dilatation of extracerebral sulcal spaces *(B),* especially in the frontal regions. *Diagnosis:* general paresis.

ever, there was some overlap. There is no correlation between severity of dementia and CT measurements of atrophy. Eighty-five percent of patients without clinical dementia had borderline or normal measurements; however, 15 percent of normal subjects had CT findings consistent with mild or moderate atrophy. Of patients with clinical evidence of dementia, CT showed these results; normal, 20 percent; mild atrophy, 11 percent; moderate to severe atrophy, 60 percent; enlarged ventricles without enlarged sulcal spaces, 9 percent.[14] The clinical course of neurological deterioration was more rapid in demented patients with CT evidence of moderate or severe atrophy (Fig. 10–2).[15] If demented patients have normal-sized ventricles, this should lead to a thorough investigation for treatable toxic-metabolic conditions. However, in some demented patients who have potentially treatable conditions, CT showed cerebral atrophy. These abnormalities normalized following treatment of the underlying disorder (Fig. 10–3).

Other linear measurements such as septum pellucidum–caudate distance, third ventricular width, cella media width, bicaudate distance, and distance between the third ventricle and sylvian fissure have been determined in normal subjects.[16] These measurements are divided by the maximum transverse diameter of the skull along that particular region, e.g., the maximum distance between frontal horns divided by the maximum transverse inner diameter of the skull to establish the ventricular brain ratio.[17, 18] Other studies utilize the planimeter to measure ventricular size at the level of the foramina of Monro or bodies of the lateral ventricles. The intracranial area is measured by tracing the circumference of the inner table at that level of the brain. Ventricular size represents the ratio of ventricular to intracranial area. This was determined in normal subjects for each decade of life. There is a gradual increase between the second to sixth decade and then a dramatic increase in ventricular size after age 69. These changes are independent of change in cortical sulcal size.[19] Sources of errors with linear measurements and planimetry include: (1) small differences in attenuation values of ventricles and brain parenchyma, (2) irregularities in ventricular configuration, (3) significant photon noise levels and (4) nonhomogeneity of tissues.

Conflicting data exist for changes in supraventricular white matter attenuation values in dementia. In some patients with dementia,

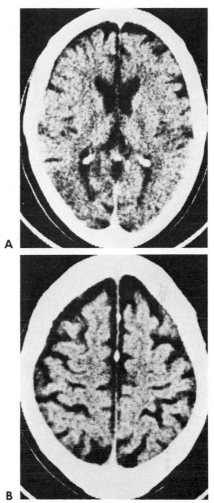

Figure 10–2. A 55-year-old man had increasing difficulty performing as an accountant. He had marked memory impairment and was very depressed. Neurological examination showed evidence of organic dementia without other neurological findings. *CT findings:* marked enlargement of ventricles *(A)* and basal cisternal and sulcal spaces consistent with presenile dementia of the Alzheimer type *(B).*

loss of gray–white matter discriminability has been reported at multiple levels, e.g., internal capsule at the level of the basal ganglia, supraventricular white matter at the level of the centrum semiovale and high parietal convexity.[20] (Discriminability is defined as visual differentiation between gray matter and white matter.) This finding has not been confirmed in all studies in which 8 mm sections and high resolution scanners have been used.

In our demented patients, linear CT measurements revealed these findings compared with control patients (matched for age and

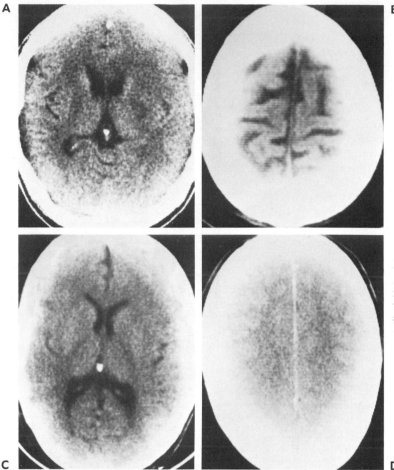

Figure 10–3. A 27-year-old woman became agitated, with paranoid ideation. She was acutely psychotic. Laboratory studies confirmed the diagnosis of hypothyroidism. *CT findings:* moderate ventricular *(A)* and subarachnoid space dilatation *(B)*. Following nine months of thyroid replacement therapy, she was neurobehaviorally normal. *CT findings:* normal ventricular *(C)* and subarachnoid space size *(D)*.

sex): (1) third ventricular–sylvian fissure ratio less than 0.59 (summation of right and left sides divided by intracranial width), (2) maximum frontal horn span greater than 20 mm, (3) four sulci larger than 3 mm, (4) bifrontal horn span intracranial ratio exceeding 0.40. Less reliable correlation was established for the number of enlarged cortical sulcal spaces; cella media width, intercaudate–internal skull diameter ratio.

With advancing age there is neuronal loss, degeneration of cell processes, increased number of senile plaques and neurofibrillary tangles. Cell loss is not uniform and there is maximal depletion in superior temporal gyrus. Brain shrinkage with age involves cerebral hemispheric gray and white matter; this causes a decrease in brain weight of 5 to 10 percent. Brain weight reduction is less than that of brain volume because there is an associated increase in brain water with age. Pathological changes in normal aging and Alzheimer's de-

mentia are similar—senile plaques, neurofibrillary tangles, granulovacuolar degeneration. Quantitative estimates of senile plaques correlates with intellectual deterioration; therefore, the number of senile plaques is usually small in intellectually intact elderly patients.[21] In these normal elderly patients, CSF space size markedly increases after the sixth decade.[19, 22–24] Attenuation values in supraventricular white matter decreases with advancing age.[25] This may result from primary change in white matter or secondary white matter phenomena caused by primary cerebral cortical tissue change. When assessing CT findings for CSF space enlargement caused by brain atrophy, certain variables must be considered. These include the age and sex of the patient, hemispheric asymmetries resulting from handedness, and associated neurological disorders such as effects of trauma or stroke. Lateral and third ventricular size is greater in men than in women.[26]

Normal Pressure Hydrocephalus (NPH).
This includes the clinical triad of *gait disturbance, incontinence and dementia.* Ventricles are symmetrically enlarged. CSF pressure is normal (but above 110 mm H_2O) and there is CSF circulatory impairment.[27] It is believed that impaired CSF circulation results from basal cisternal arachnoiditis. The specific etiologies include meningitis, subarachnoid hemorrhage, tumor, trauma and parenchymal degeneration (Alzheimer's disease). Occasionally, intracranial cysts or ectatic basilar artery aneurysm may cause CSF space compression. These two conditions may result in clinical and radiological findings to simulate NPH. Mental disturbances in NPH are varied. These include mental slowing, emotional apathy, shallow affect, memory loss, confusion and dementia. Gait impairment may be manifested by simple unsteadiness and dysequilibrium or apractic pattern. In severe forms, patients are unable to stand and have lower limb spasticity, hyperactive reflexes and Babinski signs. Incontinence may be either urinary or fecal. Patients are quite unconcerned about this incontinence. Headache is not characteristic of NPH because CSF pressure is normal. Clinical improvement may transiently occur after lumbar puncture; clinical deterioration frequently develops following air study.

When clinical features suggest a possible diagnosis of NPH, neuroradiographic studies are performed to confirm the clinical impression. Air study findings include: (1) diffuse symmetrical triventricular enlargement, (2) temporal horn dilatation, (3) nonvisualization of cortical sulcal spaces and (4) corpus callosal angle less than 120 degrees. Visualization of cortical SAS is dependent upon technical factors such as amount of air injected and head position during injection.

CT has replaced air study in the diagnosis of NPH. CT findings include: (1) symmetrical triventricular and basal cisternal enlargement, (2) bulbous and rounded shape of the frontal horns, (3) temporal horn dilatation (exceeding 2 mm), (4) nonvisualization of cortical sulcal spaces and interhemispheric fissure and (5) periventricular hypodense rims surrounding the frontal horns (Fig. 10–4). Ventricular size is greater in NPH than in atrophic processes (hydrocephalus ex vacuo). The findings of ballooned enlarged frontal horns, especially involving the temporal horn with third and fourth ventricular dilatation, is seen in 90 percent of patients with NPH but is less than

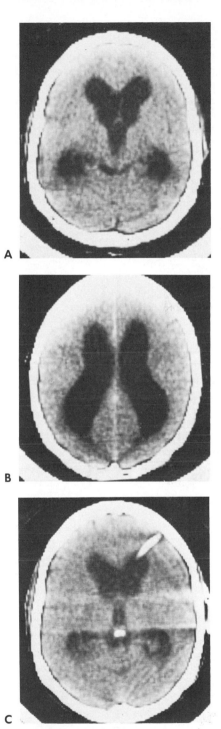

Figure 10–4. This 60-year-old woman became progressively demented but had no gait disorder. *CT findings:* bulbous enlargement of the frontal horns with triventricular enlargement *(A)* and dilated temporal horns. There are prominent basal cisterns (suprasellar, quadrigeminal) with nonvisualization of cortical sulcal spaces *(B).* Two months following diversionary shunt, she was clinically unchanged. *CT finding:* minimal change in CSF space size *(C).*

25 percent of patients with cerebral atrophy. In NPH, anterior portions of the lateral ventricles are enlarged more than posterior regions, whereas in cerebral atrophy, they are equally enlarged. Periventricular hypodensities may represent transependymal CSF resorption; these findings are consistent with active impairment of CSF circulation. These resolve after successful shunting procedures.[28]

Studies of CSF flow should complement CT to provide physiological data of CSF circulation. In the constant manometric infusion study, CSF is infused at twice the normal production rate (0.75 ml/minute) over a 90-minute interval and CSF pressure is recorded. In NPH, there is a sharp pressure rise that exceeds 300 mm H_2O. Interpretation may be difficult because normal values have not been established, especially for elderly patients. In patients with NPH, cisternographic studies (radionuclide, metrizamide) show early ventricular penetration by the tracer substance with persistent ventricular reflux; the tracer does not ascend over the parasagittal convexities. In normal subjects, cisternogram shows this sequence: (1) this tracer substance is initially seen in the basal cisterns, (2) cortical sulcal filling occurs by six hours, (3) there is minimal evidence of intraventricular metrizamide by 6 hours, (4) metrizamide blush is seen in convexity and parasagittal region by 12 hours. In NPH, persistence of metrizamide is seen in ventricles at 12 and 24 hours, and there is diminished cortical blush as metrizamide is not seen in cerebral sulcal spaces. It is not known if isotope or metrizamide cisternographic findings are more reliable indicators and prognosticators of clinical response to shunting in patients with NPH than is routine CT. Isotope cisternogram requires serial studies through 72 hours and there are 20 percent technical failures.

In some patients with clinical and neuroradiographic features of NPH, shunting is not followed by clinical improvement (Fig. 10–5). This may be related to surgical complication or associated brain atrophy. This is suggested by one report in which one third of patients who had air study evidence of NPH had CT and necropsy evidence of cerebral atrophy. However, there was no reported difference in clinical response to shunting in patients who had CT nonvisualization of cortical sulcal spaces compared to those with well-visualized cortical spaces.[29] Other patients who do not respond to shunting may have been adequately compensated. Favorable clinical response occurs in patients with these findings: (1) clinical triad of gait disturbance, incontinence and dementia is present, with gait abnormality being most prominent; (2) CT shows triventricular enlargement with temporal horn dilatation and periventricular hypodensities; (3) symptoms improve after lumbar puncture; (4) infusion studies show large pressure increment and (5) the patient has been symptomatic for fewer than six months.[30]

Vascular Disease. A common misconception is that atherosclerosis causes decreased cerebral perfusion, resulting in diffuse neuronal

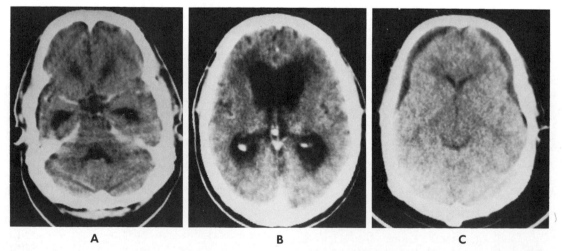

Figure 10–5. A 72-year-old man developed memory lapses and gait instability. CT findings: triventricular enlargement with temporal horn dilatation (A), periventricular hypodensities (B) and nonvisualization of sulcal spaces. Following shunt insertion, there was no clinical improvement. CT shows marked decrease in ventricular size with bilateral subdural hematoma (C).

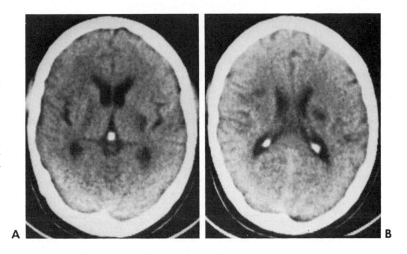

Figure 10–6. A 52-year-old hypertensive man had several prior stroke syndromes. He was demented with bilateral corticospinal tract findings and pseudobulbar palsy. *CT findings:* bilateral (right-sided, *A;* left and right, *B*) multiple lacunar infarcts with CSF space enlargement.

loss. Progressive intellectual decline and behavioral changes formerly were believed caused by "little strokes." These were believed to respond to vasodilating or anticoagulating drugs.[31] This belief is at variance with clinical-pathological realities. Clinical features of atherosclerotic multi-infarct dementia are distinct. These criteria establish the diagnosis: (1) history of systemic arterial hypertension; (2) multiple discrete episodes of sudden and usually focal neurological deterioration and (3) neurological findings of dementia and bilateral stroke syndrome (hemiparesis, pseudobulbar palsy, dysarthria and bilateral Babinski signs). In some cases multiple lacunar infarcts do not cause discrete clinical episodes, but they may summate to cause stepwise neurological deterioration.[32] We have studied 40 consecutive patients with the initial diagnosis of "arteriosclerotic dementia." In 15 cases, CT showed mass lesions or hydrocephalus; these were not disclosed by other neurodiagnostic studies. In 12 cases, CT showed diffuse but asymmetrical ventricular and cortical sulcal spaces; in seven of these cases there was superficial cortical or deep lacunar infarcts. It is sometimes difficult to differentiate multiple bilateral symmetrical enlarged cortical sulcal spaces from infarcts; however, if these superficial hypodense cortical lesions are symmetrical, this is consistent with the Alzheimer atrophic process. In nine cases CT showed multiple superficial and deep infarcts with marked asymmetry of the ventricular enlargement. In four cases, there were multiple deep lacunar infarcts with only mild ventricular enlargement (Fig. 10–6).

Subcortical arteriosclerotic encephalopathy (Binswanger's disease) is caused by involvement of the small arteries of the white matter and basal ganglia, whereas cortical vessels show less severe degenerative changes. Neuropathological findings include diffuse demyelination or focal necrosis. This is most prominent in the frontal or occipital lobes. Temporal evaluation is characterized by progressive deterioration with superimposed episodes of transient focal neurological deficit. Findings include dementia, seizures, pseudobulbar palsy and spasticity. CT findings include focal (frontal and occipital) hypodense lesions with irregular margination, minimal mass effect and no abnormal enhancement. The lesions are located in the cerebral white matter and frequently are bilateral. There may also be small basal ganglionic infarcts. The ventricles are usually enlarged. Cortical sulcal spaces are not prominent; this is consistent with relatively selective white matter involvement (Fig. 10–7). Differentiation from other white matter degenerative processes is not possible.[33]

INTRACRANIAL MASSES. CHRONIC SUBDURAL HEMATOMA (SDH). These patients may present with progressive intellectual deterioration.[34] There is usually associated focal neurological deficit; however, 20 percent of our patients had dementia without other neurological findings. The absence of signs of intracranial hypertension or focal neurological deficit in patients with dementia may falsely suggest Alzheimer's disease. In patients with chronic SDH, there are fluctuations in neurological condition. These changes reflect several possible mechanisms: (1) shifts in intracranial pressure, (2) intermittent vascular compression and (3) paroxysmal electrical activity; that is, seizures. Sudden clinical dete-

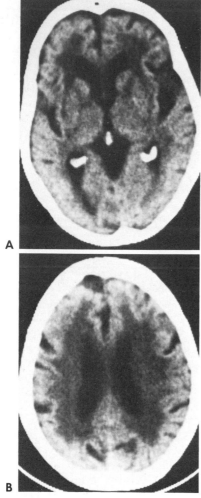

Figure 10–7. This 70-year-old woman developed progressive mental impairment. She had organic dementia and bilateral Babinski signs. *CT findings:* bilateral ventricular dilatation *(A)* with prominent periventricular hypodensities *(B)*. The cortical sulcal spaces are slightly enlarged.

rioration may simulate stroke syndrome, and in 10 percent of cases of chronic SDH, CT shows accompanying infarction.

Prior to development of CT, the diagnosis of chronic SDH was difficult to establish noninvasively. Skull x-ray may show no evidence of fracture or pineal shift. EEG findings may show focal delta activity with low-voltage pattern; however, EEG may be diffusely slow or normal. Isotope scan sometimes shows peripheral crescent-shaped uptake; this is best visualized on anterior-posterior projection. This uptake is believed caused by well-organized and highly vascularized peripheral membrane. Positive isotope scans correlated with the op-

erative finding of thick membrane. Angiography shows characteristic displacement of the peripheral cortical vessels inward away from the inner table to create an avascular region.

CT findings of chronic unilateral SDH include: (1) mass effect as manifested by ventricular compression, distortion and displacement; (2) nonvisualization of cortical sulcal spaces ipsilateral to the lesion; (3) isodense or hypodense similunar or concave-shaped lesion and (4) contrast enhancement sometimes developing in the medial capsule. The finding of small or "normal-sized ventricles" with loss of

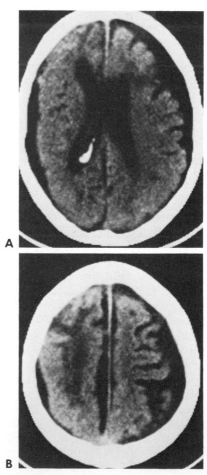

Figure 10–8. A 52-year-old man became confused following an automobile injury. He had marked memory impairment and right pronator drift. EEG and isotope scan were negative. *CT findings:* left hemispheric hypodense extracerebral lesion with compression of the left lateral ventricle *(A)* and effacement of the left sulcal spaces *(B)*. Surgical findings were consistent with liquefied chronic SDH. The hypodense lesion overlying the right hemisphere has medial interdigitation and no ventricular compression; this is consistent with cerebral atrophy and enlarged subarachnoid spaces.

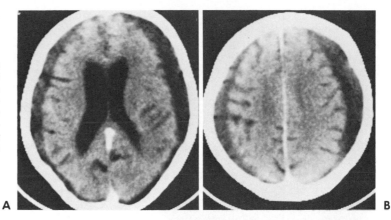

Figure 10–9. A 76-year-old man had an organic dementia with no abnormal neurological findings. EEG was diffusely slow. *CT findings:* bilateral hypodense extracerebral semilunar-shaped lesions *(A)* with ventricular dilatation *(B)*. *Operative finding:* subdural hygromas.

anterolateral divergence (straightening) in elderly patients is highly suspicious of chronic SDH (Fig. 10–8). If SDHs are bilateral and symmetrical in size and isodense-appearing, detection may not be possible by CT. However, it has been our experience that chronic SDHs are rarely equal in size or *completely* isodense. In some patients, it is difficult to differentiate the CT appearance of chronic SDH from enlarged extracerebral CSF-filled spaces, i.e., subdural, subarachnoid. The medial border of hypodense chronic SDH is smooth and may enhance; there is associated CSF space compression. In patients with hemispheric atrophy, the extracerebral spaces are enlarged. The hypodense lesions overlying the hemispheres have jagged-edged interdigitations. The enlarged CSF spaces are associated with ventricular dilatation, enlarged cortical sulcal spaces, and widened interhemispheric fissure. Subdural hygromas appear as hypodense semilunar-shaped extracerebral lesions. There is no contrast enhancement in the medial border. Mass effect is seen in almost all chronic SDHs; however, it is more variable and less marked with subdural hygromas (Fig. 10–9).

Neoplasms. These may represent the causative agent in up to 10 percent of demented patients, and many of these are benign lesions. In most patients with underlying neoplasms, other neurological abnormalities are present; however, occasionally no neurological signs occur (Fig. 10–10). Bifrontal neoplasms may cause personality change, apathy, euphoria, inattention, confusional states and memory impairment. Tumors of the anterior third ventricle and subfrontal and parasellar region may also cause dementia. Dementia may result from direct tumor compression or obstructive hydrocephalus. It is not always possible to

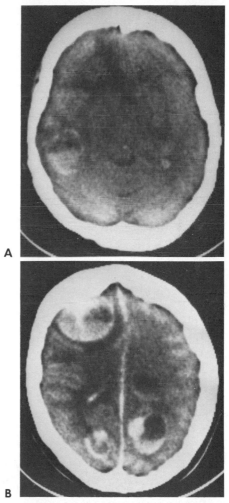

Figure 10–10. A 64-year-old woman developed memory loss and episodic confusion. For six months after diagnosis of Alzheimer's disease she had symptomatic treatment and no diagnostic studies were performed. Findings were organic dementia and right pronator drift. *CT findings:* multiple bilateral mixed-density *(A)* heterogeneous ring-enhancing lesions *(B)*. *Necropsy findings:* metastatic adenocarcinoma (primary neoplasm was never established, even at necropsy).

demonstrate a localizing neurological deficit in some demented patients, as in anosmia of a subfrontal lesion, bitemporal hemianopsia caused by a parasellar lesion, and mild hearing loss from CPA lesions. This is because of the limited attention span in some demented patients. Dementia may also result from diffuse tumor infiltration, e.g., reticulum cell sarcoma or gliomatosis cerebri.

Huntington's Disease. These patients develop chorea and mental deterioration. Mental changes may be primarily psychiatric, such as paranoia, psychosis and affective (manic-depressive) disorders, or patients may show signs of dementia. Pathological changes include degeneration of small neurons of the caudate and frontal-temporal cortex. Air study shows "squaring out" of frontal horns because of caudate atrophy and frontal sulcal space enlargement.

Sax and Menzer reported that in patients with clinical evidence of Huntington's disease, CT may demonstrate a reduced ratio of maximum frontal horn to intercaudate distance (less than 2.0). This is caused by caudate atrophy (Fig. 10–11). Cortical atrophy is also seen most prominently in the frontal-temporal region.[35] There is no correlation of severity of neurological deficit and CT abnormalities. No patient with Alzheimer's disease had CT findings similar to those seen in Huntington's disease.[36, 37] Because Huntington's disease is inherited as autosomal dominant, CT would be of high value if it showed abnormalities in patients who were clinically asymptomatic but subsequently developed clinical features of Huntington's disease. Unfortunately, this is not the case. Furthermore, in 10 percent of symptomatic patients, CT and gross necropsy show no caudate atrophy; however, microscopic examination shows small cell degeneration in the caudate. On the basis of preliminary experience, physiological disturbances in Huntington's disease may be most sensitively delineated by position emission tomography. CT has been a valuable screening study in those patients whose initial major manifestations of Huntington's disease are psychiatric; these patients have only minimal tic-like or choreiform movements (Fig. 10–12).

Pick's Disease. Patients may present initially with personality changes and behavioral disturbances; language and speech abnormalities develop at later stages. Memory loss and constructional impairment are less consistent findings than in patients with Alzheimer's disease. The characteristic pathological finding in Pick's disease is asymmetrical lobar atrophy. There is sclerosis involving the frontal and temporal lobes. This is more prominent in the left hemisphere. There is relative sparing of the superior temporal, parietal, and occipital cortex in Pick's disease. Lobar atrophy correlates with clinical features—left temporal (language and speech disturbances) and frontal (personality and behavioral changes). CT findings include: (1) dilated sylvian fissures with the left being wider than the right side, (2) widened interhemispheric fissure and dilated frontal CSF spaces, (3) temporal horn dilatation and (4) parietal-occipital sulci appearing smaller than frontal-temporal sulcal spaces.[38]

Alcohol Abuse. Several neuropsychiatric syndromes are associated with chronic alcohol abuse, including acute delirium tremens (see confusional states), withdrawal seizures, Wernicke's syndrome, Korsakoff's syndrome, alcoholic dementia and Marchiafava-Bignami disease.[39] Alcohol withdrawal seizures consist of single or multiple brief bursts of generalized seizures. These are maximal 96 hours after drinking is stopped. These seizures have no focal features; neurological examination and EEG show no focal abnormalities. Of patients with alcohol withdrawal seizures who showed focal neurological features either clinically or on EEG, 60 percent had focal lesions demonstrated by CT. If patients had no focal findings, only 4 percent had focal structural

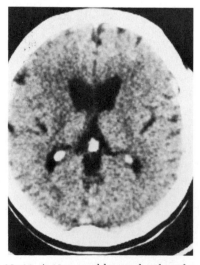

Figure 10–11. A 40-year-old man developed paranoid psychoses but no abnormal movements. His mother had had Huntington's disease. *CT findings:* abnormal shape of the frontal horn of the lateral ventricle caused by caudate atrophy.

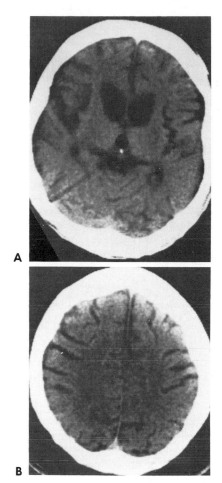

Figure 10–12. A 52-year-old man developed chorea and organic dementia with psychotic features. CT findings: squaring-out of frontal horns (A) with generalized ventricular and sulcal space enlargement (B).

pathological lesion. In one series of patients with alcohol withdrawal seizures, potentially reversible lesions were detected in 18 percent of patients with focal deficit as compared with only 1 percent of those without focal deficit.[40]

Wernicke's syndrome consists of the triad of global confusional state, ataxia and ophthalmoplegia. The confusional state may resolve; however, many patients develop residual amnesia (Korsakoff's syndrome). It is difficult to determine the natural course of memory deficit because many patients continue to drink. The prognosis for memory recovery has been reported as follows: (1) 20 percent recover completely, (2) 25 percent recover substantially but not completely and (3) 55 percent show minimal recovery. Pathological lesions causing amnesia involve mamillary bodies and dorsomedial thalamus. These lesions are not

detected by CT. An amnestic disorder identical to Korsakoff's syndrome may be seen with lesions of other etiologies such as encephalitis (herpes simplex), neoplasms, contusional injury, hypoxic-ischemic damage and bilateral hippocampal infarction.

Alcoholic dementia represents a slowly progressive disorder. It occurs in patients who drink heavily for 15 to 25 years. These patients usually manifest other alcohol-related neurological complications. Rapid deterioration may follow alcoholic binges. Pathologically, there is cerebral atrophy. This appears maximal in the frontal region. Neuropsychological studies in alcoholic patients have demonstrated significant intellectual capability impairment even if there is no clinically evident brain damage. These deficits improve if patients remain abstinent. Serial CT studies done on chronic alcoholics have showed cerebral atrophy. This is most prominent and commonly observed if CT is performed early in the abstinent period. It was sometimes "reversible" if the patient remained abstinent.[41, 42] This atrophic pattern may not result from the direct effect of alcohol; it may be caused by dehydration or protein depletion. Sequential studies need to be performed to correlate neuropsychological results and CT findings.

Infectious-Inflammatory Conditions. Neurosyphilis and chronic meningitis (fungal) are most frequent examples (see Chapter 12).

Progressive Multifocal Leukoencephalopathy (PML). This represents an inflammatory disorder caused by papovavirus. It occurs in patients with abnormal immune response, such as those with leukemia, lymphoma and other forms of cancer that are treated with cytotoxic drugs. The clinical syndrome is characterized by rapidly progressive encephalopathy or dementia. Other findings include visual hallucinations, visual field defect, seizures, spasticity and Babinski signs. The clinical pattern of PML cannot be distinguished from hematogenous tumor dissemination or other infectious-inflammatory processes in patients with underlying neoplasms. There are no neurodiagnostic studies that are specific for PML. Diagnosis is established by brain biopsy or necropsy examination; this shows multifocal demyelinated areas. These are most prominent in the parietal-occipital cerebral white matter. CT findings consist of bilateral hypodense irregularly marginated lesions located in the periventricular and corona radiata region (Fig. 10–13). They do not usually cause

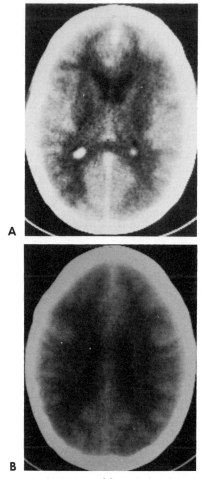

Figure 10–13. A 65-year-old man developed confusion and visual hallucinations. He was demented, with slurred speech and bilateral Babinski signs. *CT findings:* bilateral diffuse symmetrical hypodensities *(A)* seen throughout the white matter of both cerebral hemispheres *(B)*. Necropsy findings were consistent with progressive multifocal leukoencephalopathy.

mass effect or show contrast enhancement; however, rarely mass effect and enhancement are seen (Fig. 10–14).[43]

Creutzfeldt-Jakob Disease. This represents subacute spongioform encephalopathy. These patients develop dementing illness with associated myoclonus and pyramidal and basal ganglionic signs. EEG findings are quite characteristic; these consist of diffuse slowing with rhythmic bursts of triphasic slow waves synchronous with clinical myoclonic jerks. CSF shows no pleocytosis and cultures are negative.[44] CT findings include enlarged ventricles and cortical sulcal spaces, and hypodense lesions in the periventricular regions. As the clinical condition worsens, there is usually rapid progression in ventricular and cortical sulcal space size.

PSYCHIATRIC DISORDERS

In patients with neurobehavioral symptomatology to suggest primary functional psychiatric diagnosis, the possibility of underlying neurological or systemic condition must be investigated. This is necessary for two reasons: First, psychiatric patients may develop coexistent neurological or systemic diseases and second, psychiatric symptoms may be the initial indication of a neurological condition. In one series in which patients were referred for CT because of "psychiatric indications" (schizophrenia, other psychoses, depression and confusion), 4.8 percent had true positive CT findings with evidence of focal lesions that were believed to explain the neurobehavioral symptoms. These patients had focal neurolog-

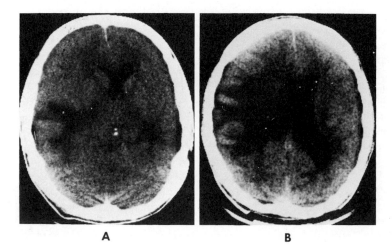

Figure 10–14. This 24-year-old man with stage IV B Hodgkin's disease was treated four years previously with irradiation and chemotherapy. In complete remission he developed headache, confusion and progressive right hemiparesis. Isotope scan showed a right temporal uptake; angiogram showed a temporal-parietal avascular mass. *CT findings:* marked left hemispheric mass effect caused by a large white matter hypodense lesion *(A)* with no abnormal enhancement but normal gyral enhancement *(B)*. Necropsy findings were consistent with leukoencephalopathy.

ical findings in addition to neurobehavioral symptoms. In 7.3 percent, CT showed focal lesions. These patients had normal neurological examination, and on the basis of clinical assessment it was probable that these represented incidental findings. Thirty-five percent of patients had CT evidence of cerebral atrophy, and CT was normal in 50 percent of patients. These findings suggest that CT should be utilized only in selected patients with neurobehavioral symptoms in whom neurological abnormalities are present as manifested by examination or EEG features.[45] In another study, the potential risk of over-reliance on CT findings was demonstrated. One patient had clinical features of affective (depressive) illness; however, diagnosis was influenced by CT findings of cerebral atrophy such that presenile dementia of Alzheimer type was considered more likely. Treatment of depression was delayed and inaccurate prognosis was given because reliance on CT findings outweighed clinical findings in this case.[46]

In patients who present with neurobehavioral symptoms with clear sensorium and normal neurological examination, we suggest that the following five features are appropriate indications for initial CT: (1) no prior psychiatric symptoms, (2) atypical age of onset for psychiatric condition considered most likely, (3) normal premorbid personality and behavior, (4) poor response to appropriate psychiatric treatment, (5) atypical clinical psychiatric features. Neurological symptoms such as seizures, dementia and confusion or abnormal neurological findings are obvious indications for CT. In patients with specific psychiatric diagnoses (schizophrenia, affective disorders), there have been conflicting reports of abnormal CT findings. Furthermore, there have been no analyses of serial CT findings in patients who have received specific psychiatric therapy such as electroconvulsive shock (ECT), antipsychotics and antidepressants.

Schizophrenia. This diagnosis is established by clinical criteria. These include: (1) abnormalities of thought process and perception, i.e., hallucination; (2) onset usually in adolescence and early adulthood and never after age 45, (3) continuous signs of illness for six months, (4) deterioration from prior level of vocational, educational and social functioning and (5) single or multiple acute psychotic episodes. There are no confirmatory diagnostic studies for this condition. There have been reports of abnormalities in schizophrenic patients, including evoked responses, cerebral blood flow, rapid eye movements and clinical neurological abnormalities.[47] On the basis of limited experience, air studies demonstrated ventricular enlargement, especially involving the third ventricle. This information is difficult to assess because of controversy concerning clinical diagnostic criteria. Necropsy studies have failed to demonstrate consistent abnormalities in chronic schizophrenic patients. CT studies have shown conflicting data in schizophrenic patients. Weinberger and Torrey reported enlarged ventricular size in 93 percent of chronic schizophrenics compared with controls.[48] Ventricular enlargement (ventricular brain ratio in which perimeters were measured with planimeter) did not correlate with patient age, duration of illness or impact of therapy (institutionalization, antipsychotics, ECT). Gluck et al. reported no difference in size of CSF-filled spaces in schizophrenic patients. In this study they utilized linear measurements, including maximal third ventricular width, anterior frontal horn width and number of enlarged cortical sulci.[49] Heath reported cerebellar vermal atrophy in chronic schizophrenic patients;[50] however, this study did not establish normal control subjects. It is important to determine if there are CT changes in chronic schizophrenia, because these patients may represent a subgroup who respond differently to antipsychotic drugs and whose prognosis is different from that of patients with normal CT.

Affective (Manic-Depressive) Disorders. CT may be of value in selected patients with initial onset of depressive symptoms in middle or later life. In certain patients depression is the major clinical manifestation of organic dementia. The presence of depressive symptoms may make clinical assessment of mental capability quite difficult.[51] The results of CT findings and psychometric testing results must be analyzed carefully. It is possible for psychological testing to be consistent with the primary affective disorder and for CT scan to show cerebral atrophy. In one study of elderly patients with affective disorders, there were patients with CT evidence of cerebral atrophy but no clinical dementia;[52] however, it is important to establish normal CT measurements in elderly patients. We have evaluated the clinical course of 20 elderly patients with depressive symptoms but no clinical evidence of dementia who had CT evidence of cerebral atrophy. These patients responded less completely and relapsed more frequently and rapidly than a similar group of patients with normal CT. Depressed patients with CT evidence of cerebral atrophy who are treated with antipsychotic drugs are more likely to develop dyskinesias than patients with normal CT. Serial studies in depressed patients with brain changes caused by ECT are in progress. Weinberger and Torrey noted that chronic schizophrenics who had received prior ECT had larger ventricles than those who had not received ECT.[48] It is not established if this is caused by schizophrenia or ECT.

Anorexia Nervosa.[53] These patients have an aversion to food and starve themselves. Patients suffer severe weight loss and appear emaciated. Clinical manifestations include bradycardia, hypotension, dry scaly skin, loss of scalp hair but usually normal body hair pattern; these changes appear to be caused by malnutrition. Endocrine studies show impaired gonadal function without evidence of hypopituitarism; however, skull x-ray and CT are sometimes performed in these patients to exclude hypothalamic-pituitary tumor. Air studies of patients with anorexia nervosa has shown cerebral atrophy; this abnormality has been confirmed by necropsy findings. CT has shown cerebral atrophy in some of these patients. This has reversed following adequate hydration and nutrition. The enlarged CSF spaces are believed to result from fluid collection in cerebral spaces resulting from malnourishment.

Acute Confusional States. These patients are disoriented; they have impaired sensorium and clouded consciousness. They may be lethargic or agitated and delerious. The severity of impaired sensorium may fluctuate throughout the day; it is usually most severe at night. Hallucinations may develop; these are usually visual or tactile but may be auditory. If the confusional state is caused by a focal pathological process, examination would be expected to show focal neurological signs such as hemiparesis, reflex asymmetry, Babinski sign, visual field defect, and intracranial hypertension signs including abducens nerve paresis and papilledema. However, there are some neuropathological conditions in which patients present with confusional state *without* focal neurological signs.

SUBARACHNOID HEMORRHAGE (SAH). Following aneurysmal SAH, some patients may become confused. This may result from diffuse cortical irritation by extravasated blood, diffuse vasospasm with cerebral ischemia, cerebral edema or hydrocephalus. These conditions are defined by CT and in these patients CT should precede lumbar puncture.

HYPERTENSIVE ENCEPHALOPATHY. There is an acute increase in systemic arterial blood pressure. Clinical features include headache, vomiting, visual blurring, seizures and confusion. There is impaired cerebral autoregulation that results in cerebral edema, petechial cerebral hemorrhage and microscopic cerebral infarction. CT may show ventricular and sulcal compression caused by cerebral edema, and excludes macroscopic parenchymal hematoma. Negative CT does not modify the clinical diagnosis or exclude gross cerebral infarction.[54]

BACTERIAL ENDOCARDITIS. Twenty to 30 percent of patients present with neurobehavioral manifestations. These are believed to result from microembolism, miliary abscesses or direct toxic effect.[55] In patients with bacterial endocarditis who present with encephalopathy, CT may show multiple abscesses, infarctions or hematomas.

CEREBRAL VASCULITIS. Neuropsychiatric disturbances are the most common manifestations of cerebral involvement in systemic lupus erythematosus. Patients may present with confusional states, psychoses, seizures or visual hallucinations. CT may show the abnormalities of multiple hypodense lesions representing multiple infarcts, cerebral atrophy and intracerebral hematoma (single or multiple).

ISCHEMIC VASCULAR DISEASE. Three ischemic vascular syndromes cause sudden onset of confusion without focal findings. Right middle cerebral artery branch occlusions cause acute confusional states. CT shows superficial parietal cortical ischemic-infarcted lesions.[56] Anterior cerebral artery occlusion causes ischemic damage in the cingulate, orbital-frontal and septal regions. These patients are quiet, apathic and inattentive. Primitive reflexes (snout, suck, palmomental) may be prominent. Posterior cerebral artery occlusion with occipital and hippocampal ischemic lesions may result in confusion, and these patients appear agitated. In another type of ischemic vascular lesion, patients become transiently confused and amnestic; this usually clears within 24 hours (transient global amnesia). This disorder is caused by bilateral posterior cerebral artery occlusion that results in bilateral hippocampal ischemia. Because symptoms resolve rapidly, CT usually shows no abnormalities.

FAT EMBOLISM. Following trauma with multiple bone fractures, confusion may develop. This may be secondary to hypoxia resulting from pulmonary embolism or fat embolism with cerebral infarction. CT may detect cerebral infarction; however, small fat droplets are not detected by CT.

Metabolic Encephalopathy. The majority of patients present with altered level of consciousness; however, some also develop focal neurological deficit. CT may be necessary to exclude an underlying pathological lesion in these latter patients.

NONKETOTIC HYPEROSMOLAR DIABETIC COMA. One third to one half of patients are initially diagnosed as having "acute stroke." There is experimental evidence that insulin may exacerbate cerebral edema and worsen neurological deficit.[57] Despite focal deficit developing in these patients, diagnostic studies and necropsy findings have shown no focal lesions. We have found CT to be normal in most cases; however, in 5 cases we have demonstrated a hypodense or isodense enhancing lesion consistent with ischemic vascular disease.

UREMIC ENCEPHALOPATHY. This results from renal impairment and associated metabolic abnormalities. Following dialysis, some of these patients become acutely confused and seizures develop (dialysis dysequilibrium syndrome). Abnormal mentation rapidly resolves within 48 hours; however, if confusion persists or focal neurological deficit develops, CT is necessary. Some dialyzed patients may develop intracranial hematoma caused by rapid intracranial fluid space shifts. These lesions are delineated by CT.[58] In some chronically hemodialyzed patients, encephalopathy develops (dialysis dementia). This is characterized by confusion, myoclonus and speech impairment. EEG shows marked slowing with superimposed spike bursts. CT has shown no characteristic abnormalities. Normal CT findings are consistent with minimal pathological findings reported in necropsy studies.

Cerebral Anoxia and Brain Death. If cerebral circulation is interrupted for several seconds or longer, brain oxygen is rapidly depleted. Following successful resuscitation, complete recovery may occur; however, in other cases cerebral hypoxia causes edema and ischemia. Postanoxic ischemia occurs following cardiac arrest in which cerebral blood flow has actually ceased. It is postulated that capillary swelling subsequently develops even if cerebral circulation is adequately restored. Ischemic brain damage may be diffuse or focal. This frequently occurs in border zone (watershed) regions such as anterior and middle cerebral arteries and posterior and middle cerebral arteries. Most pathological damage occurs in the cortical and subcortical gray matter, with relative sparing of the white matter. CT findings resulting from postanoxic ischemia reflect the effects of cytotoxic edema or cerebral infarcts. If neurological recovery occurs, CT usually shows no abnormalities. Following cerebral anoxia some patients rapidly recover consciousness but subsequently lapse into coma with spasticity, hyper-reflexia and positive Babinski signs. This delayed anoxia complication is postulated to be caused by cerebral white matter demyelination. CT may initially be normal. Follow-up CT may show bilateral symmetrical hypodense lesions located in the cerebral white matter.[59]

Cerebral death implies occurrence of irreversible loss of brain function. Clinical criteria for brain death include unresponsiveness, absence of spontaneous respiratory pattern and absent brain stem reflexes. EEG shows electrical silence. Radionuclide and angiographic studies show cessation of cerebral blood flow. In patients who show clinical signs of brain death CT has been performed to confirm impairment of cerebral blood flow and to determine causal intracranial lesion. CT findings in cerebral death may include failure of intracranial vessels (arteries, veins) to visualize on intravenous enhanced scan, and lack of enhancement of normal brain parenchyma.[60] With use of dynamic scanning following intravenous bolus injection of contrast, there is no enhancement and time-density analyses for multiple regions of interest show no increase in attenuation. The latter finding implies absent parenchymal perfusion.[61] In cerebral death, CSF-filled spaces may appear small because of cerebral edema.

REFERENCES

1. Malzberg B: Important statistical data about mental illness. In Handbook of Psychiatry, Vol 1. Basic Books, New York, 1959, pp. 161–174
2. Malamud N: Organic brain disease mistaken for psychiatric disorder: a clinicopathological study. In FB Benson and D Blumer (eds). Psychiatric Aspects of Neurologic Disease. New York, Grune and Stratton, 1975, pp. 287–305
3. Wells CE: Chronic brain disease: an overview. Am J Psychiatry 135:1, 1978

4. Strub RL, Black WF: Organic Brain Syndromes. FA Davis, Philadelphia, 1981, pp. 119–213

5. Marsden CD, Harrison MJG: Outcome of investigation of patients with presenile dementia. Br Med J 2:249, 1972

6. Post F: Diagnosis of depression in geriatric patients and treatment modalities appropriate for the population. In Depression. CDM Gallaut and CM Simpson (eds). Spectrum Pub., New York, 1976, pp. 205–231

7. Freeman F: Evaluation of patients with progressive intellectual deterioration. Arch Neurol 33:658, 1976

8. Huckman MS, Fox JH, Ramsey RG: CT in the diagnosis of degenerative diseases of the brain. Semin Roentgenol 12:1, 1977

9. Mann AH: Cortical atrophy and air encephalography: clinical and radiological study. Psychol Med 3:374, 1973

10. Gosling RH: Association of dementia with radiologically demonstrated cerebral atrophy. J Neurol Neurosurg Psychiatr 18:129, 1955

11. Nielsen R, Petersen D, Thygessen P: Encephalographic ventricular atrophy. Acta Radiol Diagn 4:240, 1966

12. Nielsen R, Petersen D, Thygessen P: Encephalographic cortical atrophy. Acta Radiol Diagn 4:437, 1966

13. Sabattini L: Evaluation and measurements of the normal ventricular and subarachnoid spaces by CT. Neuroradiology 23:1, 1982

14. Huckman MS, Fox J, Topel J: The validity of criteria for the evaluation of cerebral atrophy by CT. Radiology 116:85, 1975

15. Fox JH, Topel JL, Huckman MS: Use of CT in senile dementia. J Neurol Neurosurg Psychiatr 38:948, 1975

16. Gyldensted C: Measurement of normal ventricular system and hemispheric sulci of 100 adults with computed tomography. Neuroradiology 17:149, 1979

17. Brinkman SD, Sarwar M, Levin HS: Quantitative indexes of CT in dementia and normal aging. Radiology 138:89, 1981

18. Hughes CP, Gado M: Computed tomography and aging of the brain. Radiology 139:391, 1981

19. Barron SA, Jacobs L, Kinkel WR: Changes in size of normal lateral ventricles during aging determined by CT. Neurology 26:1011, 1976

20. George AE, de Leon MJ, Ferris SH: Parenchymal CT correlates of senile dementia. Am J Neuroradiol 2:205, 1981

21. Tomlinson BE, Blessed G, Roth M: Observations on the brains of demented old people. J Neurol Sci 11:250, 1970

22. Earnest MP, Heaton RK, Wilkinson WE: Cortical atrophy, ventricular enlargement and intellectual impairment in the aged. Neurology 29:1138, 1979

23. Roberts MA, Caird FI: CT and intellectual impairment in the elderly. J Neurol Neurosurg Psychiatr 39:986, 1976

24. Gonzalez CF, Lantier RL, Nathan RJ: CT scan appearance of the brain in the normal elderly population. Neuroradiology 16:120, 1978

25. Zatz LM, Jernigan TL, Ahumada AJ: White matter changes in cerebral computed tomography related to aging. J Comput Assist Tomogr 6:19, 1982

26. Haug G: Age and sex dependence of the size of

27. Huckman MS: Normal pressure hydrocephalus: evaluation of diagnostic and prognostic tests. Am J Neuroradiol 2:385, 1981

28. LeMay M, Hochberg FH: Ventricular differences between hydrostatic hydrocephalus and hydrocephalus ex vacuo by computed tomography. Neuroradiology 17:191, 1979

29. Jacobs L, Kinkel W: CT in normal pressure hydrocephalus. Neurology 26:501, 1976

30. Messert B, Wannamaker BB: Reappraisal of the adult occult hydrocephalus syndrome. Neurology 24:224, 1974

31. Alvarez WC: Little Strokes. Philadelphia, JB Lippincott Co., 1966, pp. 10–40

32. Hackinski VC, Lassen NA, Marshall J: Multiinfarct dementia. Lancet 2:207, 1974

33. Zeumer H, Schonsky B, Sturm KW: Predominant white matter involvement in subcortical arteriosclerotic encephalopathy. J Comput Assist Tomogr 4:14, 1980

34. McKissock W, Richardson A, Bloom WH: Subdural hematoma: a review of 389 cases. Lancet 1:1365, 1960

35. Sax DS, Menzer L: CT in Huntington's disease. Neurology 27:388, 1977

36. Barr AN, Heinze WJ, Dobben CD: Bicaudate index in CT of Huntington's disease and cerebral atrophy. Neurology 28:1196, 1978

37. Terrence CF, Delancy JF, Alberts MC: Computed tomography for Huntington's disease. Neuroradiology 13:173, 1977

38. Wechsler AF, Verity MA, Rosenschein S: Pick's disease. Arch Neurol 39:287, 1982

39. Victor M, Adams RD, Collins CH: Wernicke-Korsakoff syndrome. Philadelphia, FA Davis, 1971

40. Feussner JR, Linfors EW, Blessing CL: CT brain scanning in alcohol withdrawal seizures: the value of the neurological examination. Ann Intern Med 94:519, 1981

41. Fox JH, Ramsey RG, Huckman MS: Cerebral ventricular enlargement: chronic alcoholics examined by CT. JAMA 236:365, 1976

42. Lishman WA: Cerebral disorder in alcoholism. Brain 104:1, 1981

43. Carroll BA, Lane B, Norman D: Diagnosis of progressive multifocal leukoencephalopathy by CT. Radiology 122:137, 1977

44. Krishna Rao CVG, Brennan TG, Garcia JH: CT in the diagnosis of Creutzfeldt-Jakob disease. J Comput Assist Tomogr 1:211, 1977

45. Larson EB, Mack LA, Watts B: Computed tomography in patients with psychiatric illness: advantage of a "rule-in" approach. Ann Intern Med 95:360, 1981

46. Wells LE, Duncan GW: Danger of overreliance on computerized cranial tomography. Am J Psychiatr 134:811, 1977

47. Baldessarini RJ: Schizophrenia. N Engl J Med 297:988, 1977

48. Weinberger DR, Torrey F: Neophytides. Lateral cerebral ventricular enlargement in chronic schizophrenia. Arch Gen Psychiatr 36:735, 1979

49. Gluck E, Radu EW, Mundt C, Gerhardt P: A computed tomographic prolective trohoc study of chronic schizophrenics. Neuroradiology 20:167, 1980

50. Heath RG, Franklin DE, Shraberg D: Gross pathology of the cerebellum in patients diagnosed and treated as functional psychiatric disorders. J Nerv Ment Dis 167:585, 1979
51. Post F: Dementia, depression and pseudodementia. *In* Psychiatric Aspects of Neurologic Disease. DF Benson and D Blumer (eds). Grune and Stratton, New York, 1975, pp. 99–120
52. Jacoby RJ, Levy R: Computed tomography in the elderly. 3. Affective disorders. Br J Psychiatr 136:270, 1980
53. Enzmann DR, Lane B: Cranial computed tomography in anorexia nervosa. J Comput Assist Tomogr 1:410, 1977
54. Rail DL, Perkin GD: Computerized tomographic appearance of hypertensive encephalopathy. Arch Neurol 37:310, 1980
55. Jones HR, Siekert RG, Geraci JE: Neurological manifestations of bacterial endocarditis. Ann Intern Med 71:28, 1969
56. Mesalum MM, Waxman SG, Geschwind N: Acute confusional states with right middle cerebral artery infarctions. J Neurol Neurosurg Psychiatr 39:84, 1977
57. Arieff AI, Caroll HJ: Nonketotic hyperosmolar coma with hyperglycemia. Medicine 51:73, 1972
58. Leonard A, Shapiro FL: Subdural hematoma in regularly hemodialyzed patients. Ann Intern Med 82:650, 1975
59. Yagnik P, Gonzalez C: White matter involvement in anoxic encephalopathy in adults. J Comput Assist Tomogr 4:788, 1980
60. Arnold H, Kuhne D, Rohr W, Heller M: Contrast bolus technique with rapid CT scanning: a reliable diagnostic tool for the determination of brain death. Neuroradiology 22:129, 1981
61. Handa J, Matsuda M, Matsuda I: Dynamic computed tomography in brain death. Surg Neurol 17:417, 1982

Chapter 11

DIZZINESS AND HEARING IMPAIRMENT

Acoustic neurinomas represent 8 to 10 per cent of primary intracranial tumors. Ten per cent of patients with unilateral hearing loss are found to have acoustic neurinomas. Early diagnosis represents a challenging diagnostic problem. These tumors usually arise from the peripheral portion of the acoustic or vestibular division of the 8th nerve located within the internal acoustic canal; they may extend intracranially to the cerebellopontine angle (CPA) cistern. Less frequently, these tumors originate in the posterior fossa. The tumors are sometimes several centimeters in size before they become symptomatic. In patients with von Recklinghausen's disease, bilateral acoustic neurinomas may develop; these may occur in association with other supra- or infratentorial tumors such as meningiomas and gliomas.

The most common early symptoms of CPA tumors are otological.[1, 2] These are caused by compression of the auditory or vestibular branches of the 8th nerve; vascular compromise of the nerve may be a contributing factor. Hearing loss is the most common symptom (97 per cent); it is the initial disturbance in 67 percent. The next most frequent symptoms are dysequilibrium and unsteadiness (70 to 80 percent) resulting from disturbed vestibular function; however, true vertigo is rarely described by patients. The feeling of unsteadiness frequently occurs following rapid changes in head position.

Tinnitus is present in 70 percent of patients with small tumors; this symptom may be caused by impaired vestibulospinal reflexes. This results in cervical paraspinal muscle contraction, a reaction that represents an attempt to accommodate the barrage of aberrant vestibular impulses. In patients with large tumors, headache may be a manifestation of intracranial hypertension. Retroauricular pain

or paresthesias is believed caused by nervus intermedius involvement.

As an acoustic neurinoma expands into the posterior fossa, sensory trigeminal nerve dysfunctions (trigeminal neuralgia, facial numbness and paresthesias) are the earliest symptoms. The corneal reflex is unilaterally depressed. In patients with trigeminal neuralgia (tic douloureux) who have such abnormal neurological findings as abnormal corneal reflex, nystagmus, ophthalmoplegias and gait unsteadiness, neurodiagnostic investigation is necessary to exclude a posterior fossa lesion. However, patients with trigeminal neuralgia without abnormal neurological findings are much less likely to have an underlying mass lesion. Other symptoms of acoustic neurinomas are caused by obstructive hydrocephalus or brain stem or cerebellar compression; these include headache, vomiting, gait disturbance and altered mentation.

Neurological examination is usually normal in patients with small acoustic neurinomas; however, one third of patients with intracanalicular tumors have horizontal nystagmus. Peripheral facial weakness is present in 10 percent of patients, but the corneal reflex is abnormal in one third of patients. Hearing tests (pure tone audiometry and speech discrimination studies) and auditory (brain stem) evoked potentials are sensitive indicators of auditory nerve function; these are abnormal in 80 to 96 percent of patients with acoustic neurinomas.[1, 3] Caloric testing is the best indicator of vestibular nerve function; it is abnormal in 90 percent of patients with acoustic neurinomas.[4, 5] As the tumor expands into the CPA, neurological findings include abnormal corneal reflex and trigeminal distribution hypoesthesia. As the tumor expands within the posterior fossa, neurological abnormalities include abducens nerve paresis, limb and gait ataxia, papilledema and Babinski sign.

Diagnostic evaluation for patients who present with otological symptoms initially involves petrous bone x-rays. Small intracanalicular tumors are most reliably detected by plain skull x-ray; this demonstrates abnormalities in 70 to 95 percent.[6, 7] Multiple views including Stenver and Towne projections are most sensitive in detecting petrous bone asymmetries; however, these should be supplemented by petrous bone tomography. The characteristic radiographic finding of acoustic neurinoma is widening of the internal auditory canal; asymmetry of greater than 2 mm is consistent with tumor. There is usually bone erosion, but in 4 percent of patients with acoustic neurinomas this may be seen without canal widening. In some cases petrous bone roentgenograms are falsely positive and the presence of acoustic tumor is not confirmed by subsequent contrast studies. In rare instances, acoustic neurinomas originate in the posterior fossa and cause no abnormalities of the internal auditory canal, but there is radiographic evidence of intracranial hypertension.

Radiological contrast of the internal acoustic canal region is inherently high. This is because of the nature of the dense petrous bone, the mastoid air cells, and the CSF within the CPA cistern. This characteristic makes possible a high degree of spatial resolution with fourth-generation CT scanners such that anatomical detail for structures as small as 0.6 mm is possible in this region.[8, 9]

Several modifications of technique are necessary for high-resolution petrous bone CT. These include very thin collimation utilizing 2 mm tissue sections that reduces partial volume averaging, and algorithm that extends the range of attenuation values to 4000 H.U. With

this technique internal acoustic canals may be assessed (Fig. 11–1). The widened internal acoustic meatus appears as an angular or funnel-shaped bone defect on the medial aspect of the petrous pyramid (Fig. 11–2). The initial erosive change occurs in the posterior wall; this is optimally seen with coronal views. With optimal scanning technique it may be possible to detect tumors 0.5 cm^3 in volume, and to detect intracanalicular acoustic neurinomas with minimal (less than 5 mm) extension into the CPA cistern.[10] With high-resolution CT, bone abnormalities are seen in 77 percent of acoustic neurinomas.

Plain and intravenous contrast medium–enhanced CT is quite sensitive in detecting acoustic neurinomas that extend into the posterior fossa. If there is more than 1.5 cm extension into CPA, CT is 95 percent accurate. CT diagnosis of a CPA mass is based upon both direct findings (abnormal soft-tissue density characteristics, enhancement pattern) and indirect findings (fourth ventricular mass effect, posterior fossa cisternal asymmetries). CT criteria for diagnosis of an extra-axial posterior fossa mass include: (1) displacement of normal brain parenchyma away from bone with widening of the adjacent cisterns (CPA, ambient, quadrigeminal); (2) erosion or destruction of bone; (3) contiguity of the mass to the petrous bone; (4) extension of the mass upward through the tentorium; (5) characteristics of the lesion such as sharp margination and shape (flat, broad-based, triangular) and (6) the presence of a surrounding hypodense rim.[11] Certain small intracanalicular tumors that extend into the posterior fossa appear as enhancing lesions within the fluid-filled CPA cistern.

If the intravenous contrast medium–enhanced CT study is negative, gas (air) cisternography should be performed.[12, 13] The pres-

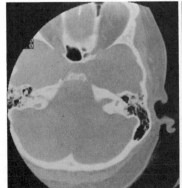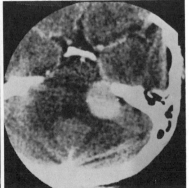

Figure 11–1. A 39-year-old woman developed right-sided hearing loss. Findings were trigeminal hypoaesthesia and decreased corneal reflex. *CT findings*: enlarged internal acoustic meatus *(A)* with isodense homogeneous enhancing CPA mass *(B)*.

A

B

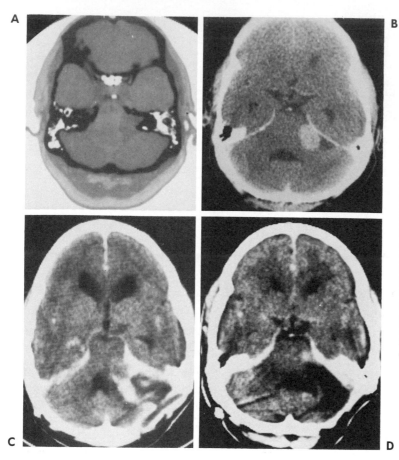

Figure 11–2. A 48-year-old man developed vertigo, gait instability and headache. Findings were right-sided deafness, right limb and gait ataxia and papilledema. *CT findings*: markedly enlarged right auditory canal *(A)* with an isodense enhancing mass in the CPA and slight distortion of the fourth ventricle *(B)*. Two weeks following surgical resection of acoustic neurinoma, he had no papilledema and minimal ataxia. *CT findings*: ring-enhancing CPA lesion with slight distortion of the fourth ventricle *(C)*. Six months later, he had minimal ataxia. *CT findings*: hypodense lesion in the right CPA with midline enlarged fourth ventricle *(D)*.

ence of gas that completely fills the internal auditory canal excludes the diagnosis of an acoustic tumor (Fig. 11–3). With gas cisternogram, it is usually possible to visualize the intracisternal portion of the facial and auditory nerves as they extend from the CPA cistern toward the internal auditory canal. The loop of the anterior-inferior cerebellar artery is sometimes also identified as it extends into the internal auditory meatus. The finding that air does not completely fill the internal auditory canal is consistent with intracanalicular acoustic tumor. If air outlines the CPA, hyperdense-enhancing tumor may be well visualized even if it was not initially seen on intravenous contrast medium–enhanced CT (Fig. 11–4). This is because air provides a high degree of contrast resolution within the CPA cistern. Technical failures are uncommon with air cisternography. At this time, there have been no diagnostic errors reported with this technique.

Another technique for demonstrating acoustic tumors is cisternography with metrizamide or Pantopaque; however, the use of these is not as safe or reliable as air-CT cisternography. Nonfilling of the canal with Pantopaque may falsely suggest acoustic tumor. It may be caused by arachnoiditis, swelling of the vestibular ganglion, narrow internal auditory canal, inflammatory changes of the vestibular nerve, or anterior–inferior cerebellar arterial loop projecting into the internal auditory meatus. This technique has been effective in detecting small (4 mm) tumors, some of which do not show radiographic enlargement of the canal.[14] If a CPA lesion is present, metrizamide cisternography shows these abnormalities: (1) filling defect of the CPA cistern, (2) widening of the CPA and ambient cisterns, (3) contralateral shift of the brain stem and (4) displacement of the fourth ventricle. Metrizamide may be superior for outlining cystic lesions (arachnoid, epidermoid); however, it is less sensitive than air-CT study for detecting intracanalicular acoustic neurinomas.[15] This is because hyperdense metrizamide provides less effective contrast relative to hyperdense bone than can be achieved with hypodense air.

In patients with suspected CPA lesions,

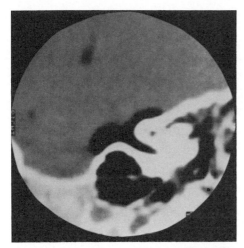

Figure 11–3. This 48-year-old woman developed progressive right-sided sensorineural hearing loss. She had decreased caloric response. Petrous bone tomograms and intravenous enhanced CT showed no abnormality. Air-CT cisternogram shows air outlining the internal auditory canal and CPA cistern.

owing to the presence of opposing vector forces. Angiography may reflect the resultant summation of these vascular displacements rather than individual vector forces.[17]

If the lesion causing vestibular or hearing impairment originates in the internal auditory canal, acoustic neurinoma is the most likely pathological lesion. Eighty percent of CPA lesions are acoustic neurinomas; the remaining 20 percent consists of other lesions. One half of these other tumors are meningiomas; less common lesions include metastases, chordoma, cholesteatoma, arachnoid cyst, arachnoiditis, granuloma (sarcoid, tuberculoma) and vascular lesion (angioma, aneurysm). In addition, tumors that originate in the fourth ventricle (ependymoma, medulloblastoma, choroid plexus papilloma), cerebellum or brain stem may grow eccentrically and exophytically into the CPA cistern to simulate acoustic neurinoma.[18]

vertebral angiography is usually reserved for special situations: (1) suspicion of a vascular lesion (angioma or aneurysm), (2) presence of intracranial hypertension that contraindicates lumbar puncture and cisternal contrast studies, (3) suspicion of a large tumor such that information concerning tumor blood supply is necessary for a surgical procedure. In approaching large acoustic neurinomas, it is crucial to demonstrate angiographically the course of vessels traversing the tumor. This is necessary to avoid the complication of brain stem hemorrhage or infarction resulting from surgical damage to the cerebellar arterial branches or draining petrosal veins.[16]

The angiographic diagnosis of extra-axial CPA tumor is based upon characteristic vascular displacements: (1) posterior displacement of the basilar and superior cerebellar arteries and anterior pontomesencephalic vein, (2) stretching and vertical displacement of the anterior cerebellar artery, (3) elevation of the petrosal vein and (4) posterior displacement of the hemispheric branches. A transient faint tumor stain may be seen in acoustic neurinomas, but the presence of markedly enlarged supplying and draining vessels with intense prolonged stain is more characteristic of meningioma or metastases. If the tumor originates in the fourth ventricle, cerebellum or brain stem and secondarily extends into the CPA, angiographic findings may be confusing

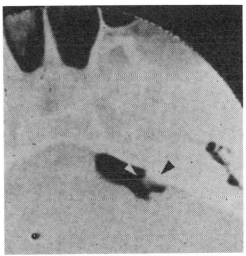

A

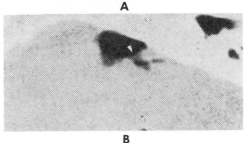

B

Figure 11–4. Air-CT cisternogram shows soft tissue mass extending into the air-filled CPA cistern from the internal acoustic canal (A). A section 2 mm lower shows inferior displacement of the facial and acoustic nerve (small white arrowhead) by the mass (B). With permission of Dr. T. Naidich, Laryngoscope 90:526, 1980.

Acoustic Neurinomas

These tumors appear isodense (60 percent) or hypodense (40 percent). The hypodense region may reflect cyst formation. The cyst may be surrounded by a thin hyperdense rim, which is maximally visualized on intravenous contrast medium-enhanced study. The central portion of the lesion may contain very low density components including negative values; this is suggestive of cyst formation containing xanthomatous (fat) material. Acoustic neurinomas are usually round in shape; less commonly, they appear triangular with the base flattened and directed toward the petrous bone. Extension is usually posterior and me-dial and, rarely, upward through the tentorium. The smaller acoustic tumors extend from the internal acoustic meatus into the CPA cistern. Larger tumors may either efface or widen the contiguous cistern (CPA, ambient, quadrigeminal). This cisternal widening is caused by compression of the normal brain parenchyma. Large tumors cause mass effect as manifested by distortion (flattening, tilting) or displacement (rotation, contralateral shift) of the fourth ventricle. Obstructive hydrocephalus caused by compression of the fourth ventricle is present in one half of acoustic neurinomas; however, only 10 percent have clinical evidence of intracranial hypertension.[19]

Most acoustic neurinomas show contrast enhancement. The pattern is usually round dense homogeneous enhancement (Fig. 11–5). Less commonly, enhancement occurs only in the peripheral rim; this pattern is seen with cystic neoplasms. The acoustic neurinomas show maximal enhancement immediately after infusion; this rapidly decreases by one hour. This pattern is contrasted with meningiomas, in which there is maximal enhancement one to three hours following infusion; however, this distinction is not reliable in the differential diagnosis (Fig. 11–6). The acoustic neurinoma appears surrounded by a hypodense rim in 10 to 25 percent of these lesions; this finding is more common in tumors that are larger than 3.0 mm. The hypodense rim is more characteristic of meningiomas (80 percent).

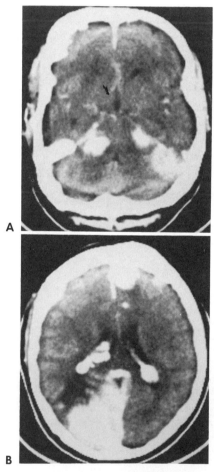

Figure 11–5. A 39-year-old man developed bilateral hearing loss. He had several small cafe-au-lait spots. He had bilateral absent caloric responses with radiographic evidence of petrous bone erosion. CT findings: bilateral enhancing CPA lesions (A) (surgically confirmed acoustic neurinomas) with right frontal, left occipital, intraventricular and right posterior fossa-enhancing (B) lesions, all of which were pathologically confirmed to represent meningiomas.

Trigeminal Neurinomas

These tumors arise from the Schwann sheath cells (schwannomas). Those originating from the gasserian ganglion are located in the middle fossa and are extradural; those arising from the trigeminal nerve are located in the posterior fossa and are intradural. Some tumors originate in one location and extend into the other fossa. Initial symptoms of middle fossa neurinomas include facial paresthesias or trigeminal neuralgia. Patients with posterior fossa neurinomas frequently present with facial paresis, hearing loss and ataxia.

Characteristic skull radiographic findings are scalloped erosion of the medial portion of the petrous bone without enlargement or bone destruction of the internal auditory canal. The lesion may be hypodense, isodense or hyperdense on noncontrast CT. It is rarely calcified. There is dense homogeneous sharply margin-

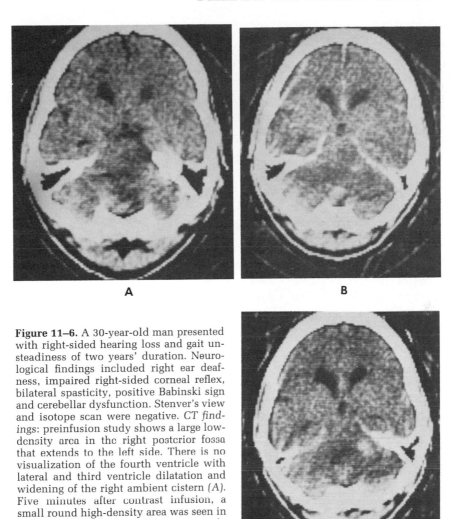

Figure 11–6. A 30-year-old man presented with right-sided hearing loss and gait unsteadiness of two years' duration. Neurological findings included right ear deafness, impaired right-sided corneal reflex, bilateral spasticity, positive Babinski sign and cerebellar dysfunction. Stenver's view and isotope scan were negative. CT findings: preinfusion study shows a large low-density area in the right posterior fossa that extends to the left side. There is no visualization of the fourth ventricle with lateral and third ventricle dilatation and widening of the right ambient cistern (A). Five minutes after contrast infusion, a small round high-density area was seen in the right CPA (B); however, repeat study one hour later showed more definite enhancement (C). Operative finding: CPA meningioma.

ated enhancement. The lesion appears confluent with the apex of the posterior petrous pyramid. The tumor may extend through the tentorium with distortion of the quadrigeminal cistern and elevation of the posterior third ventricle.[20]

Meningiomas

These tumors originate from the arachnoid villi of the venous sinus in the petrous portion of the temporal bone. The clinical findings may be identical to those of acoustic neurinomas; however, hearing loss is less severe and intracranial hypertension is more likely with meningiomas. Other unique characteristics of CPA meningiomas include: (1) petrous bone radiography shows hyperostosis or calcification, and the internal acoustic canal is normal; (2) isotope scan is frequently positive and (3) vertebral angiogram may show vascular stain pattern, and feeding vessels are derived from dural vessels.

CT findings of CPA meningiomas are quite distinctive. On noncontrast scan there is a round hyperdense broad-based lesion that is contiguous with bone. This may be a speckled-homogeneous or heterogenous-hyperdense lesion with interspersed calcified portions. Following contrast infusion there is usually dense homogeneous consolidated enhancement. Meningiomas that have undergone lipomatous degeneration may show dense homogeneous enhancement but with interspersed hypo-

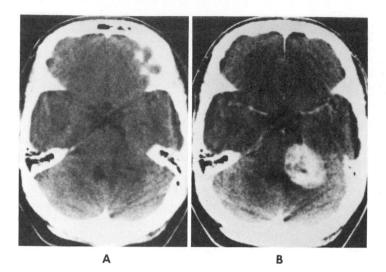

A   **B**

Figure 11–7. A 49-year-old developed left-sided facial numbness and hearing loss. Findings included right-limb ataxia and impaired corneal reflex. Skull x-ray showed enlarged and eroded porus acousticus. *CT findings:* right CPA hypodense lesion with enlargement of the ambient and CPA cistern *(A)*. There is dense nonhomogeneous round enhancement *(B)*. *Operative findings:* meningioma with lipomatous degeneration.

dense regions (Fig. 11–7). This pattern may simulate cystic acoustic neurinomas. The meningioma is sharply marginated and frequently (80 percent) surrounded by a hypodense rim. This probably represents focal atrophy rather than edema. It may be round in shape; less frequently, it appears comma-shaped as it grows upward through the tentorium to the dorsum sella. Meningiomas that are located directly contiguous with the internal acoustic meatus may enlarge this structure; however, the center of the tumor is located anterior to porus acousticus in more than 50 percent of cases. The following CT features strongly favor the diagnosis of meningioma: (1) peritumoral calcification, (2) center of the tumor located anterior to the porus acousticus, (3) extension of tumor upward and frequently above the tentorium and (4) oval or comma-shaped tumor with broad attachment to bone.[21]

Cholesteatomas

Primary cholesteatomas arise from congenital epithelial rests. They present as a lateral CPA or midline posterior fossa mass. Frequently these tumors initially compress the facial and then the acoustic nerve. These tumors are multilobulated. They contain fat and calcified elements. The CT finding is that of a homogeneously hypodense nonenhancing sharply marginated lesion. Because of fat content, density characteristics may include negative values.

Dermoid or Epidermoid Tumors

These congenital tumors occur laterally in the CPA or are midline in location. These are

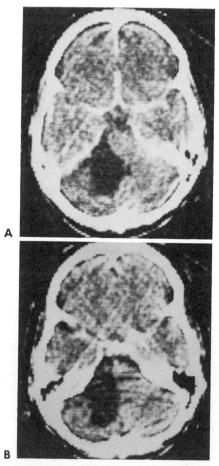

A

B

Figure 11–8. A 33-year-old woman noted impaired hearing in her left ear. Findings included left-limb ataxia and rotatory and horizontal nystagmus. Skull x-ray was normal. *CT findings:* hypodense sharply marginated nonenhancing left CPA cistern lesion *(A)* causing contralateral displacement of the fourth ventricle *(B)*. *Operative finding:* epidermoid cyst.

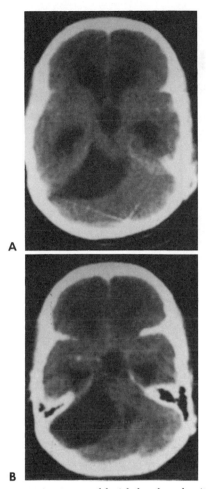

Figure 11–9. An 8-year-old girl developed gait instability and vertigo. Findings included left-limb ataxia and abducens paresis. Skull x-ray and isotope scan were negative. CT findings: left CPA sharply marginated hypodense lesion contiguous with the cistern (A) and extending upward through the tentorium (B). There is biventricular enlargement with contralateral displacement of the fourth ventricle.

usually large tumors. They distort and displace the fourth ventricle to cause obstructive hydrocephalus. The CT finding is a hypodense round sharply marginated nonenchancing lesion (Fig. 11–8) with interspersed hyperdense calcified portions. Other lesions have a hyperdense calcified capsule with a hypodense core; this reflects the presence of cholesterol and desquamated epithelial cells.

Other Lesions

Subarachnoid cysts may appear as hypodense sharply marginated CPA lesions. The hypodense appearance is consistent with their CSF content. They may be contiguous with cisternal spaces (Fig. 11–9). These cysts do not enhance. They may appear to narrow (arrowhead configuration) as they extend upward through the tentorium.

Metastatic neoplasms are rarely located in the CPA region. These usually represent cerebellar tumors that have extended exophytically. They appear as hypodense or mixed-density heterogeneous lesions with a thick irregular complex enhancing rim.

Hematomas may rarely occur in this region

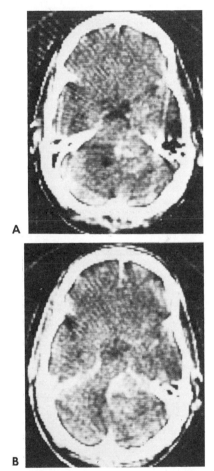

Figure 11–10. A 47-year-old man presented with progressive right-sided hearing loss and sudden development of right facial paralysis. Findings included right 5th, 6th, 7th and 8th nerve involvement with bilateral cerebellar signs. CT findings: patchy lamellated nonhomogeneous high-density lesion (A) with peripheral medial dense enhancement is seen compressing and displacing the fourth ventricle to the left side (B). Vertebral angiography showed slight mass effect in the right cerebellopontine angle (CPA) with abnormal venous pattern. Operative findings: extra-axial hematoma in the right CPA with evidence of dilated tortuous veins consistent with angioma.

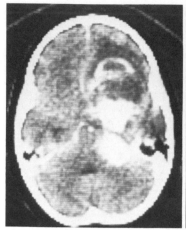

A

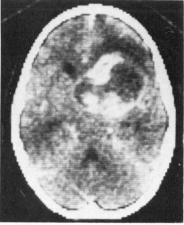

B

Figure 11–11. An 8-year-old girl had had intramedullary cervical astrocytoma surgically decompressed and irradiated three years previously. She subsequently developed right-sided hearing loss, trigeminal pain and facial paresis. *CT findings:* enhancing lesion in the right CPA displacing the fourth ventricle to the left side; it is contiguous with bone and extends to the apex of the petrous pyramid *(A)*. Other lesions are in the right middle fossa and floor of the anterior fossa. This is consistent with cisternal spread of glioma *(B)*.

and may be caused by aneurysms or angiomas. Ectatic vertebral-basilar fusiform aneurysms and berry aneurysms have been reported to cause hearing loss and other cranial nerve palsies. These lesions may cause radiographic evidence of a widened internal acoustic meatus.[22] Some patients with posterior fossa vascular malformations may present with CPA syndrome; however, their course is characterized by discrete episodes in which there is sudden neurological deterioration. CT may show evidence of CPA hematoma with tortuous enhancement pattern that represents abnormal vessels (Fig. 11–10).

Primary intra-axial neoplasms may have extrinsic exophytic extension into the CPA (astrocytoma, ependymoma, medulloblastoma) (Fig. 11–11). Accurate delineation of the location of certain of these lesions may require vertebral angiography, metrizamide cisternography CT and coronal and sagittal CT reconstructions.

REFERENCES

1. Harner SG, Laws ER: Diagnosis of acoustic neurinoma. Neurosurgery 9:373–379, 1981
2. Ojemann RG, Montgomery WW, Weiss AD: Evaluation and surgical treatment of acoustic neuroma. N Engl J Med 287:895–899, 1972
3. Johnson EW, House WF: Auditory findings in 53 cases of acoustic neuromas. Arch Otolaryngol 80:667, 1964
4. Pulec J, House WF, Hughes RL: Vestibular involvement and testing in acoustic neuromas. Arch Otolaryngol 80:677, 1964
5. Austin D: Modern diagnosis and treatment of acoustic neurinoma. Am J Med Sci 251:468, 1966
6. Valvassori GE: The abnormal internal auditory canal in the diagnosis of acoustic neuroma. Radiology 92:449–459, 1969
7. Reidy J, De Lacey GJ, Wignall BK: The accuracy of plain radiographs in the diagnosis of acoustic neurinomas. Neuroradiology 10:31, 1975
8. Hatam A, Moller A, Olivercrona H: Evaluation of the internal auditory meatus with acoustic neuromas using computed tomography. Neuroradiology 17:197, 1979
9. Valvanis A, Dabir K, Hamdi R: The current state of the radiological diagnosis of acoustic neuroma. Neuroradiology 23:7–13, 1981
10. Taylor S: The petrous temporal bone (including the cerebellopontine angle). Radiol Clin North Am 20:67–86, 1982
11. Naidich TP, Lin JP, Leeds NE: CT in the diagnosis of extra-axial posterior fossa masses. Radiology 120:333, 1976
12. Kricheff II, Pinto RS, Bergeron RT: Air-CT-cisternography and canalography for small acoustic neuromas. Am J Neuroradiol 1:57–64, 1980
13. Sortland D: CT combined with gas cisternography for the diagnosis of expanding lesions of the cerebellopontine angle. Neuroradiology 18:19–22, 1979
14. Britton BH, Hitselberger, Hurley BJ: Iophendylate examination of posterior fossa. Arch Otolaryngol 88:608, 1968
15. Dubois PJ, Drayer BP, Bank WO: An evaluation of current diagnostic radiogic modalities in the investigation of acoustic neurilemmomas. Radiology 126:173–179, 1978
16. Wolpert SM, Hammerschlag SB: Extra-axial growth of fourth ventricular tumors—angiographic changes. Neuroradiology 12:191, 1977
17. Takahashi M, Okudera T, Tomanaga M, Kitamura K: Angiographic diagnosis of acoustic neurinomas. Neuroradiology 2:191, 1971
18. Hambley WM, House WF: The differential diagnosis of acoustic neuroma. Arch Otolaryngol 80:708, 1964
19. Davis KR, Parker SW, New PFJ: Computed tomography of acoustic neuroma. Radiology 124:81, 1977
20. Goldberg R, Byrd S, Winter J: Varied appearance of trigeminal neuroma on CT. Am J Roentgenol 134:57, 1980
21. Moller A, Hatam A, Olivercrona H: The differential diagnosis of pontine angle meningioma and acoustic neuroma with computed tomography. Neuroradiology 17:21–23, 1978
22. Phelps PD, Lloyd EAS: High resolution air CT meatography: the demonstration of normal and abnormal structures in the cerebellopontine cistern and internal auditory meatus. Br J Radiol 55:19, 22, 1982

Chapter 12

INFECTIOUS INFLAMMATORY CONDITIONS

CNS infection occurs when the blood-brain barrier is impaired. This develops through four possible routes: (1) hematogenous dissemination, (2) passage through the choroid plexus, (3) rupture of parenchymal abscesses into CSF spaces and (4) contiguous spread from a source of parameningeal infection as in sinusitis, otitis media or osteomyelitis. On the basis of clinical findings, it is not possible to define the nature of pathological processes such as meningitis, cerebritis and empyema, or to characterize the infectious agent. This necessitates neurodiagnostic analyses and CSF examination, including culture and serodiagnostic studies.

Acute Bacterial Meningitis

The common causes vary with patient age; in the neonatal group are seen gram-negative enterobacilli, Streptococcus and *Staphylococcus aureus;* in children younger than five years old, *Haemophilus influenzae* and *Neisseria meningitidis;* and in patients older than five years, *Diplococcus pneumoniae* and *Neisseria meningitidis.* In purulent meningitis, inflammatory leptomeningeal (pia and arachnoid) reaction develops. Pathological response includes: (1) cerebral and pial vessels congestion, (2) meningeal thickening, (3) cerebral edema and (4) purulent exudate in basal cisterns, ependyma and cortical sulcal spaces. Clinical findings include headache, fever, vomiting and stiff neck. Neurological complications are cranial nerve palsies resulting from basal meningeal exudate, and altered consciousness and seizures caused by bacterial toxins, cerebral edema and cerebral ischemia.

Development of altered mentation, seizures, focal neurological deficit or papilledema suggests a complicating process. These processes are cerebral infarction resulting from inflammatory arteritis or cortical vein thrombosis, cerebritis or brain abscess, subdural or epidural empyema, hydrocephalus and cerebral atrophy.[1] If clinical findings suggest the occurrence of these conditions, CT is the initial diagnostic study; if meningitis is uncomplicated, initial CT is not necessary. The risk of precipitating herniation following lumbar puncture in uncomplicated meningitis is quite low, whereas delay in establishing diagnosis and initiating therapy while CT is arranged for may adversely affect outcome. In most patients with uncomplicated bacterial meningitis, CT is negative.

In some children with meningitis, CT shows small subdural effusion; this represents normal inflammatory response. There is no mass effect and usually no enhancement. Following treatment, this effusion resolves. After treatment with antibiotics, CSF formula normalizes and patients become asymptomatic. In some cases CSF formula may improve, but the patient clinically worsens. In this clinical setting CT and subdural taps are indicated.[2] Clinically symptomatic subdural effusion most frequently develops in children who are less than 2 years old. It is most common with *Haemophilus influenza* meningitis. Its incidence is not known because subdural taps and CT are not routinely performed. Development of subdural effusions is suspected if patients show these findings: (1) fever and positive CSF culture persist 48 hours after initiation of antibiotics, (2) there are abnormal neurological

229

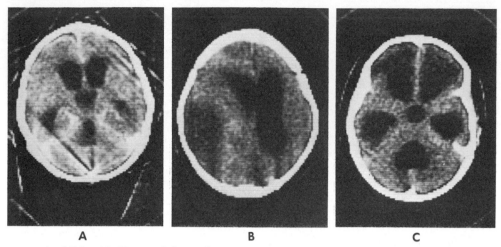

A   **B**   **C**

Figure 12–1 A child with *Haemophilus influenzae* meningitis was treated with ampicillin. *CT findings:* triventricular dilatation (A). She developed right-sided weakness and focal seizures three weeks later, although the CSF became normal. CT findings: left parietal convexity hypodense loculated nonenhancing lesion with significant mass effect (B). Following drainage of this subdural effusion, CT showed more hydrocephalus (C). She subsequently required shunt.

findings, (3) fontanelles become tense and bulging, (4) abnormal transillumination pattern is seen and (5) radiographic evidence of suture separation is present.[3] Subdural effusions contain variable amounts (5 to 150 ml) of fluid. They are unilateral or bilateral. They may appear clear or xanthochromic (because of high protein content). Subdural taps may be required. Some effusions containing 30 ml have not always been detected by CT. Routine use of CT has led to decreased utilization of subdural taps; however, if there are clinical indications taps should be performed even if CT is negative.

Subdural effusions appear as hypodense extracerebral fluid collections (Fig. 12–1); they are not isodense or hyperdense unless hemorrhage or infection has occurred. If the effusion is surrounded by densely adherent and thick membrane, surgical drainage or craniotomy may be required. Subdural effusions may rarely develop as a delayed complication of meningitis two to six weeks later. In these cases, initial CT was not completely normal and showed parenchymal lesions such as cerebritis, or infarction; the effusion was seen on subsequent scan (Fig. 12–2). These patients had delayed and progressive clinical deterioration; however, CSF did not show recurrence of meningitis. Surgical drainage was required in these patients with delayed subdural effusion.

There are some patients with bacterial meningitis who develop sudden neurological defi-

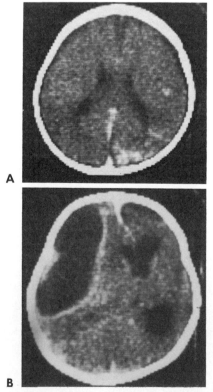

Figure 12–2. A 4-year-old with *Haemophilus influenzae* meningitis had complete recovery; however, CT showed an isodense gyral enhancing right occipital lesion (A). Four weeks later, she became lethargic and developed right hemiparesis. CT showed a hypodense subdural lesion with enhancing medial border and marked mass effect (B). At surgical drainage a thick proteinaceous subdural effusion with densely adherent membranes was removed.

cit (hemiparesis, quadriparesis, blindness, dementia). In these cases CT may subsequently show vascular lesions; that is, ischemia or infarction. This is most common with *Haemophilus influenza*, especially if there has been delay in instituting appropriate antibiotic therapy. This complication has been associated with high morbidity and mortality. It probably results from inflammatory arterial wall changes; vasospasm maybe a contributing factor. CT shows hypodense homogeneous and speckled lesions; they are sharply marginated and confined to the specific vascular (arterial) territories (Fig. 12–3). Other lesions appear isodense or hyperdense on plain scan. This may represent neovascularity rather than interspersed hemorrhage. Mass effect is not usually prominent. Enhancement develops in 66 to 80 percent of these cases. This is usually a gyral or linear pattern. It is most intense in the second to fourth week after the initial clinical ictus. Ventricular and subarachnoid space dilatation is usually present. This may be seen to increase on serial scans; however, shunting was not required in these patients.[4]

CT findings of postinflammatory vasculitis may simulate cerebritis. Cerebritis shows CT features that are not common with these vascular lesions. These include irregular margination and shape, marked mass effect, and ring enhancement. Differentiation of these two conditions has significance for patient management (Fig. 12–4). With vascular lesions, outcome is not improved by corticosteroids or extending the course of antibiotics beyond that utilized for meningitis. These vascular lesions may develop as the CSF formula improves. In cerebritis, corticosteroids and an extended course of an antibiotic (four to six weeks) is appropriate therapy. CT findings are usually distinctive enough in these two conditions that surgical biopsy is not required. In some cases angiographic findings may be helpful. The diagnosis of arteritis is established by visual-

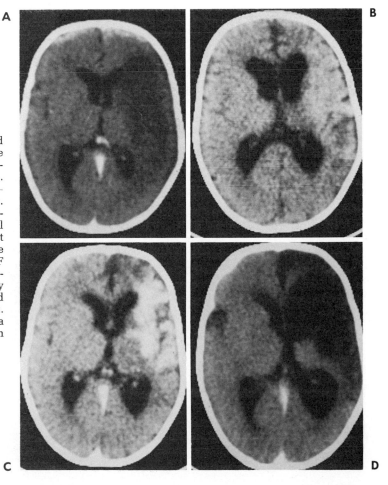

Figure 12–3. A child had prolonged febrile illness for two weeks before diagnosis of *Haemophilus influenzae* meningitis was established. During ampicillin therapy she suddenly developed left hemiparesis. *CT findings:* sharply marginated hypodense right temporal parietal nonenhancing lesion with slight mass effect (*A*). Two weeks later he was clinically improving and CSF was normal. CT showed a hyperdense (*B*) lesion with dense sharply marginated enhancing lesion and ipsilateral ventricular dilatation (*C*). Two months later, CT showed a hypodense nonenhancing lesion with ventricular dilatation (*D*).

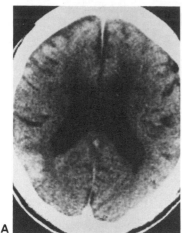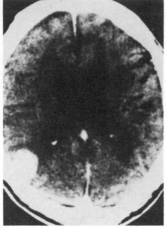

A   B

Figure 12–4. A 38-year-old man had sinusitis and bronchitis for which he received oral antibiotics for 5 days. One week later, he became febrile and confused; he had mild right hemiparesis. CSF showed sterile pleocytosis and elevated protein content. Isotope scan was negative; angiogram showed slight parietal mass effect but no evidence of vasculitis. *CT findings:* left parietal isodense lesion (A) with dense nodular enhancement but no mass effect (B). *Biopsy finding:* cerebral infarct.

ization of focal areas of arterial narrowing that alternate with arterial dilatation. The contour of the vessel wall is irregular. Angiographic findings of cerebritis may include mass effect or there may be no abnormalities.

The CT finding of enlarged basal cisterns with evidence of diffuse enhancement is consistent with basal arachnoiditis (Fig. 12–5). This is rarely seen with purulent meningitis. All patients who did show this CT finding had cranial nerve dysfunction. Seventy-five percent of patients had ventricular enlargement; 33 percent subsequently required shunting for postmeningitic hydrocephalus. Meningeal enhancement results from three possible pathological mechanisms: (1) enlargement and dilatation of meningeal vessels, (2) extravasation of contrast material into cisterns through poorly developed capillaries and (3) impaired blood-brain barrier. Meningeal enhancement is more common in chronic granulomatous meningitis (tuberculous, fungal), subarachnoid

seeding by tumor (medulloblastoma, ependymoma) and subarachnoid hemorrhage.

In purulent meningitis, cortical sulcal spaces are opacified by inflammatory exudate, and cerebral hemispheres may be swollen from cerebral edema (Fig. 12–6). CT shows nonvisualization of sulcal spaces and compression of ventricles; there may also be diffuse peripheral hemispheric enhancement pattern. This may simulate CT findings of isodense subdural hematoma or empyema. The lack of white matter inward displacement (buckling) with normal position of the cortical vessels makes subdural hematoma or empyema unlikely. These CT findings are important differentiating features to exclude extra-axial conditions. Unless a high-resolution scanner is utilized, differentiation of intra-axial lesions (sulcal exudate and hemispheric edema) from extra-axial ones may not be possible with CT.

Ependymal inflammatory reaction commmonly occurs in bacterial meningitis; how-

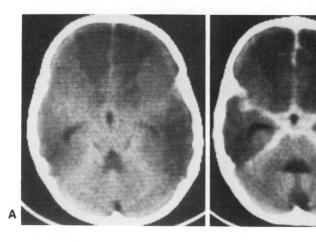

A   B

Figure 12–5. A child with purulent meningitis was treated with penicillin. Eight days later he remained obtunded and had bilateral abducens nerve palsies. *CT findings:* symmetrical hemispheric hypodense lesions (A) with dense basal cisternal enhancement (B).

Figure 12–6. A 42-year-old alcoholic developed fever, headache and stiff neck; findings were obtundation and left hemiparesis. CSF showed pleocytosis with positive culture for *E. coli. CT findings:* nonvisualization of right cortical sulcal spaces compared to left side with no inward displacement of gray-white matter interphase (*A*) with no ventricular compression (*B*). Necropsy findings showed purulent exudate over right convexity.

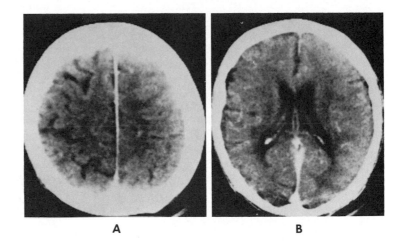

A   B

ever, the CT finding of ependymal enhancement is rare. Ventriculitis may be defined as an intraventricular abscess. This may complicate meningitis. These loculated regions containing pus-like material act as intraventricular masses to cause ventricular obstruction and impair response to antibiotics. Ventriculogram defines ventricular size and appearance. It also provides fluid for bacterial culture and antibiotic sensitivity. CT defines ventricular size and demontrates the presence of loculated intraventricular abscesses. Intervening gliotic septa separating the loculated ventricular regions may be seen as hyperdense thin peripheral rims on plain scan and these may enhance. Polycystic regions with dense ependymal and intraventricular enhancement represent a CT finding of ventriculitis (Fig. 12–7). These cysts are associated with ventricular enlargement; however, mutiple cystic lesions do not communicate. Multiloculated cysts may be demonstrated by intraventricular injection of Amipaque. These may also be cortical necrosis with dystrophic calcification.

Postmeningitic hydrocephalus most commonly develops if there has been delay in initiating appropriate antibiotic therapy or if ventriculitis has developed. Hydrocephalus usually progressively develops several weeks to months following purulent meningitis. Two thirds of patients who developed hydrocephalus showed other lesions on initial CT when ventricles were not enlarged. Hydrocephalus usually results from several factors: (1) adhesions in leptimeninges, (2) inflammatory occlusion of the fourth ventricle and (3) aqueductal gliosis. If patients do not show clinical signs of impaired CSF dynamics (bulging fonta-

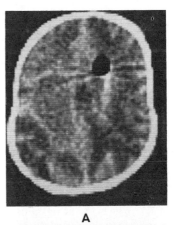

A

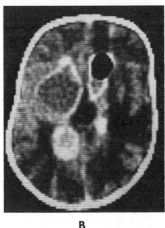

B

Figure 12–7. A child had salmonella meningitis treated with chloramphenicol. She subsequently developed multifocal seizures and increasing head size. CSF showed pleocytosis and negative culture. *CT findings:* bilateral cerebral hemispheric hypodensities with slightly hyperdense periventricular rim (*A*). There is dense ependymal enhancement and intraventricular air (*B*). *Necropsy finding:* multiloculated intraventricular abscesses.

nelles, progressive suture widening, altered mentation, gait disorder), serial CT is an alternative to immediate shunting. Ventricular enlargement may also be caused by loss of brain parenchyma resulting from cortical necrosis. When cortical necrosis develops, CT shows these findings: (1) enlarged basilar cisterns, (2) prominent sulcal pattern, (3) increased size of interhemispheric fissure and (4) normal-sized temporal horn and fourth ventricle. Because CT is not performed routinely on all patients with bacterial meningitis, the incidence of acute ventricular dilatation that decreases following treatment is not known. Factors that may increase ventricular size include dehydration and sepsis; however, cerebral edema may act to reduce ventricular size.

Acute Viral Meningoencephalitis

This illness develops rapidly. Patients show signs of diffuse or multifocal CNS involvement (seizures, altered mentation, focal neurological deficit). Previous studies have focused on specific types of encephalitis: herpes simplex, postvaccinal and postinfectious. Other common etiological agents are coxsackieviruses and arbovirus; diseases than can involve this condition are mumps, influenza and infectious mononucleosis. The diagnosis of acute viral encephalitis is established by a history of associated viral infection, abnormal CSF findings (lymphocytic pleocytosis), fourfold change in acute and convalescent serological titers (blood, CSF). If clinical findings of viral encephalitis suggest the possible occurrence of an underlying mass lesion (neoplasm, abscess, hematoma), CT should precede LP. However, most cases of viral encephalitis do not present in this manner. In most cases of acute viral encephalitis not caused by herpes simplex CT is normal, but CT may rearely show hypodense nonenhancing lesions representing necrosis. Follow-up scans in some patients with acute meningoencephalitis who have neurological sequelae may show CT findings of cortical or basal ganglionic calcification. CT findings of encephalitis may simulate those of cerebritis, contusional injury, infarction, or demyelinated lesions such as multiple sclerosis and leukoencephalitis.[5]

Herpes Simplex (HSV) Encephalitis

This causes necrotizing hemorrhagic lesion. It has predilection for the temporal, insular or orbital frontal regions. In young children involvement may be more widespread.

Initial symptoms include myalgia, fever and headache. These are followed by neurological signs caused by temporal lobe necrosis: psychomotor seizures, amnesia, confusion, aphasia and visual field defect. Psychiatric symptoms (hallucinations, psychoses, catatonia) may be initial manifestations. Intracranial hypertension and transtentorial herniation may result from hemorrhage, edema and necrosis. Surgical decompression may be necessary in these cases.

Diagnosis is established by brain biopsy; this shows characteristic histopathological findings, positive immunofluorescent HSV stains and positive viral culture. CSF findings include lymphocytic pleocytosis with red blood cells, elevated protein and decreased sugar content. EEG findings include unitemporal or bitemporal slowing but may be negative. Isotope scan may show frontal-temporal uptake. Angiography may show temporal or frontal-opercular mass effect, sometimes with localized vascular stain resulting from arterial vasodilatation or early venous opacification; abnormal tumor vessels are not seen.

In HSV encephalitis CT shows hypodense lesions that invariably involve the medial temporal regions.[6, 7] There are interspersed hyperdense portions representing hemorrhage (Fig. 12–8). Sharp transition from hypodense temporal lesion to normal density is seen at the lateral portion of the basal ganglia.[8] Edema

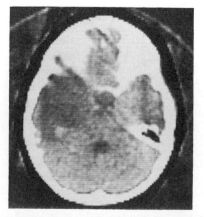

Figure 12–8. A 3-year-old girl began to act strangely. She became confused and had a right focal motor seizure. EEG showed bitemporal spike and slow wave. CSF showed sterile pleocytosis. CT findings: left frontal-temporal hypodense nonenhancing lesion with interspersed hemorrhagic component with marked mass effect. Necropsy finding: herpes simplex encephalitis.

Figure 12–9. A 13-year-old boy developed headache and lethargy; he became obtunded with right hemiparesis. CSF showed lymphocytic pleocytosis and several hundred red blood cells; culture was negative. EEG showed bitemporal delta pattern. *CT findings:* left temporal hypodense lesion (*A*) with mass effect and diffuse enhancement (*B*). *Biopsy finding:* herpes simplex encephalitis.

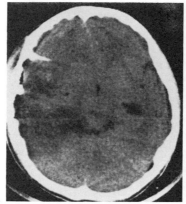 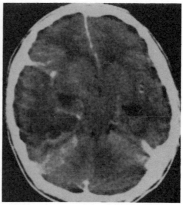

A   B

and mass effect are present in 80 percent of cases. Contrast enhancement is seen in 50 percent of cases. This is usually a diffuse or gyral pattern (Fig. 12–9); ring enhancement is not usually seen. In one third of cases, clinical findings and EEG findings were consistent with unilateral temporal involvement; CT showed bilateral temporal hypodense lesions to obviate the need for surgical biopsy. In patients with suspected HSV encephalitis, CT should be the initial diagnostic study. If patients present with clinical findings of expanding temporal mass, CT findings may exclude glioma or abscess. Although CT findings are not specific, accurate localization for surgical biopsy may be obtained. Serial scans may demonstrate progression from unilateral to bilateral temporal hypodense lesions. If the patient's level of consciousness deteriorates because of progressive mass effect, surgical decompression and biopsy may be indicated. Recent experience has shown the potential benefit of specific antiviral agents such as adenine arabinoside in treatment of HSV encephalitis, but this drug is not effective for other viral encephalitis. In some patients treated with this drug, enlargement of hypodense lesion(s) has developed. Follow-up CT scans in patients with HSV encephalitis have demonstrated decreased size of hypodense lesions and mass effect several months later.

Chronic Granulomatous Meningitis

Tuberculous Meningitis. This occurs in patients with primary pulmonary infection with hematogeneous transmission to leptomeninges. Small granulomas form in meninges or brain parenchyma; these may subsequently calcify. Tuberculous meningitis results if gran-

ulomas rupture with dissemination of tubercle bacilli into CSF spaces. There is chronic basilar granulomatous inflammatory reaction. This may involve cranial nerve perineurium, and sometimes obstruction of CSF flow occurs within ventricles and basilar cisternal spaces. The granulomatous exudate may cause inflammatory reaction in the adventitia and media of meningobasal arteries with arterial occlusion resulting in cerebral ischemia and infarction.[9]

The onset of tuberculous meningitis is insidious. Symptoms include headache, fever and nuchal rigidity; cranial nerve dysfunctions are common findings. CSF shows lymphocytic pleocytosis with elevated protein and decreased sugar content; acid-fast stain and culture are positive for tubercle bacillus. These patients usually have positive tuberculous skin reaction; chest x-ray may show primary pulmonary focus. In patients with tuberculous meningitis, CT may show dense symmetrical enhancement of basal cisterns but not convexity of sulcal spaces. The ventricles are usually enlarged unless there is cerebral edema with small-sized ventricles. All patients who showed dense cisternal enhancement had poor clinical outcome; one half had ventricular enlargement. Slight cisternal enhancement did not correlate with poor outcome. Patients with post-tuberculous meningitis hydrocephalus caused by aqueductal stenosis or obstruction of the outlet of the fourth ventricle are followed with serial CT.

In the initial stage of tuberculoma formation there is prominent inflammatory reaction containing giant cells; the limiting capsule is thin and poorly formed. During the next stage, the central portion becomes necrotic and is filled with caseating material. The surrounding cap-

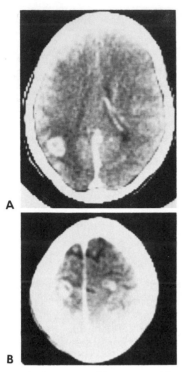

Figure 12–10. A 36-year-old woman with pulmonary tuberculosis developed headache and lethargy. EEG and isotope scan were negative. *CT findings:* left parietal hypodense lesion with multiple bilateral ring-enhancing lesions (*A*) with central hypodense lesions (*B*). These represented tuberculomas.

sule becomes thicker. The tuberculomas may be reabsorbed or calcify. Tuberculomas have unique CT findings. They have varied appearance on plain scan, including an isodense, hyperdense or calcified pattern. The majority have surrounding edema. Noncalcified lesions showed nodular or ring enhancement with a central hypodense region; this pattern represents caseating granuloma (Fig. 12–10). The finding of solitary ring-enhancing lesion is nonspecific; however, multiple small coalescing ring-enhancing lesions with central hypodense region is suggestive of tuberculomas. The ring is continuous, smooth and uniform in thickness; less frequently it is irregularly shaped and of variable thickness. Detection of a central hypodense region of the granuloma is a function of scanner spatial resolution, lesion size and tissue section thickness.[10]

Sarcoid granulomas are noncaseating; they show homogeneous and nodular enhancement. Other granulomas (cysticercosis, fungal agents or bacterial abscesses) may show CT findings identical to tuberculosis. Target lesions consist of central dense calcification with surrounding hypodense rim on plain scan with a dense surrounding rim of contrast enhancement.[11, 12] This pattern is characteristic of tuberculoma; however, it may be seen in thrombosed aneurysms, gliomas and ring-enhancing hematomas. In patients clinically suspected of tuberculosis CT shows characteristic findings such as meningeal enhancement, multiple contiguous small rings with hypodense central region and the target lesion. Presumption of the diagnosis of intracranial tuberculous should be strong enough to institute medical therapy without surgical biopsy. If CT shows multiple homogeneous nodular enhancing lesions, it is not possible to differentiate this from other infectious processes, metastatic neoplasms or sarcoidosis; diagnosis must be established by other laboratory investigations or biopsy findings.

Cryptococcal Meningitis

This causes chronic basilar granulomatous meningitis; small multiple nodules may also form. Small subcortical multiple cysts with minimal surrounding reactive gliosis or collagen capsule formation sometimes develop. One half of cases of cryptococcal meningitis occur in immunosuppressed patients; the others occur in otherwise healthy patients. The clinical course is that of subacute or chronic meningitis. Focal neurological deficit, seizures and intracranial hypertension are late findings.

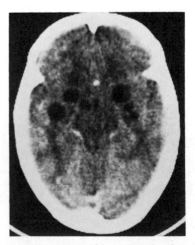

Figure 12–11. A 31-year-old woman developed headache and vomiting; findings include papilledema and right hemiparesis. CSF contained 50 lymphocytes and positive India ink stain for cryptococcus. *CT findings:* bilateral confluent sharply marginated nonenhancing hypodense ganglionic-thalamic lesions. *Necropsy findings:* multiple small confluent cysts with intervening septae.

CSF shows lymphocytic pleocytosis with decreased sugar content. Diagnosis is established by these three findings: (1) positive India ink preparations to demonstrate encapsulated organism, (2) elevated cryptococcal antigen titer and (3) positive fungal culture. In patients with uncomplicated cryptococcal meningitis, CT is negative; however, diffuse enhancement may be seen in the basal cisterns and sylvian fissure.[13] Intracranial granulomas (toruloma) appear as isodense lesions with nodular or ring enhancement. This pattern is nonspecific; pathological diagnosis requires surgical therapy.[14] The finding of multiple coalescing subcortical (ganglionic, thalamic) hypodense nonenhancing lesions represents multicysts and correlates with poor outcome (Fig. 12–11); this is characteristic for cryptococcus.

Uncommon CNS Fungal Diseases

Actinomycosis. The most common CNS tissue reaction is abscess formation. CNS involvement results from direct extension of a cervical-facial lesion or hematogeneous dissemination from thoracic or abdominal source. CT findings include hypodense or isodense homogeneous nodular enhancing lesion; this reflects abscess formation. Treatment includes penicillin and surgical excision; some lesions resolve with medical therapy alone.

Aspergillosis.[15] This fungal disorder occurs most commonly in patients with underlying disease (leukemia, lymphoma). Infection reaches the CNS by hematogeneous dissemination. Tissue pathological response includes abscess and granuloma formation; there may be vascular thrombosis with hemorrhage, necrosis and infarction. CT findings include: (1) areas of infarction, (2) hypodense irregularly marginated round lesions representing cerebritis, (3) mass effect and (4) enhancement (incomplete ring, gyral pattern). The evolution from the area of infarction that shows increased mass effect and incomplete ring enhancement on subsequent scans is suggestive of aspergillosis (Fig. 12–12). Treatment involves surgical excision; chemotherapeutic agents are not effective.

Candidiasis. This may develop in patients with diabetes mellitus, in pregnant women and in those who have received intravenous antibiotics. It occurs by hematogeneous spread from the gastrointestinal system or heart. The fungus may invade blood vessels to cause thrombosis or infarction; abscess or granuloma formation also develops. CT findings are similar to those seen in aspergillosis.

Mucormycosis. This develops in association with poorly controlled diabetes mellitus and in intravenous drug users. The fungus initially enters the paranasal sinuses; it extends through the cribiform plate to the CNS to involve the orbit and anterior fossa. The fungus invades blood vessels to cause hemorrhagic necrosis; there is usually no abscess or granuloma. CT findings are characteristic of hemorrhagic infarction or enhancing mass.

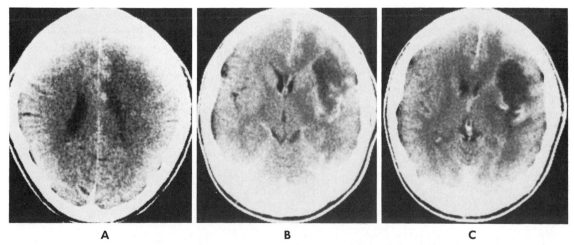

| A | B | C |

Figure 12–12. A 34-year-old intravenous drug user developed left hemiplegia. *CT findings:* 4 days later, right frontal-parietal hypodense lesion with peripheral enhancement (A). One week later he became lethargic. *CT findings:* sharply marginated ovoid hypodense lesion with peripheral incomplete rim enhancement (B). Despite treatment with corticosteroids, he did not improve clinically. *CT findings:* hypodense lesion with incomplete ring enhancement (C). *Operative finding:* aspergillosis.

Sarcoidosis. When intracranial involvement occurs (5 to 8 percent), clinical findings are usually caused by chronic basilar meningitis. CSF findings cannot be differentiated from granulomatous disease of infectious etiologies (fungal, tuberculous) or neoplastic conditions (carcinomatous, leukemic, lymphomatous). Chest x-ray shows hilar adenopathy and there is laboratory evidence of impaired liver function; diagnosis is established by lung, liver or conjunctival biopsy that shows noncaseating granuloma.[16]

Symptoms of intracranial sarcoidosis include cranial nerve palsies—most frequently, facial and abducens—and hydrocephalus caused by CSF obstruction in basal cisterns or the outlet of the fourth ventricle. There is sometimes involvement of the optic chiasm, pituitary-hypothalamic region and third ventricle; this may cause visual impairment, endocrine dysfunction and intracranial hypertension. Sarcoid granulomas are distributed in a diffuse pattern but may coalesce to form a discrete mass. CT abnormalities caused by sarcoid include: (1) diffuse basal cisternal enhancement, (2) isodense or hyperdense noncalcified lesions with dense nodular homogeneous enhancement, (3) hydrocephalus and (4) enlargement of the lacrimal gland. These lesions may be single or multiple (Fig. 12–13). Sarcoid granulomas do not calcify. Following treatment with corticosteroids, symptoms resolve and follow-up scans show a decrease in size and density of enhancing lesions. After corticosteroids are discontinued, CT should be repeated to exclude recurrence.[16, 17]

Focal Suppurative Cerebritis and Brain Abscesses

Suppurative reaction within brain parenchyma may result from local contiguous exten-sion (sinusitis, mastoiditis), hematogeneous dissemination of systemic infection (endocarditis, bronchiectasis) or sepsis without specific systemic infection. Hematogeneous dissemination frequently results in multiple noncontiguous lesions or in a single lesion, whereas direct local extension almost always causes a solitary focus. The earliest pathological change of focal suppurative cerebritis is characterized by tissue necrosis with polymorphonuclear cellular response and petechial hemorrhages. This is surrounded by edema in the white matter and astrocytic microglial proliferation with endothelial hyperplasia and lymphocytic-venous cuffing in surrounding vessels. At this stage focal cerebritis is not clearly delineated from normal brain parenchyma and no definite surrounding capsule has formed.[18]

Early symptoms include meningitic syndrome; there may be focal neurological deficit. CSF findings include pleocytosis, elevated protein content, normal sugar content and negative bacterial culture. EEG shows focal slow-wave pattern. Isotope scan shows spherical homogeneous or annular doughnut-shaped uptake. The heterogeneous uptake with a central empty core was initially believed specific for brain abscess; it is seen with other lesions with central necrosis, such as metastasis. Angiography sometimes shows an avascular mass, but infrequently no mass effect is demonstrated. If the source of cerebritis is bacterial endocarditis, angiography may demonstrate embolic arterial occlusion. The diagnosis of cerebritis may be established by surgical biopsy but may be negative in rare instances.

CT has become a sensitive and reliable diagnostic procedure for establishing the diagnosis of cerebritis. In our experience all lesions of cerebritis or abscess that were larger than 10 mm were detected; however, lesions less than 9 mm are not always detected,

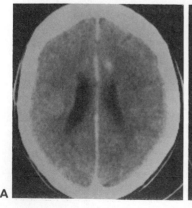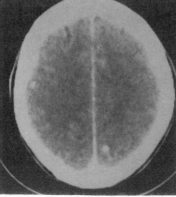

Figure 12–13. A 39-year-old man with sarcoidosis developed confusion and headache. CSF was normal. *CT findings:* multiple isodense homogeneous nodular enhancing lesions.

A

B

especially if the scan is degraded by motion artifact. We have necropsy confirmation of a 5 mm nodular enhancing lesion with a small amount of surrounding edema. Noncontrast scan shows these features: First, the hypodense region is heterogeneous owing to the relative contribution of edema, necrosis, petechial hemorrhage, gas-forming bacteria and collagen formation and second, there is marked mass effect and vasogenic edema. On postcontrast scan, enhancement patterns may be seen, including incomplete ring formation, thin but complete ring formation and speckled or gyral pattern. Fifteen percent of lesions do not enhance.

Treatment of focal suppurative cerebritis includes intravenous antibiotics; this is usually supplemented by corticosteroids to reduce cerebral edema. Following medical treatment clinical recovery is expected, with normalization of CT scan; however, the suppurative area may become an encapsulated abscess (Fig. 12–14). During the stage of suppurative cerebritis, the infected region is not sharply delineated from surrounding brain parenchyma. If surgical intervention is performed, herniation may occur into the surgically decompressed area, causing further tissue necrosis. During the stage of cerebritis there is beginning capsule development. This subsequently becomes complete to form an encapsulated abscess. The capsule thickness may vary from 1 to 4 mm. It is thicker on the

superficial cortical surface than on the less well-formed thin ventricular surface. This pattern is due to the abundant gray matter vascular supply; therefore, capsule formation is slower to form and weaker on the white matter region. This explains the propensity of abscesses to rupture into ventricles. Capsule formation develops within two to four weeks. The capsule may contain secondary daughter or satellite abscesses. The central portion of the abscess contains necrotic material and bacteria (causing gas formation); this is surrounded by a hypodense region representing edema with marked mass effect.[19, 20]

In our studies, solitary brain abscesses showed these patterns on noncontrast scan: (1) hypodense lesion, (2) hypodense lesion with surrounding hyperdense rim, (3) hypodense irregularly marginated lesion with eccentric hyperdense nodule, and (4) central very low density core reflecting the presence of gas-forming bacteria. Following contrast infusion, abscesses enhanced. Enhancement patterns included: (1) thin peripheral ring (complete or partial), (2) dense nodular, (3) multiple contiguous rings (Fig. 12–15) and (4) thin complete ring with small contiguous rings or nodules (Fig. 12–16). There is enhancement in the capsule; this is regular in shape and better formed on the surface adjacent to the cortex or deep nuclear masses (basal ganglia, thalamus). It is important not to interpret enhancement that results from normal structures such

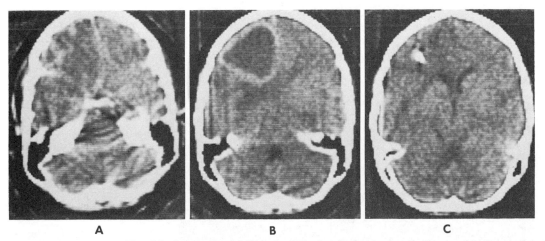

A   **B**   **C**

Figure 12–14. A 10-year-old girl had periorbital cellulitis and had right focal seizure. She was febrile, confused and had papilledema. *CT findings:* left frontal hypodense lesion compressing the left lateral ventricle. Following contrast infusion, the falx is bowed and there is patchy enhancement (*A*). Following treatment with antibiotics and corticosteroids, she developed right hemiparesis. *CT findings:* hypodense lesion with thick but regular rim of enhancement that is thinner on the medial aspect (*B*). Following surgical evacuation, there is a residual hypodense lesion, and an indwelling catheter is seen (*C*).

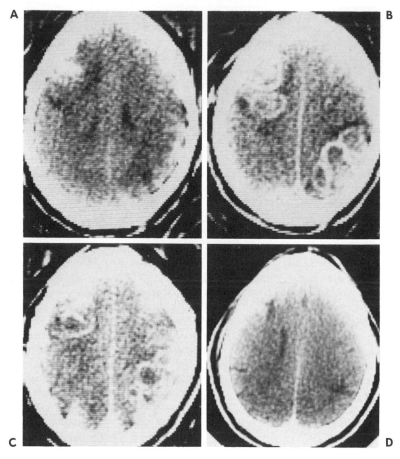

Figure 12–15. This 30-year-old man with *Staphylococcus aureus* endocarditis had generalized seizure and developed right hemiparesis. Isotope scan showed right parietal uptake. *CT findings:* left frontal and parietal mixed-density lesion (*A*) with multiple ring-enhancing lesions and contiguous right hemispheric ring-enhancing lesions (*B*). Following treatment with antibiotics, he became neurologically asymptomatic. CT shows decrease in size and enhancement (*C*). Three months later without any further treatment, CT scan shows no enhancing lesions (*D*).

as falx, tentorium and blood vessels contiguous with a hypodense lesion with enhancing abscess capsule rim. All patients with brain abscesses showed enhancement; however, this may be reduced in patients treated with corticosteroids.[21-23]

In patients who show systemic signs of pyogenic infection and develop neurological symptomatology, the CT finding of a ring-enhancing lesion is characteristic of brain abscess. Additional information provided by CT includes: (1) number of intracranial lesions, (2) presence of satellite lesions contiguous to the major lesion, (3) periventricular enhancement,

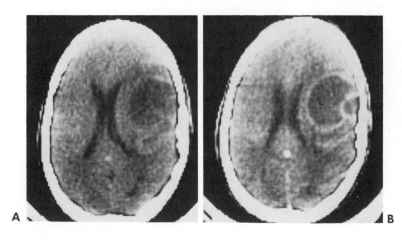

Figure 12–16. A 21-year-old man developed low-grade fever and progressive left-sided weakness. CSF was acellular; isotope scan showed right parietal uptake. *CT findings:* right parietal mixed-density lesion (*A*) with ring enhancement and surrounding peripheral nodular and ring enhancement (*B*). *Surgical findings:* encapsulated abscess with contiguous satellite abscesses.

(4) completeness of peripheral enhancing rim, (5) severity of mass effect and (6) presence of hydrocephalus. If serial CT scans show evolution from cerebritis, that is, a hypodense lesion with minimal enhancement to encapsulated abscess (ring-enhancing lesion), this is the diagnostic pattern. This evolution occurs within three to four weeks. An abscess may develop despite adequate medical treatment with antibiotics and corticosteroids. In these cases surgical drainage may be necessary. Lesions that are larger than 3 cm and have a thick capsule usually require surgical drainage.

In 20 percent of patients with brain abscess, the source of infection is not established. These patients present with neurological deficit and intracranial hypertension, but fever and meningeal signs are absent.[24] The CT finding of a ring-enhancing lesion cannot be considered in isolation of clinical features. The enhancing ring of an abscess is quite uniform in shape and thickness, whereas those associated with neoplasms are more complex-shaped and are irregularly marginated, variable in thickness and better formed on the deeper white matter surface. An abscess shows dense enhancement and significant mass effect, whereas infarcts have characteristic ovoid or wedge shape and minimal mass effect for lesion size; they conform to specific vascular territories. Abscesses may have mixed-density appearance on noncontrast scan with peripheral ring enhancement; this is contrasted with ring-enhancing hematoma, which shows a more dense central hematoma with a thin peripheral enhancing rim. We have had several cases in which serial scans or angiography was necessary to differentiate intracerebral hematoma from abscess. Samson reported angiographic findings in abscesses:[24] (1) avascular masses (80 percent), (2) midline shift only (16 percent) and (3) normal (4 percent). Abscesses may show abnormal vascular patterns: a vascular rim of hyperemia in the capsular wall seen in the early venous phase, and concentric bands alternating with radiolucent areas at the periphery believed to represent bowing of the vascular gyral pattern that is separated from compressed edematous parenchyma. The vascular rim of abscesses is believed to result from fibroblastic vascular proliferation within the capsule.

Before CT was developed, it was not possible to differentiate focal suppurative cerebritis from abscess on the basis of clinical diagnostic findings. Since operative mortality for brain abscesses remained high (30 to 40 percent) despite therapeutic advances, it was hoped that lower mortality would result from improved diagnostic sensitivity utilizing CT.[25] In the stage of edema and hyperemia with minimal necrosis, complete clinical recovery and CT resolution may result from antibiotics and corticosteroids. If the patient clinically improves but CT evolves to a ring-enhancing lesion, surgical intervention may be delayed and scan may subsequently appear normal.[26] The findings of a large lesion with thick ring enhancement in patients who show no clinical improvement indicates the need for surgical drainage. Other patients showed completely formed ring-enhancing lesion, but clinical recovery and CT resolution occurred with medical management only (Fig. 12–17). This indicates that antibiotics have penetrated to the suppurative region despite CT evidence of a completely formed ring. Antibiotics may stop the spread of infection and sterilize the suppurative region to allow healing without surgery. This would explain continued change in the CT scan even after antibiotics and corticosteroids are discontinued. Antibiotics are usually continued for four to six weeks, and it is hoped that patients will be neurologically asymptomatic and the ring-enhancing lesion will have decreased in size at this time. Complete CT normalization usually occurs; however, this may not be seen until two to six months after completion of therapy. As nonsurgical management of these patients becomes more widespread and pathological confirmation is lacking, it is important to remember that CT differentiation of cerebritis and abscess is not always accurate.

If the abscess is large and surrounded by a thick capsule, corticosteroids and antibiotics may stabilize patients initially, but subsequent surgical intervention (drainage, excision) is usually required. If CT shows a solitary lesion that has a well-formed and complete enhancing rim, surgical intervention may be safely performed with low mortality. Claveria et al. reported that after surgical drainage the finding of peripheral rim enhancement indicates spread or persistence of abscess.[6] Other investigators differ with this and believe that some ring enhancement may persist for several weeks in the postoperative state.[27] This may represent granulation tissue or reactive gliosis. Multiple noncontiguous abscesses should be treated medically.

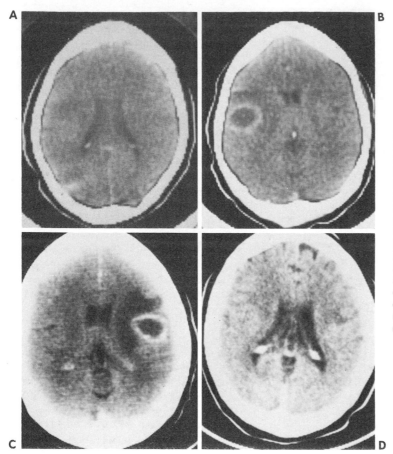

Figure 12–17. A 32-year-old woman, a drug addict, became confused and developed right hemiparesis. CSF showed sterile pleocytosis; blood culture was positive for *Staphylococcus aureus*. CT showed left parietal hypodense nonenhancing lesion (*A*). Following two weeks of antibiotics therapy, complete ring-enhancing lesion is seen (*B*). Within six weeks her hemiparesis resolved and antibiotics were discontinued. CT still shows ring-enhancing lesion (reader's right) (*C*). Six months later, CT is normal (*D*).

Epidural and Subdural Empyema

Collections of pus form in either epidural or subdural spaces. These may occur without underlying brain abscess. Epidural empyema may complicate craniotomy or result from infection in the frontal sinus or frontal bone (osteomyelitis). The epidural empyema is well localized and flattened between dura and bone.[28] CT shows an extracerebral lenticular-shaped hypodense lesion that is directed inwardly convex and compresses underlying brain parenchyma. Lott et al. have reported that epidural lesions extend across the midline in the frontal region, and there is posterior compression and bowing of the falx (Fig. 12–18).

Subdural empyema may result from these conditions: (1) penetration of dura by frontal sinusitis, (2) septic thrombophlebitis involving emissary veins allowing organisms to enter the dural space and (3) infection of subdural effu-

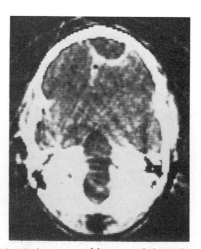

Figure 12–18. A 22-year-old man with frontal sinusitis developed headache, fever and right leg paresis. Skull x-ray showed frontal bone osteomyelitis. *CT findings:* bifrontal hypodense lenticular-shaped lesion with hyperdense nonenhancing medial capsule with posterior displacement of the falx. *Surgical finding:* epidural empyema.

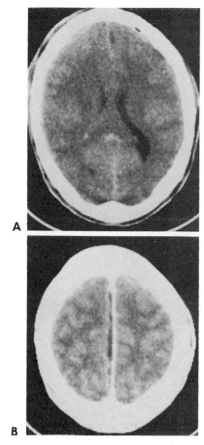

sion. Clinical findings of subdural empyema may be directly related to meningeal involvement or to the presence of an expanding subdural mass. Important diagnostic studies are plain skull x-ray demonstrating osteomyelitis or clouding of paranasal sinuses, EEG showing focal delta pattern or bilateral slowing, isotope scan showing peripheral crescent uptake, and CSF findings usually showing sterile pleocytosis. Definitive diagnosis is established by angiography; this shows the scalloped appearance of terminal branches of the middle cerebral artery with irregular displacement from the inner table by an avascular mass. Other findings include vascular stain with prominent meningeal vessels surrounding an avascular mass and cortical vessel spasm. Subdural empyema may spread diffusely over both hemispheres or become loculated by the formation of surrounding granulation tissue over the convexity or parafalcial region.[29, 30]

The high mortality of subdural empyema has been related to diagnostic error. This results in late surgical intervention after focal neurological deficit and intracranial hypertension have developed. The most common initial diagnosis is meningitis or abscess. The clinical presentation may be predominantly meningitic. Unless subdural empyema is considered, lumbar puncture may precipitate herniation syndrome.

CT has been highly accurate in defining the presence of subdural empyema even in patients without focal neurological deficit. CT findings reflect pathological changes caused by

Figure 12–19. A 19-year-old man developed purulent sinusitis. He subsequently developed headache, fever, lethargy and stiff neck. CSF showed sterile pleocytosis. *CT findings:* left hemispheric isodense lesion with marked mass effect (*A*) and small hypodense interhemispheric lesion (*B*). *Necropsy findings:* parietal convexity and interhemispheric subdural empyema.

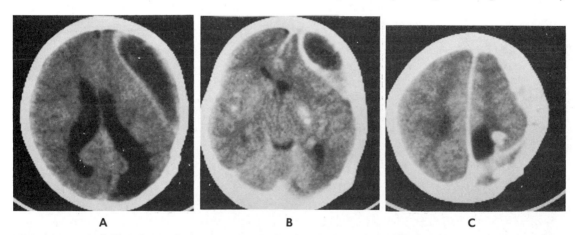

Figure 12–20. A child with *H. influenzae* meningitis developed left hemiparesis during treatment with ampicillin. *CT findings:* right convexity hypodense lesion with hyperdense rim (*A*) that densely enhances (*B*). There is a parietal-occipital hypodense lesion with dense nodular enhancement (*C*). *Operative findings:* subdural empyema and parenchymal abscess.

subdural empyema.[31] In the initial stages, there is fluid collection consisting of inflammatory exudate. Underlying cerebral edema is present that may result from associated cortical vein thrombosis. CT shows prominent hemispheric mass effect usually without abnormal density or enhancement (Fig. 12–19). Because of isodense hemispheric swelling and the small amount of exudate, there may be no evidence of abnormal subdural fluid collection. At this stage differentiation from focal cerebritis is not usually possible on the basis of CT findings. Angiography is sometimes more reliable than CT in detecting subdural empyema at this state.

Within several weeks surrounding membranes become developed and are highly vascularized. CT shows a lens-shaped or semilunar extracerebral lesion. The empyema is usually hypodense. If it is highly proteinaceous or thick because of pus, it may appear isodense or hyperdense. Isodense empyema may not be detected unless it causes mass effect and unless postcontrast scan demonstrates enhancing membrane. If subdural empyema is bilateral there may be no midline shift, but there is usually compression and collapse of contiguous lateral ventricles. CT may also detect the presence of an underlying parenchymal lesion (cerebritis, abscess, infarction) (Fig. 12–20). Treatment consists of antibiotics and surgical drainage. Following complete surgical evacuation by repeated subdural taps or craniotomy, the subdural lesion and enhancing membranes disappear.[32] If the lesion persists, further surgical treatment may be necessary. It is sometimes difficult to differentiate medial enhancing membrane of subdural empyema from diffuse peripheral gyral enhancement of inflamed cortex in meningitis (Fig. 12–21).

Protozoan CNS Infections

These are single-celled organisms that may cause encephalitis syndrome. These include malaria, trypanosomiasis, toxoplasmosis and amebic encephalitis.

Toxoplasmosis. This occurs in infants as a result of congenital infections. The mother acquires infection during pregnancy and transmits it to the fetus. Clinical findings of congenital CNS toxoplasmosis include chorioretinitis, microcephaly, cataracts and seizures. Intracranial calcifications are scattered throughout the brain. These cluster in the caudate, choroid plexus and subependymal regions; none are located in the posterior fossa. CT demonstrates calcified lesions (Fig. 12–22); however, similar findings are seen with cytomegalovirus (Fig. 12–23), rubella, tuberous sclerosis and cysticercosis. Toxoplasmosis may occur in immunologically suppressed adult patients. This presents with subacute meningoencephalitis, and in some cases multiple necrotic granulomas scattered throughout the cerebral hemispheres (Fig. 12–24). CT findings may show those as nodular or ring-enhancing lesions that simulate pyogenic abscesses, tuberculomas or sarcoidosis. Diagnosis is established only by brain biopsy.

Malaria. Coma may develop because of diffuse cerebral edema or disseminated intravascular coagulation. CT findings would be expected to show ventricular compression caused by edema. Multiple infarcts or hematomas reflect the effects of coagulopathy.

Amebic Meningoencephalitis.[33] The free-living forms (Euglena and Naegleria) cause CNS invasion through the nasal cavity. Other free-living forms may cause subacute meningoencephalitis. This may be characterized by granuloma formation and vasculitis. CT may show

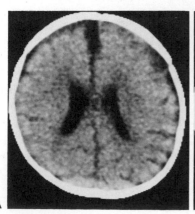
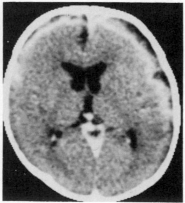

Figure 12–21. A 1-year-old child with *H. influenzae* meningitis showed improvement in CSF but progressive head enlargement. *CT findings:* thin hypodense bifrontal lesion (*A*) with dense underlying enhancement (*B*). *Operative findings:* dense purulent material overlying both hemispheres with inflamed cortex but no definite empyema.

A   B

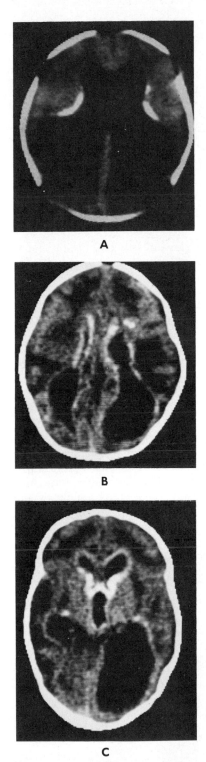

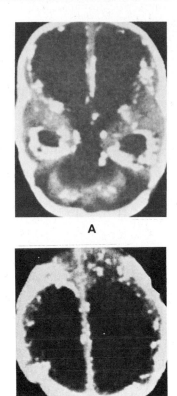

Figure 12–23. A child had delayed development and increased head size. *CT findings:* marked ventricular enlargement outlined by periventricular (A) and cortical calcification (B). *Necropsy findings:* cytomegalic inclusion-body disease.

basal cisternal enhancement or gray matter enhancement. Another form, *Entamoeba histolytica,* causes abscesses in intestine and liver; these may spread hematogeneously to cause brain abscess. CT findings are consistent with pyogenic abscess. The diagnosis is established by demonstrating amebic antibodies in CSF or immunofluorescent tissue staining.

Helminthic CNS Infections

These are animals with formed organ systems. They cause focal intracranial masses or calcified lesions. The most common CNS infection is cysticercosis; less common infections are caused by Trichinella, Echinococcus and *Strongyloides.*

Cysticercosis. This affects man in its larval form as the intermediate host of the pork tapeworm *(Taenia solium).* Areas of CNS involvement are intraventricular, parenchymal, arachnoidal or mixed forms. Clinical findings depend on the form of the disorder: (1) arach-

Figure 12–22. A 2-month-old had increasing head size and delayed neurological development. *CT findings:* hydrocephalus with periventricular calcification (A). Two weeks later CT shows calcification to be widespread (B) with hemispheric hypodensities. Six months later, calcification encompasses the ventricles (C). *Necropsy findings:* toxoplasmosis.

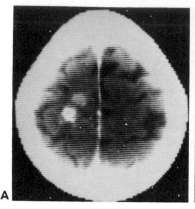
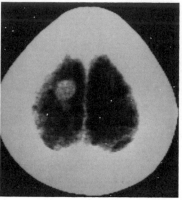

A

B

Figure 12–24. A 52-year-old man with histiocytic lymphoma became febrile and confused. CSF showed sterile pleocytosis with elevated protein content. *CT findings:* multiple cerebral hemispheric calcified lesions (A) with left parietal enhancing lesion (B). *Necropsy findings:* toxoplasmosis.

noidal (meningobasilar) causes meningitic syndrome and intracranial hypertension, (2) ventricular causes obstructive hydrocephalus and (3) parenchymal causes mental deterioration and seizures. Cysts that are contiguous with blood vessels may cause arteritis that results in infarction. Skull x-ray may show intracranial calcification. Subcutaneous nodules may be palpable. In patients with arachnoidal involvement CSF pressure is elevated and sterile pleocytosis, including elevated eosinophil count, is demonstrated. Serologic titers for cysticercosis showed elevated indirect hemagglutination levels in serum and CSF.

CT findings reflect the stage of the pathological process (parenchymal, ventricular or arachnoidal).[34, 35] In the arachnoidal-cisternal form, there may be dense cisternal enhancement. With ventricular involvement cysts develop that may be of the same density as CSF;

CT may show obstructive hydrocephalus without direct visualization of a cyst. These are most common in the fourth ventricle. Parenchymal lesions appear as irregularly marginated hypodense lesions with nodular or peripheral ring enhancement or as isodense nodular enhancing lesions. In the chronic form, larvae die; cystic formation and calcification occur. Multiple small intracranial calcifications are consistent with cysticercosis. The characteristic finding is central calcification that represents scolex; this is surrounded by a curvilinear calcified band in the cyst wall. CT is more sensitive than skull radiography in detecting intracranial calcification. We have detected calcified lesions that were 5 mm in size. The cystic lesions are quite small, with intervening septae; they appear as hypodense irregularly marginated nonenhancing lesions (Fig. 12–25). Calcified lesions are located in

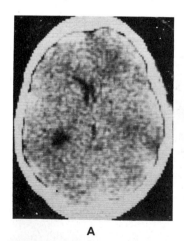
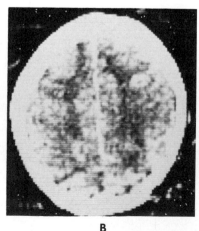
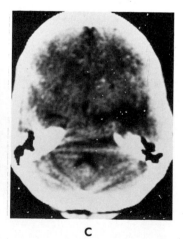

A

B

C

Figure 12–25. This 25-year-old woman with cysticercosis developed headache and was found to have papilledema. *CT findings:* biventricular ventricular compression and small left temporal hypodense lesion (A) with bilateral hemispheric enhancing lesions (B). Following treatment with corticosteroids she became aphasic. *CT findings:* multiple punctate periventricular calcifications with left (reader's right) temporal hypodense nonenhancing cyst (C). *Necropsy finding:* temporal lobe cysticercosis cyst.

the cortex (cortical, cerebellar) or may be periventricular. CT may show evolution from the meningobasal form, which shows ventricular compression and basal cisternal enhancement, to parenchymal lesions with hypodense or isodense multiple nodular or ring-enhancement lesions. As the cyst forms, a hypodense lesion with or without ring enhancement may develop. When the cyst dies, there may be rapid deterioration of the patient's condition caused by rapid cyst enlargement. Subsequently the cyst may decrease in size and CT shows multiple calcifications. There is no evidence to support the use of surgical excision of parenchymal cysts.

Syphilis

Neurosyphilis usually initially causes subacute meningitis. Diagnosis is established by CSF examination; CT is normal in this stage. Syphilitic endarteritis involves the intracranial blood vessels to cause infarction. Clinically these patients present with acute stroke syndromes. CT findings are consistent with cer-

ebral infarction. Syphilitic gummas represent inflammatory noncaseating granulomas secondary to syphilitic infection. CT shows an isodense or hyperdense noncalcified enhancing mass. Characteristic angiographic findings of gummas are avascular mass and vasculitis. Paretic neurosyphilis (dementia paralytica) is a late complication. Pathologically, the gyral pattern is narrowed and the sulci are widened, especially in the frontal and temporal region. CT shows cerebral atrophy, and diffuse paraventricular hypodense regions are seen in the subcortical white matter.[36]

Granuloma of Noninfectious Etiology

Certain collagen vascular diseases cause cerebral vasculitis. These result in single or multifocal infarcted areas.[37] Because vascular lesions may affect small intracranial vessels, CT may show no abnormality; however, if larger vessels are involved CT may show the characteristic findings of infarction. In other disorders (necrotizing angiitis, granulomatous giant cell angiitis, temporal arteritis and rheu-

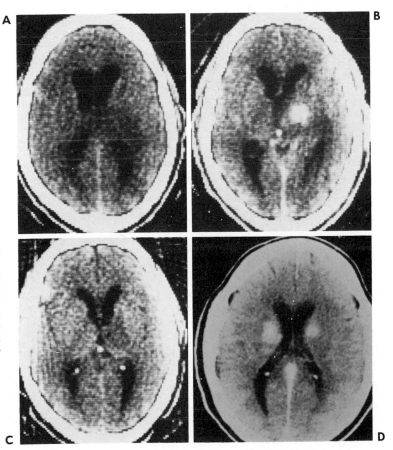

Figure 12–26. A drug addict with a scrotal abscess became febrile and confused. CSF showed sterile pleocytosis. *CT findings:* hypodense ganglionic-thalamic lesion (*A*) with nodular enhancement (*B*). Following treatment with corticosteroids and antibiotics he improved. CT was performed three weeks after medication stopped and showed a residual hypodense nonenhancing lesion (*C*). Two years later, he became febrile and confused. Blood culture grew *Staphylococcus aureus.* CT showed hypodense and dense nodular (*D*) enhancing lesions. Following antibiotics and corticosteroids, hypodense thalamic-ganglionic lesions remained. *Necropsy findings:* vasculitis with necrosis and granuloma formation.

matoid arthritis), vasculitis causes infarction sometimes with granuloma formation. Granulomas are usually multiple. They are located throughout both cerebral hemispheres and the subcortical region. CT findings include hypodense lesion with dense nodular enhancement. These lesions may simulate pyogenic abscess, sarcoidosis, tuberculoma, metastases or multiple sclerosis. Angiographic findings include: (1) multiple vascular occlusions, (2) vessel wall irregularity and (3) alternating areas of narrowing and dilatation. These patients clinically improve following treatment with corticosteroids. CT may show resolution of the lesions (Fig. 12–26). There is nothing specific about CT findings. The diagnosis depends on clinical features, CT findings and angiographic features; however, brain biopsy is the only way to confirm this diagnosis. We had two patients who had this diagnosis but were initially treated with corticosteroids and antibiotics because multiple brain abscesses was the initial diagnosis.

REFERENCES

1. Swartz MN, Dodge PR: Bacterial meningitis—a review of selected aspects. II. Special neurological problems, postmeningitic complications and clinical-pathological correlations. N Engl J Med 272:954–1003, 1965
2. Cockrill HH, Dreisbach J, Lowe B: Computed tomography in leptomeningeal infections. Am J Roentgenol 130:511–515, 1978
3. Menkes JH: Textbook of Child Neurology. Lea and Febiger, Philadelphia, 1974, pp. 213–220
4. Dunn DW, Daum RS, Weisberg L: Ischemic cerebrovascular complications of *H. influenzae* meningitis: the role of CT scan. Arch Neurol 37:650, 1982
5. Kennard C, Swash M: Acute viral encephalitis. Brain 104:129–148, 1981
6. Claveria LE, duBoulay GH, Moseley IF: Intracranial infections; investigation by computerized tomography. Neuroradiology 12:59–71, 1976
7. Dutt MK, Johnston IDA: Computed tomography and EEG in herpes simplex encephalitis. Arch Neurol 39:99, 1982
8. Zimmerman RD, Russell EJ, Leeds NE: CT in the early diagnosis of herpes simplex encephalitis. Am J Radiol 134:61–66, 1980
9. Rovira M, Romero F, Torrent D: Study of tuberculous meningitis by CT. Neuroradiology 19:137–141, 1980
10. Whelan MA, Stern J: Intracranial tuberculoma. Radiology 138:75–81, 1981
11. Welchman JM: Computerized tomography of intracranial tuberculomata. Clin Radiol 30:567–573, 1979
12. Bhargava S, Gupta AK, Tandon PN: Tuberculous meningitis—CT study. Br J Radiol 55:189, 1982
13. Enzmann DR, Norman D, Mani J: Computed tomography of granulomatous basal arachnoiditis. Radiology 120:341–344, 1976

14. Tress B, Davis S: Computed tomography of intracerebral toruloma. Neuroradiology 17:223–226, 1979
15. Grossman RI, Davis KR, Taveras JM: Computed tomography of intracranial aspergillosis. J Comput Assist Tomogr 5:646, 1980
16. Peyton D: Neurologic manifestations in sarcoidosis. Ann Intern Med 87:336–345, 1977
17. Bahr AL, Krumholz A, Kristi D: Neuroradiological manifestations of intracranial sarcoidosis. Radiology 127:713–717, 1978
18. Heineman HS, Braude AI, Osterholm JL: Intracranial suppurative disease: early presumptive diagnosis and successful treatment without surgery. JAMA 218:1542–1547, 1971
19. Weisberg LA: Nonsurgical management of focal intracranial infection. Neurology 31:575–580, 1981
20. Weisberg LA: Cerebral computerized tomography in intracranial inflammatory disorders. Arch Neurol 37:137–142, 1980
21. Whelan MA, Hilal SK: Computed tomography as a guide in the diagnosis and follow-up of brain abscesses. Radiology 135:663–671, 1980
22. New PFJ, Davis KR, Ballantine HT: Computed tomography in cerebral abscess. Radiology 121:641–646, 1976
23. Enzmann DR, Britt RH, Yeager AS: Experimental brain abscess evolution: computed tomographic and neuropathologic correlation. Radiology 133:113–122, 1979
24. Samson DS, Clark K: A current review of brain abscess. Am J Med 54:201–210, 1973
25. Shaw MDM, Russell JA: Value of computed tomography in the diagnosis of intracranial abscess. J Neurol Neurosurg Psychiatr 40:214–220, 1977
26. Berg B, Franklin G, Cunco R: Nonsurgical cure of brain abscess: early diagnosis and follow-up with computerized tomography. Am Neurol 3:474–484, 1978
27. Feely MP, Dempsey PJ: Assessment of the postoperative course of excised brain abscess by computerized tomography. Neurosurgery 5:49–52, 1979
28. Lott TK, El Gammal T, Dasilva R: Evaluation of brain and epidural abscesses by computed tomography. Radiology 122:371–376, 1976
29. Kaufman DM, Miller MH, Steigbigel NH: Subdural empyema: analysis of 17 recent cases and review of the literature. Medicine 54:485–498, 1975
30. Hitchcock E, Andreadis A: Subdural empyema. J Neurol Neurosurg Psychiatr 27:422, 1964
31. Luken MG, Whelan MA: Recent diagnostic experience with subdural empyema. J Neurosurg 52:764–771, 1980
32. Sadhu VK, Handel SF, Pino R: Neuroradiologic diagnosis of subdural empyema and CT limitations. Am J Neuroradiol 1:39–44, 1980
33. Lam AH, deSilva M, Procopis P: Primary amoebic meningoencephalitis. J Comput Assist Tomogr 6:620, 1982
34. McCormick GF, Zec CS, Heiden J: Cysticercosis cerebri: review of 127 cases. Arch Neurol 39:534, 1982
35. Carbajal JR, Patacios E, Azar B: Radiology of cysticercosis of the central nervous system. Radiology 125:127–131, 1977
36. Godt P, Stoeppler L, Wischer U: The value of computed tomography in cerebral syphilis. Neuroradiology 18:197–200, 1979
37. Ferris EJ, Levine HL: Cerebral arteritis: classification. Radiology 109:327–341, 1973

Chapter 13

HEAD INJURY

There are more than 400,000 patients per year in this country with head injuries who are admitted to the hospital, and a larger number who suffer head injury are not hospitalized. The sequelae to these injuries represent the major cause of neurological disability. Efficient utilization of diagnostic studies and appropriate management in these cases requires an understanding of the clinical and pathological aspects of head trauma. It is not economically feasible to perform CT scan on all head-injured patients.[1] Factors that determine clinical outcome in head injury include: (1) age of the patient, (2) duration of unconsciousness, (3) neurological findings (level of responsiveness, pupillary reactivity, spontaneous and reflex eye movements, motor response, (4) presence of a specific pathological lesion as determined by CT and surgical findings, (5) intracranial pressure and (6) extracranial complications.

The value of CT is well established in diagnosis of intracranial hematoma, cerebral edema, contusional injuries, diffuse white matter injury, hydrocephalus, and cerebral atrophy. CT can be more accurate than clinical examination, angiography or air studies.[2-7] Angiography is necessary if these post-traumatic conditions are suspected: arterial occlusion, venous sinus occlusion, carotid-cavernous fistula, aneurysm, and arterial spasm. It should be remembered that if CT is not available, direct-puncture carotid angiography may be performed very quickly to demonstrate trauma-related extracerebral and intracerebral lesions.

Three criteria define significant craniocerebral trauma: a definite history of blow to the head, a period of altered consciousness, and amnesia for a portion of the episode. Not all these patients require CT scan. In one study of head-injured patients, only one third required CT; one half of these patients had normal CT. Eighty-five percent of patients scanned because of impaired consciousness and focal neurological deficit had abnormal findings.[5]

If the patient has been unconscious for a short period of time and is neurologically normal except for a brief period of amnesia, CT is usually not necessary at that time. It is important to be aware that results from different centers may reflect the effects of sampling bias, as there may be marked variations in type of patients and severity of head injury.

CLINICAL ASSESSMENT

Immediately following head injury, many patients do not have altered consciousness or focal neurological signs. Other patients develop nonfocal neurologic deficits (altered consciousness, seizures, amnesia) or focal findings (hemiparesis, aphasia). On the basis of clinical findings, it is not always possible to determine if there has been gross structural pathological damage such as contusion or intracranial hematoma or if the neurological findings represent the effects of concussion. In cerebral concussion, recovery generally occurs rapidly and completely. However, necropsy studies of patients who were diagnosed as having "concussion injury" sometimes show unsuspected lesions.[6] Also, delayed neurological deterioration may develop in some patients initially diagnosed as having "concussion injury."[8] In some children who have suffered only mild head injury without altered consciousness, subsequent rapid neurological deterioration may develop several hours later: this may include impaired consciousness, vomiting, headache and blindness. These children usually recover rapidly within 24 hours;

however, emergency CT is usually performed to exclude intracranial hematoma. The negative result is very reassuring in these children. The pathophysiology of these clinical disturbances is not known; however, it is possible that this represents transient cerebral dysfunction. This is supported by EEG evidence of reversible occipital slowing in children who have transient blindness.

We have examined one hundred consecutive patients with the clinical diagnosis of "concussion." In this series, CT showed abnormalities in six who were studied 24 hours to 7 days after injury. These six patients had small contusions and superficial or subcortical hematomas; mass effect was minimal or absent. None of these patients showed delayed deterioration; therefore, medical or surgical treatment was not required. Follow-up scan showed spontaneous resolution. In another series of 500 consecutive patients who had clinical diagnosis of "postconcussive syndrome," diagnosis was based upon symptomatology that included headache, dizziness, poor memory and visual blurring. CT was performed two weeks to two years after head injury. Abnormalities were seen in six patients (porencephalic cyst, small chronic subdural hematoma, ventricular dilatation); however, none required surgical intervention. Their clinical symptoms resolved without change in CT findings. This suggests that CT is of limited value in patients with "postconcussive syndrome" who have no abnormal neurological signs.

Other acutely head-injured patients recover more slowly. This suggests gross structural brain damage. The mechanisms of brain damage in head injury include: (1) mechanical injury to neurons and axons, (2) intracranial hemorrhage, (3) edema and (4) ischemia resulting from brain swelling or an expanding mass.[1] These may be exacerbated by systemic complications such as hypotension, hypoxia, infection, and metabolic derangements.

Clinical deterioration can follow several temporal patterns: (1) initial alteration of consciousness with rapid improvement (lucid interval) followed by subsequent altered mentation, usually with pupillary and motor abnormalities; (2) normal consciousness immediately after injury with delayed neurological deterioration; (3) initial change in consciousness with subsequent focal or diffuse neurological worsening and (4) fluctuations in level of consciousness. None of these patterns is characteristic of specific pathological injury. Failure of the head-injured patient to recover consciousness may be influenced by factors not directly attributable to head injury: one of these factors is seizure causing the injury and producing the postictal state, another is stroke that has caused the fall and subsequent head injury. Extracranial factors that alter consciousness in the trauma patient include drugs (alcohol, analgesics) and systemic disorders (hypoxia, hypotension, hypercapnia).

Other head-injured patients develop focal neurological deficit with normal levels of consciousness. This is characteristically seen with small cerebral contusions. Motor dysfunction or aphasia may occur after a blow to the side of the head; hemianopsia may develop with a blow to the back of the head. Hemiparesis may indicate a structural lesion located in the cerebral hemispheres. Other possible causes include spinal cord injury, postictal state, and nontraumatic lesions (stroke, neoplasm). Certain cranial nerve dysfunction such as optic neuropathy, facial paresis, trigeminal anesthesia and ophthalmoparesis may be caused by lesions at multiple sites: cerebral hemisphere, brain stem, base of skull and extracranial locations. For example, facial paresis may be caused by petrous bone fracture or cerebral hemispheric injury; fixed dilated pupil may result from orbital injury or transtentorial herniation.

Indications for skull x-ray in head-injured patients include: (1) an established history of unconsciousness, (2) penetrating head injury, (3) skull depression established by physical examination, (4) otorrhea or rhinorrhea, (5) blood in the middle ear, (6) raccoon eyes, (7) Battle's sign, (8) foreign bodies in the wound, (9) altered mentation and (10) focal neurological signs.[9] Clinical findings suggesting basal skull fracture (periorbital hematoma, rhinorrhea, mastoid hematoma, otorrhea) are indications for tomography of the skull base if routine x-rays are normal; however, these tomograms may be performed on an elective and not an emergency basis. Basilar skull fracture increases the risk of intracranial infection occurring as meningitis, epidural empyema or brain abscess. Depressed skull fracture frequently is associated with an underlying contusion. These radiographic abnormalities suggest the need for emergency CT scan: (1) skull fracture, linear or depressed; (2) intracranial air; (3) intracranial foreign body and (4) pineal shift.

PERFORMANCE OF CT

Certain precautions are taken in acutely head-injured patients. Initial cervical spine x-ray is performed because neck manipulation may be needed to position the head for CT. This may be accomplished with a single lateral view, including the C–7 to T–1 region. Respiratory depression, potential risk of aspiration, and upper airway or lower respiratory tract abnormalities may necessitate inserting an oropharyngeal airway or intubating the patient. If the patient is intubated with controlled-assisted ventilation, intravenous diazepam may be utilized to control excessive motion artifact; however, short-acting paralysis or narcotic medication whose effects may be rapidly reversed by antagonistic drugs, e.g., naloxone (Narcan), is preferred. In acutely head-injured patients, sedation may depress respiratory drive. The effect of hypercapnia is to increase intracranial pressure. This complication may be avoided by controlled ventilation. Motion artifact may degrade image quality. The presence of head tilt may falsely suggest midline shift. These remain problems despite rapid scan time. If patients have suffered multiple traumatic injuries, limited head CT that includes the posterior fossa, lateral and third ventricles and vertex is adequate. In patients with acute craniocerebral trauma, contrast material may cause renal failure, shock or worsen brain function to produce seizures or encephalopathy. In the acute stage, contrast infusion CT study adds minimal diagnostic information.

STRUCTURAL PATHOLOGICAL LESIONS

Acute Cerebral Swelling and Brain Edema. Immediately following head injuries, diffuse generalized brain swelling may occur. This is not related to severity of the primary head injury. This acute cerebral swelling is a pediatric disorder. It is caused by transient loss of vasomotor tone (vasoparalysis). There is acute vasodilatation and vascular engorgement (hyperemia) that results in increased brain blood volume. The cerebral swelling may cause ventricular and subarachnoid space compression. These patients may rapidly progress to coma. If diagnosis is established and patients are treated with hyperventilation, rapid recovery usually occurs.

CT findings in diffuse brain swelling include:[8, 10, 11] (1) bilateral compression of ventricles, (2) nonvisualization of cortical sulcal spaces, (3) effacement of basal cisterns, (4) normal position of gray-white matter interface and (5) normal brain density pattern on plain scan. Diffuse enhancement is sometimes seen on postcontrast scan. The prominent enhancement may represent blood in acutely vasodilated blood vessels. Isodense bilateral subdural hematoma or cerebral edema may simulate CT findings of diffuse cerebral swelling; angiography may rarely be necessary to exclude subdural hematoma.[12] Acute cerebral swelling must be differentiated from cerebral edema in which there are hypodense regions representing edema fluid. In patients with acute diffuse brain swelling, clinical and CT abnormalities usually rapidly improve following hyperventilation. Mannitol increases blood flow; this may worsen acute diffuse brain swelling, although it may produce improvement in the other circumstance of cerebral edema.

Cerebral (vasogenic) edema probably occurs to some extent in all cases of head trauma. However, it is not always of sufficient magnitude to cause clinical disorders. Focal edema usually accompanies contusions and surrounds intracranial hematomas. Cerebral edema may develop rapidly following craniocerebral injury. Patients have generalized (altered consciousness) and/or focal (hemiparesis, aphasia, visual defect) neurological dysfunction. EEG usually shows bilateral slowing; however, this finding may reflect initial concussive injury. In cerebral edema the most constant CT finding is decreased tissue density. This represents increased water content (Fig. 13–1). Hypodense regions may be well-circumscribed or diffuse. These are usually irregularly marginated with frond-like projections. Mass effect is usually seen. The process may be unilateral or bilateral (symmetrical or asymmetrical). Because of impairment in the blood-brain barrier, there may be diffuse contrast enhancement (Fig. 13–2). If there is bilateral hemispheric edema, the entire ventricular and subarachnoid spaces system may be effaced, with nonvisualization of suprasellar and perimesencephalic cisterns (Fig. 13–3). Following treatment (hyperventilation, mannitol, corticosteroids), follow-up scans usually show better visualization of ventricles and subarachnoid spaces with resolution of hypodense lesions.[13] In several patients with necropsy-confirmed

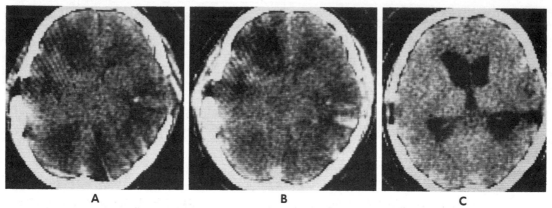

A   **B**   **C**

Figure 13–1. A 33-year-old man was severely beaten with a metal object. He was comatose with bilateral Babinski signs. Following surgical evacuation of bilateral subdural hematoma, he remained obtunded. *CT findings:* biparietal craniotomy defects are seen. There are diffuse hypodensities throughout both hemispheres causing ventricular compression that represent edema fluid *(A).* There is right parietal gyral enhancement. This represents edema and parietal contusion *(B).* Six months later he had severe memory impairment. CT showed ventricular dilatation and right parietal hypodense atrophic lesion *(C).*

bilateral diffuse cerebral edema, CT showed no abnormality; therefore, normal scan does not exclude this diagnosis.[14]

Contusions. Focal brain contusions (bruises) and lacerations (tearing of brain parenchyma) may develop directly at the impact point or contrecoup to the injury. Contusions are frequently found directly underneath a depressed skull fracture. Contusions occur in regions at which the skull moulds to cerebral convolutions, such as the anterior-inferior or lateral temporal lobe or frontal lobe. Cerebral gyral crests are bruised by jagged-edged bones at the skull base. Bilateral or multiple contusions are common; they are usually asymmetrical.[15] Predominant pathological lesions are subpial hemorrhage, necrosis and edema. This damage usually involves the gyral crest but

may extend into the gyral depths. If hemorrhagic foci are multiple and confluent, they may coalesce to form a cortical hematoma.

Patients with small cerebral contusions may present with focal deficit with normal consciousness. This usually develops immediately following injury. Subsequent clinical deterioration may result from edema and secondary mass effect. Surgical decompression or treatment of surrounding edema may be necessary. Other patients improve spontaneously. Skull x-ray frequently shows linear or depressed skull fracture. EEG demonstrates focal slow wave and spike wave discharge. Isotope scan may show abnormal uptake resulting from blood-brain barrier breakdown. Angiogram may show an avascular mass with stretching and loss of undulation of cortical vessels. An-

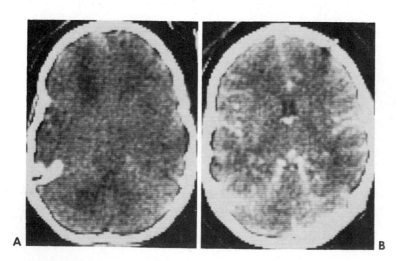

A   **B**

Figure 13–2. A boy fell out of a truck and became unresponsive. He sustained right occipital fracture. Burr hole exploration showed no evidence of extracerebral hematoma. *CT findings:* bilateral symmetrical ventricular compression with bilateral frontal hypodense lesions *(A).* There is prominent diffuse enhancement *(B).* These findings are consistent with cerebral edema.

Figure 13–3. This 35-year-old man remained lethargic 48 hours after hitting his head on a steering wheel. He had bilateral Babinski signs. *CT findings:* bilateral ventricular and basal cisternal effacement *(A)*. There is no abnormal tissue density and gray-white matter interphase is preserved *(B)*. Following treatment with corticosteroids, he markedly improved and ventricles were normal in size (not shown). This is consistent with cerebral edema.

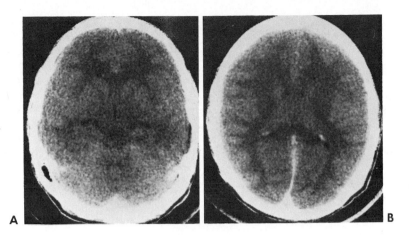

giography may be negative if contusions are superficial or small.

With CT, hemorrhagic contusions appear as heterogeneous hyperdense lesions. These are surrounded by an irregularly marginated hypodense component (Fig. 13–4). A hyperdense portion represents hemorrhage; a hypodense component reflects edema and necrosis. This mixture creates a mottled or salt-and-pepper pattern. Contusions are usually superficial. They are frequently multiple. Edema has irregular margination and extends across the vascular territories. This differentiates contusional injury and traumatic hematomas from infarction caused by traumatic vascular occlusion. The presence of a large superficial contusion may mask a thin superficial subdural or epidural clot (Fig. 13–5). In rare instances, high-resolution CT may show a contusion in the brain stem. This occurs in association with other lesions; an isolated brain stem contusion usually does not occur. Postcontrast study in contusional injuries adds no unique diagnostic information. Enhancement may occur because of impaired blood-brain barrier or rarely vasoparalysis. This may occur in diffuse, gyral or peripheral ring configuration (Fig. 13–6). It is most intense 7 to 14 days after injury, and it usually decreases in intensity after that time but may persist for as long as one month after injury. In hemorrhagic contusions, CT findings of hyperdense lesion and mass effect resolve within 10 to 14 days. Hemorrhagic contusion may evolve into an irregularly marginated hypodense lesion, whereas others completely normalize without residual hypodense lesion. There may be CSF space enlargement. It has been reported that small hemorrhagic contusions can mature into larger hypodense lesions;[3] however, we have not seen examples of this change.

Intracerebral Hematomas (ICH). Traumatic hematomas result from shearing or rapid deceleration injuries. Blood vessels are torn and blood is extravasated into brain parenchyma. The majority occur in the frontal and temporal region; less frequently, they are seen in the parietal or occipital region. They are usually

Figure 13–4. A 23-year-old man was hit by an automobile while riding his motorcycle. He was lethargic and right hemiparetic. *CT findings:* left frontal multiple contiguous hemorrhagic areas *(A)* with surrounding hypodense regions *(B)* consistent with hemorrhagic contusion.

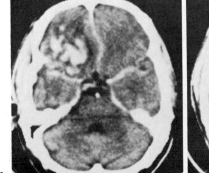
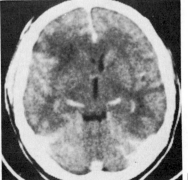

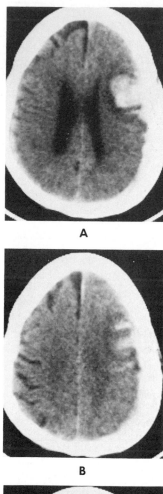

A

B

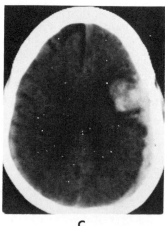

C

Figure 13–5. A 42-year-old man was hit in the right parietal region. He became confused and left hemiparetic. *CT findings:* right parietal superficial hyperdense intracerebral lesion *(A)* with effacement of contiguous sulcal spaces *(B).* Utilizing wide window width, a thin hyperdense extracerebral crescent is seen separate from bone *(C). Surgical findings:* hemorrhagic contusion with accompanying acute subdural hematoma.

superficial in location, rarely occurring in such deep structures as the internal capsule. If hemorrhage occurs in the pituitary fossa in association with basilar skull fracture extending through the sella turcica, it is usually fatal. Disseminated intravascular coagulation may complicate severe head injury in which there is release of tissue thromboplastin. This may result in reduction of coagulation factors and a generalized bleeding tendency such that intracerebral hematoma may develop.

Intracerebral hematoma usually develops immediately following head injury; however, delayed neurological deterioration may develop as long as two weeks later.[16, 17] Delayed hematomas result from damage to blood vessels in association with local hypoxia and hypercapnia, which increase cerebral blood flow. Because of impaired cerebral autoregulation, hemorrhage evolves into edematous and necrotic brain. Post-traumatic aneurysms may rupture to cause subarachnoid or intracerebral hemorrhage; this may develop months after initial head injury. In patients with intracerebral hematoma, neurological deficit and outcome are related to four factors: location, size, mass effect and accompanying injuries (subdural or epidural hematoma). Angiography shows an intracerebral avascular mass with cortical vessels draping around the lesion. Angiography may not detect multiple intracerebral hematomas and may lead to underestimation of hematoma size or it may be negative if the hematoma is small.[18]

CT is the most reliable diagnostic study for detecting traumatic ICH (Fig. 13–7). These areas appear as homogeneous hyperdense lesions with smooth but irregular margination. A hypodense region caused by edema may surround the hematoma. Large hematomas cause mass effect and extend into the ventricles. Peripheral ring enhancement is seen in 20 to 30 percent. This is maximal 7 to 21 days later and subsequently diminishes in intensity but may still be present two months after the injury. It may be difficult to differentiate subtemporal subdural hematoma from traumatic intratemporal hematoma; this may require coronal sections. Traumatic hematomas involving the brain stem, cerebellum and pituitary gland are now detected with high-resolution scanners (Fig. 13–8). If there is suspicion that hematoma is not directly related to trauma, postcontrast scan is necessary to exclude hematomas of other etiologies, e.g., neoplasm, angioma and aneurysm.

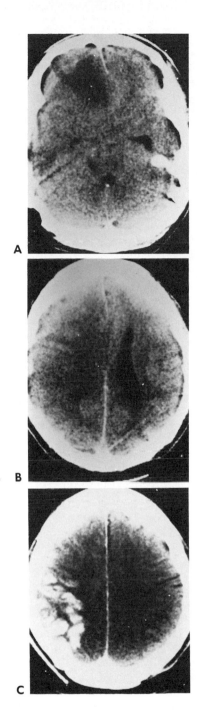

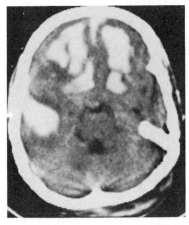

Figure 13–7. A 25-year-old man was beaten with a wooden club. He was comatose and right hemiplegic. *CT findings:* bifrontal and left temporal confluent superficial intracerebral hematoma with evidence of cisternal blood. There is left hemispheric mass effect.

Figure 13–6. A 40-year-old man was severely beaten. He was comatose and the left pupil was dilated. *CT findings:* left hemispheric hypodense intracerebral lesions *(A)* with overlying mixed-density subdural hematoma. There is lateral ventricular distortion and medial (inward) displacement of gray-white matter interface *(B)*. He was found to have subdural hematoma with underlying contusion. One week later he was clinically improved. *CT findings:* isodense left hemispheric gray matter enhancement with resolution of mass effect *(C)*. This is consistent with secondary ischemic lesion.

The indications for surgery in patients with intracranial hematoma have been modified by CT. In one series, less than one half of patients with ICH required surgery; this correlated with increased intracranial pressure rather than clinical or CT findings such as hematoma size and midline shift.[4, 14, 17] The major indication for surgical intervention is evidence of diffuse edema with marked mass effect and compartment shift, e.g., transtentorial herniation. If patients in stable condition without evidence of intracranial hematoma show deterioration several days after trauma, this is consistent with delayed traumatic ICH (Fig. 13–9); however, this occurrence may be caused by other disorders such as post-traumatic infarct or edema. Other possible explanations for delayed worsening include: (1) post-traumatic rupture of angioma or aneurysm, (2) hemorrhage into cerebral neoplasm, (3) delayed occurrence of subdural or epidural hematoma and (4) secondary hemorrhage into cerebral infarct.

Diffuse White Matter Lesions. Certain head-injured patients have no skull fracture or intracranial hematoma; however, they are in deep coma with bilateral extensor rigidity and impaired brain stem reflexes. This may result from white matter shearing injury.[19] Pathological findings include: (1) eccentric and asymmetric hemorrhages in deep white matter and corpus callosum, (2) hemorrhage in the superior cerebellar peduncle, (3) bilateral diffuse cerebral edema, (4) intraventricular and subarachnoid hemorrhage and (5) focal hemor-

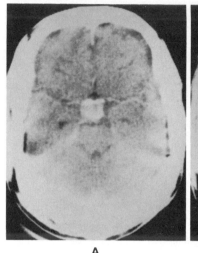 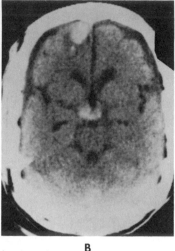

A   B

Figure 13–8. A 40-year-old alcoholic was beaten severely. He had Battle's sign and raccoon eyes. Skull x-ray showed basilar skull fracture. *CT findings:* left frontal *(A)* and pituitary hematomas *(B)* and accompanying extracerebral hypodense subdural lesions.

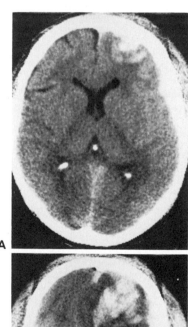

A

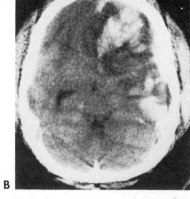

B

Figure 13–9. A 24-year-old man was struck in the right frontal region. He was lethargic but had no focal deficit. *CT findings:* small superficial intracerebral hematoma *(A)*. Three days later he became obtunded and left hemiparetic. *CT findings:* marked enlargement of two contiguous intracerebral hematomas with surrounding edema and marked mass effect *(B)*.

rhagic areas contiguous to the third ventricle. If patients survive for several weeks, cerebral atrophy may develop.

CT findings in diffuse white matter injuries include: (1) bilateral ventricular and cisternal compression and effacement, (2) bilateral eccentric and asymmetric hemorrhages contiguous to corpus callosum, (3) intraventricular and cisternal blood and (4) focal hyperdense hemorrhagic lesions adjacent to or within the third ventricle (Fig. 13–10). If patients survive, repeat CT scan shows ventricular dilatation and diffuse cerebral white matter hypodensities. Before CT became available, head-injured patients who were comatose with bilateral decerebration and impaired brain stem reflexes who had no evidence of an intracranial hematoma or mass effect were diagnosed as having "primary brain stem contusion." Experimental and neuropathological studies have shown that isolated brain stem injury does not occur; these patients probably have suffered white matter shearing injuries.

Extradural Hematoma. Epidural hematoma represents a collection of blood located between the inner skull table and dura. This may result from laceration of the middle or posterior meningeal artery while other epidural hematomas result from damage to the meningeal emissary veins or venous sinus. The most common locations are the temporal, frontal and occipital regions. Extradural hematomas also occur in the posterior fossa. These hematomas consist of a firm solid clot located external to the dura. Blood extravasates from the meningeal vessels with a force sufficient to strip the dura from skull. An ovoid mass

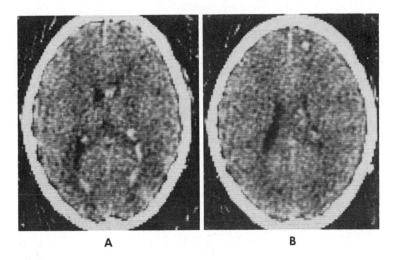

Figure 13–10. Immediately following a motorcycle accident, a man became comatose and decerebrate with miotic pupils and absent brain stem reflexes. Skull x-ray showed no fracture. *CT findings:* bilateral ventricular compression *(A)* with callosal and intraventricular hemorrhage *(B)* consistent with diffuse white matter shearing injury.

A   B

forms in the epidural space, compressing the underlying brain. The hyperdense lesion is sharply delineated from the underlying brain and is confined to a localized region because the marginal dura is adherent to the skull.

The clinical pattern includes the following sequence: there is an initial period of unconsciousness followed by a lucid interval, after which rapid neurological deterioration (altered consciousness, hemiparesis, pupillary dilatation) develops. However, the lucid interval is seen in only 20 percent of patients with epidural hematomas. Clinical worsening is more rapid with arterial epidural hematomas than with venous ones. Skull x-ray usually shows a linear fracture, most often traversing the middle meningeal artery groove. Bone fragments shear or lacerate this artery. Angiography shows an avascular mass located between normal parenchyma and the skull inner table.

There is displacement of the middle meningeal arteries and dural sinus away from the skull, with stretching and attenuation of the underlying arteries. These lesions are unilateral and usually cause midline shift. The presence of an accompanying intracerebral lesion may decrease the signs of mass effect and may lead to underestimation of hematoma size.

In acute epidural hematoma, CT shows a well-localized hyperdense extracerebral lesion (Fig. 13–11). The hematoma has a biconvex or lenticular shape with sharp margination as a result of the fact that dura remains adherent at both edges. Arterial pressure causes the lesion to bulge inward toward the brain parenchyma. Arterial epidural hematoma is most common in the temporal region. There is evidence of mass effect with early transtentorial herniation. Subacute epidural hematomas become symptomatic 48 hours to 2 weeks after

Figure 13–11. A 20-year-old man was struck in the left parietal region. He was immediately unconscious after injury. He regained consciousness transiently but became obtunded 18 hours later. *CT findings:* left parietal well-localized hyperdense lenticular-shaped lesion with surrounding edema and small parenchymal hematoma *(A)*. The fracture is seen with bone settings *(B)*.

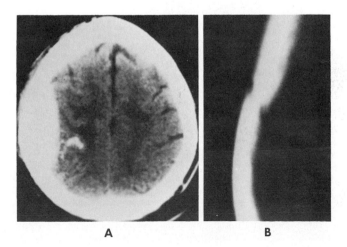

A   B

injury. These have a venous origin. Large hematomas may result if the major dural sinuses are lacerated. If the transverse sinus or torcular is torn, the epidural hematoma may involve the posterior fossa. In subacute epidural hematomas, CT shows a biconvex mixed-density lesion caused by clot liquefaction and retraction (Fig. 13–12). The dura may be inwardly displaced. This is best visualized on postcontrast scan; however, dural membrane may be seen on plain scan.

Nearly all epidural hematomas require surgical treatment. Prognosis is dependent upon several factors: (1) patient age, (2) location and size of the hematoma, (3) neurological status, (4) associated intracranial injuries, (5) extracranial injuries and (6) duration of clot. Mortality is highest with epidural hematomas causing midline shift exceeding 7 mm and with those patients in whom there was significant delay in diagnosis. Before CT came into use, 22 percent of epidural hematomas were associated with other lesions; this has been shown to be 40 to 48 percent on the basis of CT findings.[20] Certain epidural hematomas caused by venous bleeding are small. These patients may be asymptomatic; CT may demonstrate spontaneous resolution of these lesions. In other cases, slow venous leak may show delayed development of epidural hematoma. Initial CT may not demonstrate the lesion, but repeat scan shows it.

Subdural Hematoma (SDH). These have been classified on the basis of the interval following injury: acute, within 3 days; subacute, 4 to 14 days later and chronic, several weeks to months later.

Extravasated subdural blood remains as solid clot for several days and then liquefies. Most of these hematomas are primarily solid for two weeks; this precludes removal through burr hole trephination alone. In the second and third week, the hematoma contains some solid clot mixed with a variable amount of liquefied blood. After this time it is a liquefied collection with subdural membrane. Surgical studies in which the characteristics of SDH have been analyzed have shown the following: (1) hematoma was completely liquefied (57 percent); (2) hematoma was solid (15 percent) and (3) hematoma contained solid and liquid components (28 percent). These findings are a function of the time of surgery. Blood dissects arachnoid away from the dura. Since there are few thick fibrous bands to confine the blood extravasation, subdural hematoma may be more extensive than epidural hematoma.[21] The subdural type is slower to develop and this allows the underlying brain to accommodate.

Extravasated subdural blood results from tears in the superficial veins or venous sinuses or brain contusion. The blood spreads over the cerebral hemispheres. There may be associated parenchymal tissue damage. Subdural hematomas without an underlying cerebral lesion may be caused by bleeding from the superficial veins that extend from the cortex to the sinuses. Initially, extravasated blood is solid; however, if the arachnoid has been torn, blood may sometimes be mixed with CSF. Clot subsequently liquefies and there is hematoma organization. The inner dural membrane thickens and fibroblastic proliferation occurs. This becomes highly vascularized as capillaries grow into the dural membrane. There may be repeated episodes of hemorrhage from the fragile capillaries that causes expansion of SDH. This dural membrane requires approximately three weeks to form, but this is highly variable. This capsule is found at operation in one third of patients with hematomas believed to be of shorter duration; this was not identified in 10 percent of cases in which patients were symptomatic for at least four weeks. Calcification may occur within thick dural membrane. This occurs most commonly in children and young adults. It is usually associated with underlying cortical atrophy, which develops as a secondary phenomenon.

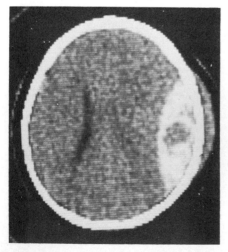

Figure 13–12. An 8-year-old boy fell out of a swing. He was immediately dazed and remained lethargic. Five days later he became left hemiparetic. *CT findings:* well-localized heterogeneous hyperdense right parietal lesion with associated mass effect. *Operative findings:* epidural hematomas with clot retraction.

One third of patients with SDH have an initial lucid interval with subsequent neurological deterioration. Forty percent of patients with acute SDH were not initially unconscious after head injury. Motor dysfunction and pupillary dilatation that developed after the initial stable period were characteristic of intracranial hematoma but not specific for SDH. Patients with chronic SDH may present with several clinical patterns. One is severe head injury with initial improvement and subsequent neurological deterioration several weeks later; a second is none or only trivial head injury but patients subsequently develop headache, altered consciousness, dementia, or motor dysfunction several months to years later.

Skull x-ray may show a linear skull fracture in patients with acute SDH: however, fracture is rarely seen in chronic SDH. Pineal shift

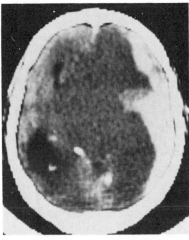

Figure 13–14. A 25-year-old man was hit with a brick in the right parietal region. He was immediately unconscious and subsequently developed status epilepticus. *CT findings:* bilenticular hyperdense right hemispheric extracerebral lesion with bulging at the pterion. There is extensive hypodense edema and intraventricular hemorrhage.

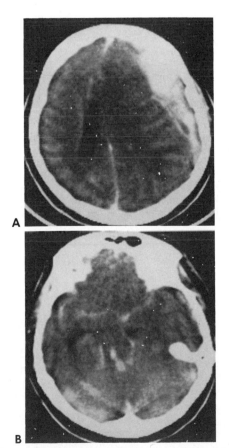

Figure 13–13. A 23-year-old man suffered multiple injuries in a motorcycle accident. He was comatose with fixed and dilated pupils. *CT findings:* right hemispheric hyperdense widespread lenticular-shaped subdural hematoma (A) causing mass effect and brain stem hemorrhagic contusion (B).

may not occur if SDH is located in certain locations such as posterior fossa or the subfrontal or subtemporal region. Isotope scan is rarely reliable in diagnosing SDH. Scalp injuries and linear skull fracture may cause superficial uptake to simulate SDH. In some cases isotope scan may show evidence of SDH. This consists of crescent-shaped uptake visualized on an anterior-posterior view, and this uptake may not be seen on lateral projection. Angiography had been the most reliable procedure prior to the CT era. Acute SDH appears as an avascular extracerebral mass located between the cortical vessels and the inner skull table. This is seen on anterior-posterior and tangential views; however, the lesion may be thin and seen only on oblique views with the head turned away from the lesion. Angiographic findings do not always permit differentiation of subtemporal subdural hematoma from temporal intracerebral hematoma because of the paucity of cortical vessels in this region.

Since the introduction of high-resolution scanners, subdural hematomas are routinely detected with CT. Angiography is not usually necessary except to identify accompanying vascular lesions. Acute subdural hematomas appear as hyperdense crescent-shaped lesions located between the calvarium and underlying cortex (Fig. 13–13). They may extend from the vertex to the skull base (Fig. 13–14). Less commonly, these hematomas are loculated by fibrous dural bands to appear circumscribed to simulate epidural hematoma. Localized SDH collections appear lenticular in shape; they are frequently multiloculated. If hyperdense SDH is located in the temporal fossa, it may be difficult to differentiate from overlying bone. Much of the mass effect seen with acute SDH is caused by brain injury and not the hematoma itself. Some acute SDH have associated intracerebral lesions or contralateral SDH (Fig. 13–15). Enhanced scan usually provides no additional diagnostic information in acute SDH.

As hematoma liquefies, there are changes in CT density pattern, lesion shape and enhancement. Within 7 days, partially liquefied hematoma appears as a heterogeneous mixed-

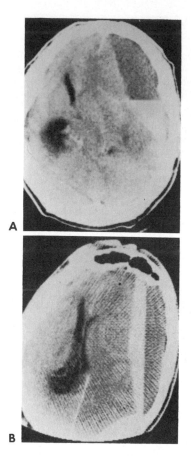

Figure 13–16. This man fell 30 feet and struck the right parietal region. He was unconscious for 30 minutes. Seven days later he became lethargic and developed left hemiparesis. *CT findings:* right parietal extracerebral mixed-density lesion with layering effect *(A)*. There is a second more localized lesion located posteriorly *(B)*. *Operative findings:* subacute subdural hematoma and epidural hematoma.

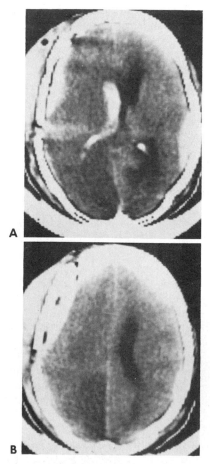

Figure 13–15. A 15-year-old boy was hit by an automobile. He was deeply comatose with fixed dilated pupils. Skull x-ray showed left parietal depressed fracture. *CT findings:* left parietal and contracoup right parietal hyperdense lenticular-shaped subdural hematoma *(A)*. There is overlying scalp hematoma with evidence of fracture and intraventricular hemorrhage *(B)*.

density lesion. A solid hyperdense area is located in the most dependent portion owing to gravitational effect (Fig. 13–16). By the second to fifth week after injury, the hematoma may be isodense with underlying brain parenchyma.[22, 23] Isodense SDH is detected by these *indirect* signs: (1) effacement of ipsilateral cortical sulcal spaces, (2) ipsilateral ventricular compression (Fig. 13–17), (3) diffuse enhancement (Fig. 13–18) or enhancement in the medial wall[24] and (4) medial displacement of gray-white matter interface.[25] If isodense SDH is unilateral, asymmetry of these findings may establish the diagnosis. With bilateral SDH there is no midline shift, and cortical sulcal spaces are symmetrically effaced. The bodies of the lateral ventricles are narrowed and the anterior frontal horns are sharply

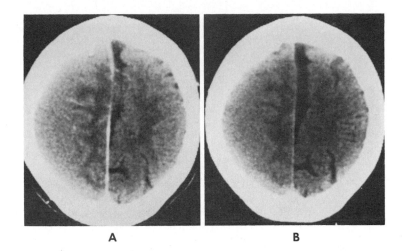

Figure 13–17. A 52-year-old woman developed headache and intermittent confusion. EEG and isotope scan were negative. *CT findings:* left hemispheric isodense lesion *(A)* with medial displacement of gray-white matter interface *(B).* *Operative finding:* subdural hematoma.

| A | B |

pointed (hare's ear sign) because of lateral ventricular compression.[26] Bilateral and symmetrical isodense subdural hematomas are sometimes detected only by angiography.

Chronic subdural hematomas are liquefied. They appear hypodense and crescent-shaped (Fig. 13–19). Lateral ventricles are medially displaced; cortical sulcal spaces are effaced. The medial membrane of SDH may consist of thickened dura. These may be visualized on plain scan (Fig. 13–20); however, it is more clearly seen on postcontrast scan. Some of these lesions may undergo multiple rebleeding episodes. This leads to formation of membranes; therefore, these multiple membranes may be recognized by CT.[27, 28] Calcification of medial hematoma wall is a rare complication; this is well seen on CT and plain skull x-ray (Fig. 13–21). Calcified hematoma may be associated with mass effect or cortical atrophy.[29]

Four conditions that may simulate CT findings of chronic SDH include: (1) subdural hygroma (Fig. 13–22), (2) enlarged extracerebral space caused by cerebral atrophy, (3) middle fossa arachnoid cysts and (4) middle cerebral artery infarction. Hygromas consist of CSF collections resulting from laceration of the arachnoid membrane. The torn arachnoid functions as a ball valve to permit CSF to leak into the subdural space during periods of increased intracranial pressure such as coughing and sneezing. CSF becomes loculated in the subdural space, and the lesion may increase in size. Subdural hygromas are most common in young children and elderly patients; they may develop following head trauma or craniotomy. These hygromas are located over the lateral convexity region and may extend from the frontal to the occipital region and into the interhemispheric fissure.

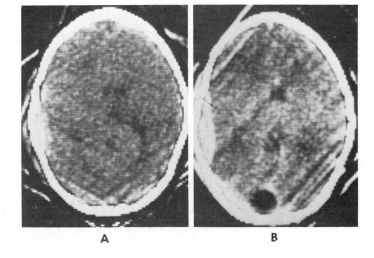

Figure 13–18. One month following head trauma, this young girl developed headache and episodic confusion. Skull x-ray and EEG were negative. *CT findings:* plain scan shows left hemispheric mass effect *(A).* Postcontrast scan shows enhancement within the left temporal extracerebral lesion and medial membrane *(B).*

| A | B |

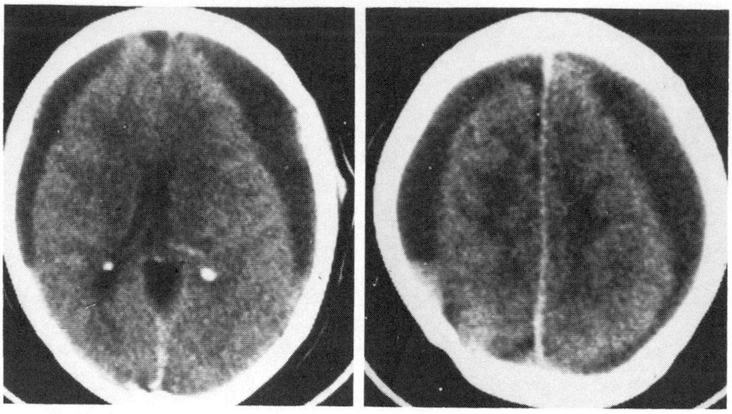

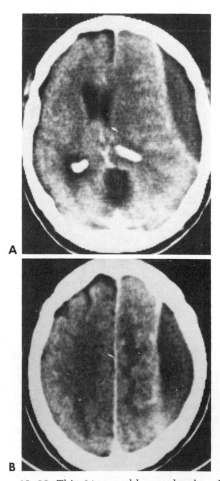

Figure 13–19. A 40-year-old man developed headache and episodic confusion one month after falling off a horse. EEG and isotope scan were negative. *CT findings:* bilateral hypodense subdural lesions *(A)* with the right-sided lesion being larger. There is ventricular compression. The posterior component of left-sided subdural hematoma has a hemorrhagic component *(B)*.

CT shows a semilunate-shaped hypodense extracerebral lesion. Mass effect may be manifested by ventricular distortion or displacement; however, sulcal spaces are not usually effaced. There is no enhancement within the medial membrane. They may enlarge, and these lesions may require surgical drainage. Others spontaneously resolve within months. It is not usually possible to differentiate SDH from subdural hygroma with angiography. Focal brain atrophy may cause CSF spaces to enlarge. CT shows a hypodense extracerebral lesion with ipsilateral enlargement of ventricles and cortical subarachnoid spaces. The gray-white matter interface is normal in position, and interdigitating enlarged sulcal spaces are prominent. Middle fossa arachnoid cysts may be associated with SDH. These appear as hypodense lesions. An accompanying SDH

Figure 13–20. This 64-year-old man developed confusion and left-sided weakness one week after falling in the shower. EEG was diffusely slow. *CT findings:* hypodense extracerebral lesion *(A)* with medial hyperdense nonenhancing medial border. Lateral ventricles are displaced to the left and gray-white matter interface in medially displaced *(B)*. *Operative findings:* liquefied subdural hematoma with thick neomembrane.

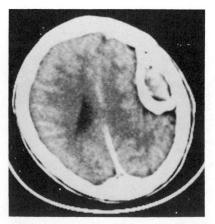

Figure 13–21. An 18-year-old man developed intermittent headache; examination was normal. Skull x-ray showed a calcified superficial lesion. *CT finding:* calcified subdural hematoma.

is sometimes detected only if the density of the SDH is different from a hypodense arachnoid cyst.[30] Large hypodense subdural hematomas may have straight or rounded medial borders to simulate middle cerebral artery infarction. These chronic lesions are separated from the lateral ventricle by intervening brain parenchyma, whereas infarction extends contiguous to the lateral ventricles. Subdural air appears hypodense. The density of air is quite different from CSF; therefore, this should never be confused with hypodense SDH (Fig. 13–23).

The usual management of SDH is surgical. Following craniotomy or trephination, CT

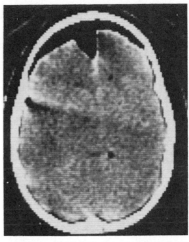

Figure 13–23. A child fell out of a swing. Two days later, he developed headache and nausea. Skull x-ray showed basilar skull fracture. *CT findings:* air is seen in the subdural, cisternal and ventricular spaces.

should demonstrate a decrease in lesion size and mass effect and patients should show clinical improvement. In some patients who clinically improve, CT shows mass effect that may resolve slowly. Certain patients show poor clinical response following surgery. This may result from several causes: (1) reaccumulation of SDH, (2) cerebral infarction, (3) postsurgical cerebral hemorrhage, (4) hydrocephalus and (5) cerebral atrophy caused by brain parenchymal compression. These complications are delineated by CT findings.

Nonsurgical management of some patients with SDH has utilized corticosteroids. Serial CT scans may be helpful in monitoring resolution of SDH in these patients. Significant reduction of mass effect usually occurs within one week of initiation of high-dosage corticosteroids; disappearance of SDH may take up to two months in patients who are treated nonsurgically. If lesion size or mass effect increases, surgical intervention is usually necessary.

UNUSUAL LOCATION OF EXTRACEREBRAL HEMATOMA

Epidural and Subdural Hematoma of Posterior Fossa. Epidural hematomas are usually more common than subdural hematomas in the posterior fossa; however, in neonates subdural hematomas are more common.[28, 31] These hematomas often follow a blow to the

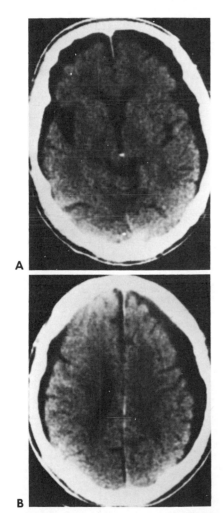

Figure 13–22. A 65-year-old man became confused two months after falling. He had organic dementia. EEG was diffusely slow. *CT findings:* bilateral semilunar hypodense lesions with prominent sulcal spaces *(A)*. Ventricles are symmetrical and slightly dilated; however, the right sylvian cistern is not visualized *(B)*. *Operative findings:* bilateral subdural hygromas.

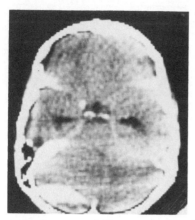

Figure 13–24. A 10-year-old boy was hit by a baseball in the occipital region. He was unconscious briefly but was neurologically normal within 24 hours. Skull x-ray was normal. *CT findings:* heterogeneous hyperdense lenticular-shaped left posterior fossa extracerebral lesion with nonvisualization of the fourth ventricle.

back of the head. SDH caused by tentorial laceration may occur in newborns following difficult obstetrical procedures. Epidural hematomas originate from a tear in the meningeal branch of the occipital or vertebral arteries or from the transverse sinus. If epidural hematoma is arterial in origin, signs of increased intracranial pressure and brain stem compression may develop very rapidly, whereas with venous bleeding, patients may become symptomatic (neck pain, nausea, vomiting, altered consciousness) within 3 to 10 days. These hematomas are frequently associated with vertical linear fracture extending across the lateral sinus toward the foramen magnum. The CT finding of epidural hematoma is that of a lenticular-shaped hyperdense posterior fossa extracerebral lesion. The hematoma may efface or displace the fourth ventricle anteriorly. Supratentorial extension is well visualized by CT. A hyperdense lesion may be heterogeneous with interspersed hypodense portions; this results from clot retraction (Fig. 13–24). Subdural hematomas result from a tear in either lateral sinus wall, emissary vein or brain injury. CT findings of subdural hematoma may be similar to those of epidural hematoma or the finding may be a crescent-shaped lesion extending along the tentorium conforming to the available space. There may be an accompanying intracerebellar hematoma.[32]

Interhemispheric Subdural Hematoma. These are caused by laceration of veins between the parietal-occipital cortex and the superior sagittal sinus. Therefore, these lesions are most extensive in the posterior interhemispheric fissure. They may extend inferiorly to the layer over the tentorium (Fig. 13–25). They are usually unilateral. The shape is that of a crescent, with the flat surface being medial along the falx. Chronic subdural hematomas appear as hypodense lesions in the parietal-occipital cortex. This may simulate cortical atrophy. The interhemispheric region is the common location for subdural bleeding in children who have suffered child abuse in the form of shaking injury.

Subtemporal Subdural Hematoma. Subdural hemorrhage may occur in the floor of the middle fossa. The lesion may extend posteriorly to the tentorial surface. Axial CT shows a thin layer of hyperdense blood, but this may be difficult to differentiate from the hyperdense appearance or bones of the middle fossa. The lesion causes the temporal horn to be elevated and displaced medially and anteriorly. Subtemporal SDH is best visualized by coronal sections.

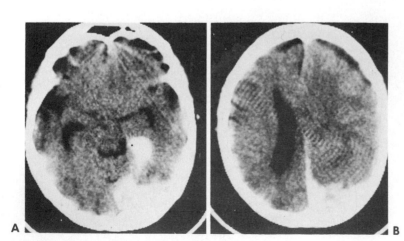

Figure 13–25. A 35-year-old woman with coagulation disorder became lethargic and was noted not to be moving her left side. *CT findings:* right tentorial (A) and posterior interhemispheric hyperdense subdural hematoma (B).

CEREBROSPINAL FLUID LEAKAGE

Rhinorrhea or otorrhea results from a basilar skull fracture that produces a tear in the dura and arachnoid. This allows CSF to drain from the nose or ear. Intracranial air (pneumocephalus) may initially enter the cisternal spaces and the ventricles. The potential risk in patients with CSF leakage is development of bacterial meningitis. CSF leakage occurs with fractures in three common locations: (1) fracture through the posterior wall of the frontal sinus with CSF leakage into the nasal cavity, (2) cribriform plate fracture with CSF leakage into the nasal cavity and (3) temporal bone fracture with leakage of CSF from the ear. Conventional tomograms are necessary to demonstrate a fracture site in the frontal sinus, cribriform plate and temporal bone. CT may demonstrate intracranial air. Metrizamide cisternal CT study may demonstrate the precise point of leakage of CSF into the nasal cavity.[33]

PENETRATING HEAD INJURIES

These may result from bullet injuries or other foreign bodies such as nails, knife blades or wood. Bullets fired from military weapons are encased in a steel jacket. These pass through the skull and brain parenchyma without shattering; however, other types of bullets shatter on impact to produce multiple intracranial metal fragments. The missile may damage intracranial structures by several mechanisms: (1) by producing cerebral edema and mass effect, (2) by causing intracranial hemorrhage, (3) by damaging cerebral blood ves-

sels and (4) by causing intracranial tracking (Fig. 13–26). Skull x-ray may demonstrate the location of the bullet and the intracranial metallic fragments and the presence of skull fracture. The quality of CT scan is frequently degraded by artifact emanating from the metallic fragments; however, the presence of intracranial hematoma and pneumocephalus is usually still detected. The presence of a linear hypodense band may represent a bullet track. Intracranial foreign bodies are a potential source of infection, especially at a later stage. CT is most reliable to detect abscess formation.

SECONDARY BRAIN INJURY

With severe head injury, there may be a rapid increase in intracranial pressure. This may lead to intracranial shift and herniation, with vascular damage in the form of ischemia, infarction and hemorrhage. These secondary brain injuries caused by vascular lesion(s) may persist after intracranial hypertension has been reduced. With brain swelling and shift, the following may be seen: (1) parahippocampal and cingulate gyrus necrosis and hemorrhage, (2) medial occipital cortex infarction caused by posterior cerebral artery occlusion and (3) brain stem rotation and hemorrhage. Traumatic brain stem hemorrhages are usually petechial. If they coalesce to form a macroscopic lesion, they may be seen on CT. Ischemic brain injury following trauma may be focal or diffuse. For example, focal ischemia may occur in the region of the cerebral contusion or subdural hematoma. Diffuse ischemic lesions frequently result from intracranial hypertension. These ischemic lesions

Figure 13–26. A woman was shot in the left temporal region. She was confused and had right hemiparesis. *CT findings:* intracranial air and a bone fragment is seen *(A)* with blood in the left sylvian cistern *(B)*.

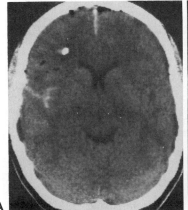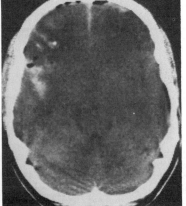

A   B

usually involve gray matter structures such as the basal ganglia, hippocampus and vascular border zone regions.

LATE EFFECTS OF HEAD INJURY

Post-traumatic hydrocephalus may result from extravasation of blood or purulent material into the basal cisterns with subsequent fibrosis and adhesion formation. Blockade may be extraventricular (communicating) or intraventricular (obstructive). The reported incidence of post-traumatic ventricular enlargement caused by hydrocephalus or atrophy (focal or diffuse) has varied from 1.5 to 29 percent. Ventricular enlargement usually develops within 90 days of head injury.[34] The ventricles may dilate early and then return to normal size; therefore, early ventricular dilatation does not have prognostic value.

Localized encephalomalacia may develop in regions of contusions or intracranial hematomas. CT shows a hypodense nonenhancing lesion with adjacent ventricular dilatation and enlarged cisternal spaces. Cavities may also develop in the brain parenchyma. These may communicate with ventricular and subarachnoid spaces. These subsequently enlarge because of CSF pulsatile force. CT may show a hypodense lesion with ventricular dilatation. The hypodense lesion may appear to communicate with the ventricles, but this communication is usually not confirmed by metrizamide CT. Leptomeningeal cysts form when the arachnoid becomes lacerated and entrapped under the fracture site. A loculated CSF collection causes localized bone erosion and enlargement of the fracture line because of CSF pulsatile erosion. CT demonstrates a defect in bone continuity with localized bone erosion caused by a hypodense cyst located beneath the fracture line. Skull x-ray shows enlargement of the fracture line.

REFERENCES

1. Langfitt TW, Gennarelli TA: Can the outcome from head injury be improved? J Neurosurg 56:19, 1982
2. Merino de Villesante, Taveras JM: CT in acute head trauma. Am J Roentgenol 126:765–778, 1976
3. Roberson FC, Kishori PRS, Miller JD: The value of serial CT in the management of severe head injury. Surg Neurol 12:161–167, 1979
4. Jennett B, Teasdale O: Management of Head Injuries. F. A. Davis, Philadelphia, 1981
5. French BN, Dublin AB: The value of CT in the management of 1000 consecutive head injuries. Surg Neurol 7:139–151, 1977
6. French BN: Limitations and pitfalls of CT in the evaluation of craniocerebral injury. Surg Neurol 7:139–151, 1977
7. Clifton GL, Grossman RG, Makela ME: Neurological course and correlated CT findings after severe closed head injury. J Neurosurg 51:611, 1980
8. Blackwood W, McMenemcy WA, Meyer A: Greenfield's Neuropathology. Williams and Wilkins, Baltimore, 1963, p. 440
9. Jennett B: Skull x-rays after recent head injury. Clin Radiol 31:463, 1980
10. Zimmerman RA, Bilaniuk LT, Bruce D: Computed tomography of pediatric head trauma: acute general cerebral swelling. Radiology 126:403–408, 1978
11. Bruce DA, Alavi A, Bilaniuk L: Diffuse cerebral swelling following head injuries in children: the syndrome of malignant brain edema. J Neurosurg 131:381–383, 1981
12. Hayman LA, Evans RA, Hinck VC: Rapid high-dose contrast computed tomography of isodense subdural hematoma and cerebral swelling. Radiology 131:381–383, 1979
13. Weisberg LA: Computed tomography in acute head trauma. Comput Tomogr 3:14–28, 1979
14. Snock J, Jennett B, Adams JH: CT after recent severe head injury in patients without acute intracranial hematoma. J Neurol Neurosurg Psychiatr 42:215–225, 1979
15. Zimmerman RA, Bilaniuk LT, Dolinskas C: Computed tomography of acute intracerebral hemorrhagic contusion. Comput Axial Tomogr 1:271–280, 1977
16. Diaz FG, Yock DH, Larson D: Early diagnosis of delayed post-traumatic intracerebral hematomas. J Neurosurg 50:217–223, 1979
17. Galbraith S, Teasdale G: Predicting the need for operation in the patient with an occult traumatic intracranial hematoma. J Neurosurg 55:75–81, 1981
18. Sweet RC, Miller JD, Lipper M: Significance of bilateral abnormalities on the CT scan in patients with severe head injury. Neurosurgery 3:16–21, 1979
19. Zimmerman RA, Bilaniuk LT, Genneralli T: Computed tomography of shearing injuries of the cerebral white matter. Radiology 127:393–396, 1978
20. Cordobes F, Lobato R, Rivas JJ: Observations on 82 patients with extradural hematoma. J Neurosurg 54:179–186, 1981
21. Markwalder TM: Chronic subdural hematomas: a review. J Neurosurg 54:637–645, 1981
22. Scotti G, Terbrugge K, Melanon D: Evaluation of the age of subdural hematomas by CT. J Neurosurg 47:311–315, 1977
23. Moller, A, Ericson K: CT of isoattenuating subdural hematomas. Radiology 130:149–152, 1979
24. Tsai FY, Huprich JE, Segall HD: The contrast-enhanced CT scan in the diagnosis of isodense subdural hematoma. J Neurosurg 50:64–69, 1979
25. Barmeir E, Dubowitz B: Grey-white matter interface displacement: a new sign in the CT diagnosis of subtle subdural hematomas. Clin Radiol 32:393–396, 1981
26. Mareu H, Becker H: Computed tomography of bilateral isodense chronic subdural hematomas. Neuroradiology 14:81–83, 1977
27. Yamada H, Watanabe T, Murata S: Developmental process of chronic subdural collections of fluid

based on CT scan findings. Surg Neurol 13:441–448, 1980

28. Zimmerman RD, Danriger A: Extracerebral trauma. Radiol Clin North Am 20:105, 1982

29. Debois V, Lombaert A: Calcified chronic subdural hematoma. Neurosurgery 14:455–459, 1980

30. Auer LM, Gallhofer B, Ladurner G: Diagnosis and treatment of middle fossa arachnoid cysts and subdural hematomas. J Neurosurg 54:366–369, 1981

31. Stone JL, Schaffer L, Ramsey RG: Epidural hematomas of the posterior fossa. Surg Neurol 11:419–424, 1979

32. Tsai FY, Teal JS, Itabashi HH et al: Computed tomography of the posterior fossa in trauma. J Comput Assist Tomogr 4:290, 1980

33. Naidich TP, Moran CJ: Precise anatomic localization of atraumatic sphenoethmoidal CSF rhinorrhea by metrizamide CT cisternography. J Neurosurg 53:222, 1980

34. Gudeman SK, Kishori PRS, Becker DP: CT in the evaluation of incidence and significance of post-traumatic hydrocephalus. Radiology 141:397–402, 1981

Chapter 14

GAIT AND MOVEMENT DISORDERS

Disturbances of gait and posture maintenance and abnormal adventitious movements may result from pathophysiological disturbances at multiple levels of the neural-axis: spinal cord, cerebellum, brain stem, basal ganglia and frontal lobe. In some patients multiple mechanisms may be involved. If the patient initially presents with nonspecific dysequilibrium and gait unsteadiness without specific cerebellar or corticospinal tract findings, a vermal lesion should be suspected.[1] Vermal tumors such as medulloblastoma and metastases usually cause mass effect and obstructive hydrocephalus by early compression of the fourth ventricle; therefore, gait disturbance and intracranial hypertension are early clinical features. The mechanism of gait disturbance is believed to result either from cerebellar system dysfunction or hydrocephalus; however, gait may improve after diversionary shunting alone. The mechanism is not known by which abnormal ventricular dilatation causes gait disturbance: This may be caused by involvement of the frontopontocerebellar pathway. In one third of patients with medulloblastomas, gait ataxia is the early symptom; however, in one half of these, lateral ventricles are not markedly dilated, although the temporal horns may be quite prominent.

Patients with other posterior fossa tumors such as acoustic neurinoma and tentorial meningioma (Fig. 14–1) may initially present with gait ataxia and dysequilibrium. In six patients with these tumors, gait abnormality was quite bizarre and could not be classified. Because there were no accompanying neurological signs, initial diagnosis of hysterical gait disturbance had been established prior to the diagnosis of tumor being made by CT. Because of lack of accompanying abnormal neurological findings and negative noninvasive diagnostic studies (EEG, skull x-ray, isotope scan), it is unlikely that invasive contrast radiographic procedures would have been performed in these patients before the advent of CT. The mechanism of gait disturbance in patients with tentorial meningiomas is believed to be cerebellar involvement, whereas in acoustic neuromas, gait dysfunction may result from cerebellar, vestibular or brain stem involvement. In certain small acoustic neuromas, gait impairment may be caused by impaired vestibular mechanism without cerebellar or brain stem involvement.

In other patients the initial gait disturbance symptom is that of stiffness, awkwardness and impaired posture maintenance. These patients have a broad-based small-stepped bradykinetic gait with impaired postural stability and poor righting reflexes. They assume a stooped posture; however, they have no difficulty initiating gait or evidence of festination quality to the gait. The gait disturbance of these patients is similiar to that seen in patients with normal pressure hydrocephalus, parkinsonism and evidence of bilateral corticospinal tract involvement. These patients are all older than 65 years and have normal mentation and no urinary incontinence. CT shows the following: (1) lateral ventricular enlargement as manifested by increased measurements of the following distances, i.e., bifrontal and bicaudate; (2) normal-sized temporal horns, (3) enlarged third ventricle, (4) normal-sized fourth ventricle and (5) no enlargement of cerebral or cerebellar sulcal pattern. Isotope or metrizamide cisternogram does not show CSF flow abnormalities. These findings have suggested that "senile gait" disorder is related to the ventriculomegaly itself.[2] The ventricles were most prominently enlarged in the frontal region. Five patients with "senile gait" under-

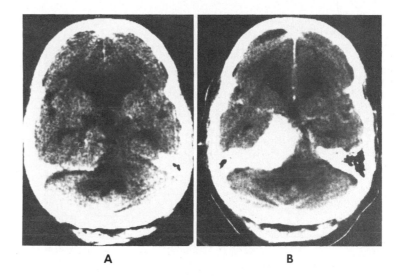

Figure 14–1. A 48-year-old woman developed gait instability. Findings were broad-based unsteady gait with normal heel-to-shin movements. Skull x-ray and isotope scan were negative. *CT findings:* hyperdense sharply marginated left tentorial (A) densely enhancing lesion with comma-shaped extending into the middle fossa (B). *Operative finding:* tentorial meningioma.

A   B

went diversionary shunting procedure because CT showed triventricular enlargement without visualization of cortical sulcal spaces; however, cisternogram did not show ventricular reflux pattern of NPH. In these patients, clinical gait disturbance did not improve after shunt, but ventricles decreased in size.

In normal pressure hydrocephalus (NPH), gait disorder is described as magnetic or apractic. These patients experience difficulty in using their legs to ambulate, although similar leg movements that are performed when the patient is lying in bed with his legs raised in the air are more dexterous. These patients have difficulty raising their legs off the floor (magnetic gait). This gait disorder is believed to result from transcortical innervatory paresis of the legs because of involvement of the anterior corpus callosal fibers.[3, 4] The gait disturbance of NPH may precede clinical onset of dementia and urinary incontinence. CT findings in NPH include: (1) triventricular enlargement with frontal horns being enlarged to a greater extent than occipital horns, (2) the presence of a periventricular hypodense rim surrounding the anterior frontal horns, (3) temporal horn dilatation and (4) nonvisualization of cortical sulcal spaces. All of our patients with gait disturbance who did not show evidence of dementia had CT findings of ventricular enlargement without visualization of any cortical sulcal spaces. Isotope and metrizamide cisternogram were performed in certain of these patients; these studies showed that tracer material refluxed into the ventricular system, confirming the impression of impaired extraventricular CSF circulation (Fig. 14–2).

There was clinical improvement in gait in 85 percent of these patients, with decrease in ventricular size following diversionary shunting. In 15 percent of patients there was no clinical improvement, and ventricular size remained unchanged after the shunt was inserted and appeared to be functioning.

Gait ataxia may be caused by superficial or deep frontal lobe lesions (pseudocerebellar signs). In his analysis Brun divided patients into two groups: those with gait ataxia that involves both legs and that caused by bifrontal lesions, and those with unilateral ataxia that involves the leg contralateral to the lesion. Although frontal lobe lesions may cause findings identical to those of cerebellar lesions, e.g., ataxia and dysmetria, nystagmus is rarely present. Pseudocerebellar signs are postulated as caused by functional impairment of the frontopontocerebellar pathways. The frontal lesions causing pseudocerebellar findings are usually neoplastic or traumatic in etiology; less commonly they are caused by vascular occlusion.[5] Prior to CT, patients with these findings represented a difficult diagnostic problem and four-vessel angiography would have been necessary.

Gait ataxia is most commonly a manifestation of cerebellar pathological disorder. Cerebellar atrophy occurs with toxic agents (alcohol, phenytoin), aminoacidurias (maple syrup urine disease), hypothyroidism, Wilson's disease, systemic carcinoma and a varied group of degenerative disorders (familial or sporadic) of unknown etiologies. There is loss of Purkinje cells with advancing age that causes cerebellar atrophy. This is most marked

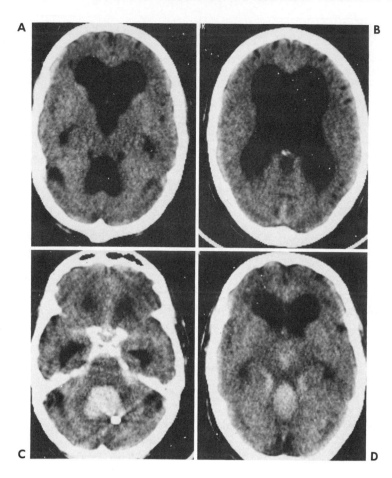

Figure 14–2. A 60-year-old man became progressively unable to walk. Findings were spastic paraparesis with urinary incontinence and normal mentation. *CT findings:* triventricular dilatation with marked fourth ventricular (A) and temporal horn dilatation. Cortical sulcal spaces are nonvisualized (B). Metrizamide cisternogram shows contrast in basal cisterns (C) and ventricles (D) with none in cortical sulcal spaces.

in the anterior lobe and superior vermis and is independent of supratentorial cerebral atrophy.[6] There are functional anatomical subdivisions within the cerebellum. The archicerebellum consists of a flocculonodular lobe with functional connections with a vestibular system; clinical abnormalities include gait instability, dysequilibrium and horizontal nystagmus. The paleocerebellum includes the anterior vermis; clinical dysfunction includes gait ataxia and truncal instability. The neocerebellum consists of lateral cerebellar hemispheres. Clinical findings include limb ataxia and other cerebellar signs (dysmetria, intention tremor, hypotonia, dysdiodokinesia).

In patients with cerebellar atrophic disorders, the relationship between air studies and clinical findings has been investigated. LeMay established that the finding of cerebellar sulci that appear 2 to 4 mm in width is consistent with mild to moderate atrophy and sulci that are greater than 4 mm in size is consistent with marked cerebellar atrophy.[7, 8] The size of the cerebellar sulci correlated with the sever-

ity of cerebellar dysfunction. Robertson reported that fourth ventricular height correlated better with clinical signs than cerebellar sulci width.[9] Utilizing midline tomography in the sagittal plane, Kennedy measured the following dimensions: vermal midline folial pattern, fourth ventricular height, and size of brain stem and posterior fossa cisterns. There was good correlation between the findings of prominent folial vermal pattern, enlarged fourth ventricles and posterior fossa cistern with severity of clinical cerebellar signs; however, one half of patients with pneumographic findings of cerebellar atrophy had no clinical cerebellar dysfunction.[10]

We have used the following CT criteria for cerebellar atrophy: (1) visualization of the lateral cerebellar folial pattern that is consistent with cerebellar hemispheric cortical atrophy; (2) visualization of the superior and midline cerebellar folial pattern that is consistent with vermal atrophy; (3) enlargement of the fourth ventricle as manifested by anteroposterior height in excess of 4 mm representing hemispheric atrophy and (4) enlargement of the cerebellopontine, superior cerebellar, cisterna magna and quadrigeminal cisterns.[11–13] The brain stem size may be represented as the ratio of the prepontine cistern divided by the distance between the posterior clinoid and the anterior-superior aspect of fourth ventricle.

In alcoholic-induced cerebellar atrophy, the initial and most severe pathological changes occur in the anterior-superior vermis.[14] CT findings are: (1) midline folial prominence resulting from vermal atrophy (90 percent), (2) lateral folial prominence caused by hemispheric atrophy (40 percent), (3) enlarged superior cerebellar cistern (90 percent) and (4) enlarged basal cisterns including the cerebellopontine and quadrigeminal cistern (33 percent). All patients who had hemispheric atrophy had accompanying vermal atrophy (Fig. 14–3).[12, 15] In patients with cerebellar atrophy, one half had cerebral atrophy; only 5 percent showed clinical evidence of dementia and one third had Korsakoff syndrome. It is not unusual for alcoholic patients without cerebellar dysfunction to show CT evidence of vermal atrophy. Follow-up studies and subsequent necropsy results will determine the prognostic significance of this CT finding in neurologically clinically asymptomatic alcoholic patients.

In carcinomatous cerebellar degeneration, vermis and cerebellar hemispheres are usually equally affected. These patients have clinical evidence of gait and limb ataxia. In several patients with systemic carcinoma who had gait ataxia, CT was performed to exclude cerebellar metastases; it showed cerebellar atrophy (Fig. 14–4). In patients with gait ataxia and CT evidence of cerebellar atrophy, thorough investigation for a systemic neoplasm should be pursued. CT findings confirm the evidence of pancerebellar atrophy as manifested by vermal and hemispheric atrophy. This is different from the study reported by Koller, in which vermal rather than hemispheric atrophy was characteristic of carcinomatous cerebellar degeneration.[12] This study suggests that CT may detect early changes that have not been appreciated in previous pathological studies.

Continuing phenytoin therapy may lead to Purkinje cell degeneration. Patients with acute phenytoin intoxication present with gait ataxia; however, with continuing drug therapy these patients usually do not show cerebellar dysfunction. Purkinje cells are very sensitive to hypoxic damage that may occur during seizures, and this may complicate assessing the exact etiology of cerebellar atrophy in chronic seizure patients on phenytoin therapy. McLain has reported irreversible cerebellar syndrome in patients on phenytoin therapy without evidence of episodes of systemic hypoxia, and these patients had elevated phenytoin blood levels.[16] Koller reported eight patients on continuing phenytoin therapy who had no clinical cerebellar deficit but had CT evidence of cerebellar atrophy.[12] CT findings of phenytoin-induced cerebellar atrophy include: (1) enlarged superior cerebellar cistern (75 percent), (2) enlarged cisterna magna (50 percent), (3) enlarged CPA cistern (63 percent), (4) vermal atrophy (37 percent) and (5) enlarged fourth ventricle. The marked enlargement of the cisternal magna was not seen in patients with other types of cerebellar dis-

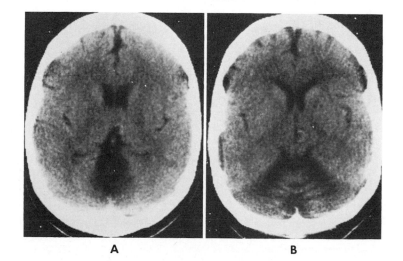

Figure 14–3. A 42-year-old alcoholic became increasingly unable to walk. Findings were gait and truncal ataxia with normal upper extremity movements. *CT findings:* superior vermal (A) and hemispheric cerebellar atrophy (B).

A   B

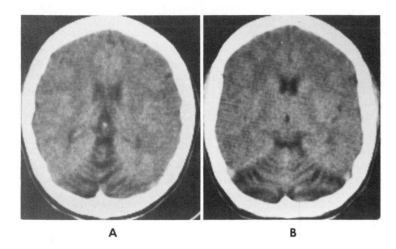

Figure 14–4. A 40-year-old man with bronchogenic carcinoma developed gait instability. Findings were gait, truncal and limb ataxia. *CT findings:* cerebellar vermal (*A*) and hemispheric atrophy (*B*).

orders; however, it was seen as an isolated finding in patients with no cerebellar disturbances.

In the primary genetically determined cerebellar degenerative disorders, CT may be utilized as one of multiple diagnostic parameters to indicate areas of the pathological involvement, e.g., vermis, cerebellar hemisphere and brain stem. Patients with clinical features consistent with olivopontocerebellar (OPC) degeneration (Fig. 14–5) may show these CT findings: (1) hemispheric atrophy with minimal vermal atrophy; (2) enlarged cisterns, including superior cerebellar, quadrigeminal and ambient; (3) enlarged fourth ventricle that results from hemispheric atrophy and (4) decrease in size of the brain stem. These are consistent with pathological findings

in these disorders, including loss of neurons in the cerebellar hemisphere, basis pontis and inferior olivery nuclei.[17, 18] Some patients with OPC develop other neurological abnormalities such as dementia and parkinsonism. In these cases CT may show cerebral atrophy and basal ganglia abnormalities such as calcification or hypodense lesions, and pathological findings confirm neuronal dropout in these regions. Ataxia telangiectasia is a disorder of unknown etiology with cutaneous and neurological manifestations (gait ataxia, head tremor, impaired vibration and position sensation, choreoathetosis). There are prominent cutaneous and conjunctival telangiectasias; however, intracranial vascular malformations are not usually seen in this syndrome. CT findings include prominent vermal atrophy with less severe

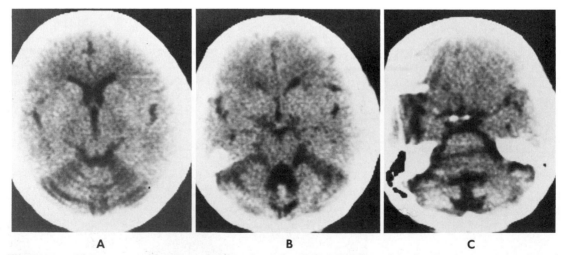

Figure 14–5. This 52-year-old woman developed gait instability and dysarthria. Findings were gait and limb ataxia, dysarthria, impaired gag reflex and rigidity. *CT findings:* enlarged cerebellar vermal and folial pattern (*A*), fourth ventricles and basal cisterns (*B, C*).

hemispheric involvement. This pattern of cerebellar involvement is confirmed by necropsy findings.[19] In patients with other disorders (Friedreich's ataxia, Charcot-Marie-Tooth syndrome), pathological lesions are predominantly in the spinal cord and peripheral nerve; therefore, CT is expected not to show evidence of cerebellar atrophy.

If gait ataxia is caused by demyelinating disease such as multiple sclerosis, pathological lesions may be in the spinal cord, cerebral white matter, cerebellum, brain stem. Gait impairment caused by cerebellar involvement is a common clinical finding. It is usually accompanied by other neurological abnormalities such as visual loss, paresthesias, spasticity, dysarthria and ophthalmoplegias due to other demyelinated lesions. Demyelinated lesions are uncommon in the cerebellum; they are more common in cerebral white matter, optic nerve, brain stem and spinal cord. Pathological studies have shown that most demyelinated lesions (plaques) are located in white matter. Forty percent are periventricular; they are usually located contiguous with the anterior and posterior lateral ventricular region (Fig. 14–6). The demyelinating process may result in supratentorial and infratentorial atrophy; this has been confirmed by pneumographic and necropsy studies.

In patients with a clinical diagnosis of probable multiple sclerosis, CT has shown a high incidence of cerebral atrophy. In one study this CT finding was present in 81 percent of patients with chronic and well-established multiple sclerosis.[20] Other CT findings in patients with MS include sharply marginated hypodense lesions located contiguous with the trigone, anterior or posterior ventricular region. It is believed that these represent demyelinated lesions. In other patients with severe gait ataxia caused by cerebellar–brain stem demyelinated lesions, CT showed hemispheric cerebellar atrophy, enlarged fourth ventricle, and enlarged ambient and cerebellopontine angle cisterns.

In patients with acute exacerbations of multiple sclerosis, CT may show enhancing lesions. These lesions are usually isodense on plain scan. There is no evidence of mass effect or edema, and the lesions show nodular enhancement.[21, 22] The enhancement may be dense and nodular or subependymal. The lesions are usually multiple (Fig. 14–7); in rare instances the demyelinated lesion is solitary (Fig. 14–8). Some demyelinated lesions appear hypodense with associated mass effect (Fig. 14–9), and there is diffuse peripheral edge enhancement.[26] The location of enhancing lesions does not always correlate with clinical neurological signs. We have seen several patients with enhancing periventricular or deep white matter lesions with active MS but without symptoms referable to these lesions. These enhancing lesions represent active demyelination with extravasation of contrast medium through the impaired blood-brain barrier. The mechanism of contrast enhancement seen with CT is similar to that causing positive isotope scan uptake. There may be resolution in enhancement if patients are treated with corticosteroids even in the absence of clinical improvement. There is more gradual spontaneous resolution of the

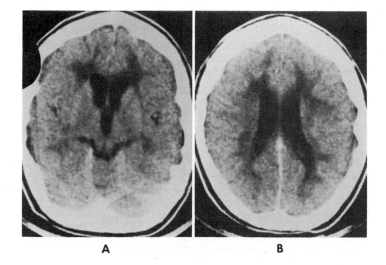

Figure 14–6. A 21-year-old woman developed gait instability, diplopia and dysarthria. Findings were bilateral internuclear ophthalmoplegia, Babinski sign and right-limb ataxia. *CT findings:* bilateral symmetrical frond-like hypodense (A) periventricular lesions (B).

A   B

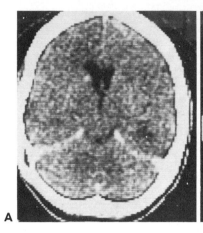
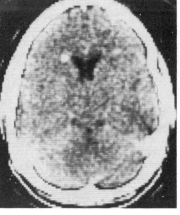

A

B

Figure 14–7. A 35-year-old woman had several episodes of diplopia and vertigo. Findings were gait ataxia and internuclear ophthalmoplegia. *CT finding:* isodense multiple periventricular enhancing lesion *(A, B).*

enhancement that develops within several months even without corticosteroid therapy. Certain hypodense lesions remained unchanged and others became isodense.[24]

The clinical diagnosis of multiple sclerosis is based upon dissemination of symptoms temporally (multiple clinical episodes of neurological deterioration) and spatially (multiple levels of the neural axis). The diagnosis is established upon clinical findings, although certain diagnostic studies are helpful. These include: (1) abnormal gamma globulin content, presence of oligoclonal gamma globulin bands; (2) abnormal evoked potentials such as visual, brain stem and somatosensory. Demyelinated lesions appear to be more sensitively detected by nuclear magnetic resonance than by CT. The diagnosis of multiple sclerosis should be always made with great caution, because this condition may simulate other disorders. Huckman et al. have reported detection of tentorial meningiomas in several patients initially diagnosed as having multiple sclerosis.[25]

Abnormal Involuntary Movements

Chorea. These are defined as semipurposeful random and nonrhythmical movements; they may involve the extremities and the trunk and oral-facial regions. These are usually symmetrical; rarely, chorea may be unilateral. Etiologies include Huntington's disease, rheumatic fever, Wilson's disease, systemic lupus erythematosus, pregnancy, vascular occlusion, and drug effects. In Huntington's disease, CT is quite useful diagnostically. It shows that the ratio of maximum distance between frontal horns compared with intercaudate distance has been reduced; this results from caudate atrophy. In rare instances, chorea develops suddenly and the movements are unilateral;

chorea is not accompanied by hemiparesis. This is probably caused by vascular ischemia involving deep penetrating lenticulostriate vessels. CT shows a hypodense or isodense

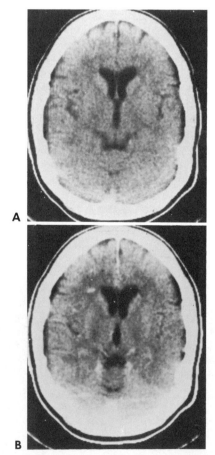

A

B

Figure 14–8. An 18-year-old woman developed difficulty walking. Findings were spastic paraparesis and optic atrophy. CSF showed elevated gamma globulin. *CT findings:* left periventricular isodense (A) enhancing lesion (B).

ebellum, cerebral cortex. CT findings in Wilson's disease include: (1) symmetrical hypodense lesions within the putamen and globus pallidus, (2) dilatation of frontal horns resulting from caudate atrophy, (3) hypodense regions within the cerebellum, (4) cerebellar atrophy and (5) brain stem atrophy as manifested by widening of surrounding perimesencephalic cisterns. The hypodense lesions in the lenticular nucleus reflect necrosis and reactive changes; these are usually seen only in patients with neurological deficit.[26] There is no CT evidence of hyperdense lesions in the basal ganglia or cerebellum despite the presence of heavy metal accumulation in this disorder. Because of the similarity of copper and calcium with heavy metals, it was originally speculated that hyperdense lesions would be

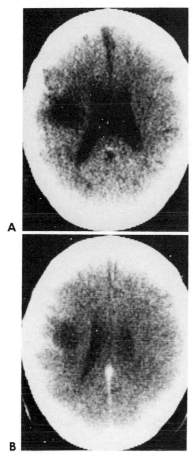

Figure 14–9. This 28-year-old woman developed visual blurring and right-sided numbness. EEG, CSF and evoked potentials were normal. *CT findings:* left parietal hypodense (A) nonenhancing lesion (B) with no mass effect. Angiogram showed left parietal avascular mass. *Operative finding:* demyelinated lesion.

enhancing lesion involving the caudate and lenticular nuclei with sparing of the internal caspule (Fig. 14–10).

Wilson's Disease. This is a disorder characterized by abnormal retention of copper in specific body areas such as liver, cornea, and brain. The diagnosis is established by the following laboratory results: decreased serum ceruloplasmin, decreased serum copper and increased urinary copper excretion. Manifestations of neurological involvement include postural tremor, dystonia, chorea and parkinsonism. The patient is frequently incoordinated and falls because of gait ataxia. Necropsy studies have shown bilateral necrosis and cysts in the lenticular nuclei. Atrophic changes have been reported in other areas: thalamus, subthalamus, substantia nigra, red nucleus, cer-

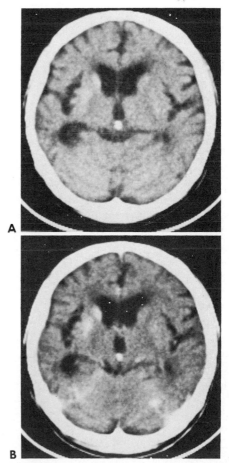

Figure 14–10. A 59-year-old man awakened with intermittent jerking movements of the right arm. Findings were right upper extremity hemichorea without hemiparesis or reflex abnormality. *CT findings:* left caudate isodense and putamenal (A) enhancing lesion with sparing of internal capsule (B).

seen by CT in patients with Wilson's disease; however, hypodense basal ganglionic CT lesions are identical to necropsy findings in these patients. CT is expected to be normal in patients without neurological findings, and this has been the experience in all series reported to date. In some cases, CT abnormalities may progress despite effective therapy with penicillamine.[27]

Hemiballism. These consist of irregular random and nonrhythmical flailing movements that are usually unilateral and involve arms more than legs. The condition results from a focal lesion in the subthalamus. The most common lesions are hemorrhage, neoplasm and infarction. In patients who demonstrate hemiballistic movements there may be no accompanying hemiparesis. CT visualizes the lesion in the thalamic region; however, coronal views are usually required to differentiate subthalamic from posterior thalamic lesions.

Parkinsonism. The clinical characteristics of gait disturbance in patients with Parkinsonism (festination, stooped simian posture, rigidity, bradykinesia) can usually be differentiated from those caused by NPH or "senile gait." However, if the parkinsonian patient has no resting tremor or cogwheel rigidity, differentiation from NPH is not always possible. In early stages of idiopathic parkinsonism, CT is usually normal. Good clinical response is usually seen in patients with normal CT. Certain patients with parkinsonism do not respond adequately to drug therapy, and CT has frequently shown abnormalities in these patients.[28, 29] These abnormal CT findings are basal ganglia basal calcification, a communicating hydrocephalus and a cerebral atrophic process. Those patients with evidence of communicating hydrocephalus would be expected to show clinical improvement following insertion of a diversionary shunt. Patients with CT evidence of basal ganglia calcification or cerebral atrophy show poor response to drug therapy; this reflects the severity of the degenerative process. In patients with parkinsonism, CT findings of cerebral atrophy correlated with severity of gait and movement disturbance but not with clinical dementia. The incidence of psychiatric symptoms that developed during drug therapy was higher in parkinsonian patients who had CT evidence of cerebral atrophy.

In rare instances, there is an underlying focal lesion causing parkinsonian syndrome such as basal ganglia tumor or cerebral hemiatrophy. This is most common if the patient has unilateral parkinsonian syndrome; however, parkinsonism frequently begins asymmetrically. We have detected five basal ganglia tumors in patients with unilateral parkinsonism. We have seen *no* tumors in patients with bilateral (symmetrical or asymmetrical) neurological findings.

Progressive Supranuclear Palsy (PSP). This represents degenerative brain disease of unknown etiology. Findings include supranuclear ophthalmoplegia (especially involving vertical gaze), pseudobulbar palsy, dysarthria, and dystonic rigidity (trunk, neck). There is disturbance of gait and equilibrium; this is probably caused by truncal ataxia and dystonia. The neurological findings have a superficial similarity to parkinsonism; however, resting tremor is not present. In PSP, there is nerve cell degeneration predominantly involving the midbrain, basal ganglia and cerebellum. Air studies may show atrophy of midbrain, pontine tegmentum, superior colliculus, cerebellum and cerebral cortex. To delineate CT abnormalities in this condition, coronal and sagittal reconstructions should supplement axial projections. CT findings include the following: (1) small size of superior

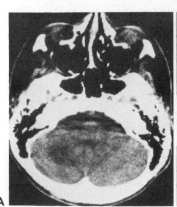 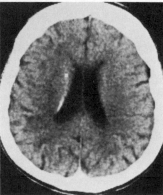

Figure 14–11. A 10-year-old developed difficulty walking, hearing loss and heart block. Findings were gait ataxia, absent reflexes, bilateral deafness and retinitis pigmentosa. CT findings: hypodense left cerebellar lesion (A) with periventricular calcified lesion (B).

A

B

colliculus, (2) enlargement of certain cisterns (interpeduncular, quadrigeminal, ambient, superior cerebellar), (3) cerebellar atrophy and (4) cerebral atrophy.[30]

Other Disorders

Oculocraniosomatic Disease (Kearns-Sayre Syndrome). Progressive external ophthalmoplegia may be associated with pigmentary retinal degeneration and heart block (Kearns-Sayre syndrome). Other neurological abnormalities (gait ataxia, deafness, parkinsonian features, muscle weakness) and somatic dysfunction (short stature, delayed sexual development) have been described. Muscle biopsy shows evidence of mitochondrial cytopathy. CT findings (Fig. 14–11) include: (1) intracranial calcification (basal ganglion, thalamus, cerebral hemispheres), (2) hypodense regions located within the cerebral white matter, (3) cerebellar hypoplasia and (4) hypodense lesions within the cerebellar hemispheres, midbrain and thalamus.[31]

REFERENCES

1. Maurice-Williams RS: Mechanism of production of gait unsteadiness by tumors of the posterior fossa. J Neurol Neurosurg Psychiatr 38:143, 1975
2. Koller WC, Glatt SC, Wilson RS: Senile gait: correlation with computed tomographic scans. Ann Neurol 12:87, 1982
3. Petrovici I: Apraxia of gait and trunk movements. J Neurol Neurosci 7:229, 1968
4. Chawla JC, Woodward J: Motor disorders in normal pressure hydrocephalus. Br Med J 1:485, 1972
5. Haymaker W: Bing's Local Diagnosis in Neurological Diseases. C. V. Mosby, St. Louis, 1969, pp 289–291
6. Koller WC, Glatt SL, Fox JH: Cerebellar atrophy; relationship to aging and cerebral atrophy. Neurology 31:1486, 1981
7. LeMay M, Abramowicz A: Pneumographic findings in various forms of cerebellar degeneration. Radiology 85:284, 1965
8. LeMay M, Abramowicz A: Encephalography in the diagnosis of cerebellar atrophy. Acta Radiol (Diagn) 5:667, 1966
9. Robertson EG: Diagnosis of cerebellar atrophy in pneumoencephalography. Charles C Thomas, Springfield, 1967, pp 155–161
10. Kennedy P, Swash M, Wylie IG: The clinical significance of pneumographic cerebellar atrophy. Br J Radiol 49:903, 1976
11. Allen JH, Martin JT, McLain LW: Computed tomography in cerebellar atrophic processes. Radiology 130:379, 1979
12. Koller WC, Glatt S, Perlik S: Cerebellar atrophy demonstrated by computed tomography. Neurology 31:405, 1981
13. Rothman SL, Glanz S: Cerebellar atrophy; the differential diagnosis by computerized tomography. Neuroradiology 16:123, 1978
14. Victor M, Adams RD, Mancall EL: A restricted form of cerebellar cortical degeneration in alcoholic patients. Arch Neurol 1:579, 1959
15. Haubek A, Lee K: Computed tomography in alcoholic cerebellar atrophy. Neuroradiology 18:77, 1979
16. McLain LW, Martin JT, Allen JH: Cerebellar degeneration due to chronic phenytoin therapy. Ann Neurol 7:18, 1980
17. Konigsmark BW, Weiner LP: The olivopontocerebellar atrophies; a review. Medicine 49:227, 1970
18. Caplan L, Thomas C, Patel D: Nonfamilial olivopontocerebellar atrophy: clinical and CT features. Ann Neurol 8:116, 1980
19. Gilman S, Bloedel JR, Lechtenberg R: Disorders of the cerebellum. F. A. Davis, Philadelphia, 1981, pp 231–262
20. Gyldensted C: Computer tomography of the cerebrum in multiple sclerosis. Neuroradiology 12:33, 1976
21. Weisberg LA: Contrast enhancement visualized by computerized tomography in acute multiple sclerosis. Comput Tomogr 5:293, 1981
22. Sears ES, Tindall RSA, Zarnow H: Active multiple sclerosis. Arch Neurol 35:426, 1978
23. Velden M, Bots GT, Endtz LJ: Cranial CT in multiple sclerosis showing a mass effect. Surg Neurol 12:307, 1979
24. Weinstein MA, Lederman RJ, Rothner AD: Interval computed tomography in multiple sclerosis. Radiology 129:689, 1978
25. Huckman MS, Fox JH, Ramsey RG: CT in the diagnosis of degenerative disease of the brain. Semin Roentgenol 12:63, 1977
26. Kendall BE, Pollock SS, Bass NM: Wilson's disease: clinical correlation and cranial computed tomography. Neuroradiology 22:1, 1981
27. Harik CI, Donovan Post MS: Computed tomography in Wilson's disease. Neurology 31:107, 1981
28. Sypert GW, Leffman H, Diemann GA: Occult normal pressure hydrocephalus manifested by Parkinsonism-dementia complex. Neurology 23:234, 1973
29. Koller WC, Cochran JW, Klawans HL: Calcification of the basal ganglia: computerized tomography and clinical correlation. Neurology 29:328, 1979
30. Haldeman S, Goldman JW, Hyde J: Progressive supranuclear palsy: computed tomography and response to antiparkinsonian drugs. Neurology 31:442, 1981
31. Seigal RS, Seeger JF, Gabrielson TD: Computed tomography in oculocraniosomatic disease (Kearns-Sayre syndrome). Radiology 130:159, 1979

Chapter 15

HEAD AND FACE PAIN

Headache may be the initial symptom of intracranial pathological processes, but this is usually accompanied by other neurological abnormalities. It is neurological findings rather than headache that herald the need for neurodiagnostic investigation. The majority of headache syndromes evaluated by neurologists are "chronic" and recurrent. These are caused by vascular or muscular contraction mechanisms. Neurodiagnostic studies such as skull x-ray, EEG and isotope scan have been utilized to screen patients for the remote possibility of a focal lesion; however, positive diagnostic yield is quite low and these tests are not cost-efficient. When focal pathological lesions are detected in patients who present with chronic headache only, review of clinical details usually indicates that other neurological abnormalities are present but not initially elicited or that the lesion is unrelated to the headache. In other patients who present with "acute" onset of headache as the only neurological disorder, neurodiagnostic studies are somewhat more cost-effective. With increasing availability of CT, the absolute number of patients with "acute" and "chronic recurrent" headache referred for CT has increased steadily and progressively at our scanning facility during an eight-year interval. This has afforded the opportunity to assess the role of CT in patients with head pain.[1, 2]

In patients with "chronic recurrent" headache or nonmigraine type who have a normal neurological examination, CT showed abnormalities in less than 0.5 percent of cases. These patients who had CT lesions had been symptomatic for 6 months to 17 years. All lesions were demonstrated on noncontrast scan; supplemental findings were obtained from enhanced scan in some cases. These lesions included subfrontal meningioma, subdural hematoma, subarachnoid cyst, porencephalic cyst, ventricular and subarachnoid space enlargement and basal ganglionic calci-

fication. It seems clear that many of these CT lesions were incidental to the headache. Following removal of those surgically remediable lesions in those patients in whom it was probable that the lesion was causally related, headache persisted. It is possible that if diagnosis had been established earlier, outcome would have been more favorable; however, an alternative explanation is that the lesion was an incidental finding.[3]

In 9 percent of patients with "chronic recurrent" headache, EEG was initially performed and showed abnormal findings. It was the abnormal EEG that led to referral for CT. This is an expected occurrence because 5 to 8 percent of normal persons have nonspecific EEG abnormalities. If EEG showed bitemporal slowing or was mildly diffusely slow, CT showed no abnormalities. If EEG showed focal slow wave pattern, CT showed focal lesions. Skull radiographic abnormal findings such as intracranial calcification, sella turcica enlargement and erosion led to performance of CT in other patients. In these cases, CT scan delineated the nature of the calcified lesion (meningioma, subdural hematoma, glioma, pituitary adenoma). In three patients with headache only, isotope scan was reported to show an abnormality; CT showed a lesion that represented metastatic lesion. The source was primary lung carcinoma, which was readily detected by routine chest x-ray.

We have analyzed retrospectively the clinical details in nine patients with "chronic recurrent" headache who were reported to have "negative" neurological examination and in these cases CT showed focal lesion; however, these patients were assessed by physicians without formal neurological training. Subsequent examination by neurologists demonstrated "soft" focal neurological deficit such as pronator drift, reflex asymmetry and Babinski sign in all cases. Seven patients had abnormal focal EEG findings and in two others

278

EEG was normal. Seven patients had CT evidence of surgically accessible lesions; they were asymptomatic following surgery. These patients suggest that careful neurological examination and EEG are excellent screening procedures prior to CT in patients with chronic recurrent headache.

In patients with "acute" headache (symptomatic for less than 2 months), CT showed focal lesions in 2 percent. Sixty percent of these patients had abnormal neurological findings on examination. In 80 percent of these cases, EEG and isotope scan findings were consistent with supratentorial lesion. In the other 20 percent EEG and isotope scan were negative; however, CT demonstrated focal lesions—neoplasm, angioma, hematoma and cyst. In these patients, headache was relieved promptly by surgical treatment of the tumor or cyst. In 6 percent of these patients with acute headache, initial CT was performed and was negative. Subsequent lumbar puncture demonstrated findings consistent with meningitis or subarachnoid hemorrhage. This emphasizes that CSF examination is mandatory if these disorders are suspected, and unless there are complicating pathological conditions, CT is likely to show no abnormalities. Despite the potential of CT for detection of subarachnoid blood and cisternal enhancement, CSF remains the definitive diagnostic study for subarachnoid hemorrhage and meningitis.

SPECIFIC HEADACHE TYPES

Migraine. Because migraine is almost always benign, little information concerning pathological changes is available other than that inferred from EEG findings.[4, 5] Two thirds of migraine patients have EEG abnormalities. These findings include generalized slow wave pattern; less commonly they include focal spike or slow wave pattern. The vascular disturbances in migraine syndrome are usually reversible, but it has been postulated that multiple and frequent attacks cause ischemia, which may result in atrophic brain changes. This may be manifested by EEG abnormalities and in rare instances epilepsy. During migraine attacks, EEG may show focal lesions. These are usually localized to the occipital region but may be more widespread. Angiographic and cerebral blood flow studies performed during acute attacks have shown arterial spasm. This results in decreased cortical blood flow; this may cause cerebral ischemia and result in cortical atrophy. These angiographic changes are consistent with reports of neurological complications in patients studied during acute attacks.[6, 7] There have usually been no predisposing factors to cerebrovascular disease; however, certain of these patients with migraine have used ergot medication, which has vasoconstrictive properties.

In assessing the role of CT in migraine, two issues should be considered: First, incidence of misdiagnosis of patients who have other intracranial lesions such as angioma and neoplasm and second, the type of lesion that results from arterial spasm and vascular occlusion. In patients with cerebral angioma, headache is usually intermittent and recurrent but always localized to one side, whereas in migraine, headache may alternate sides or initially be bilateral.[8] In patients with headache caused by angioma, visual phenomena persist throughout the course of the headache rather than disappearing as headache develops, and this latter pattern is characteristic of migraine. Occipital angiomas may cause focal seizures that result in visual phenomena such as flashing light extending across the visual fields; this is quite distinct from scintillating scotomas and fortification spectrum reported in patients with migraine. In one study performed in the era before development of CT, 2 of 33 "migraine" patients were subsequently found to have underlying angioma and in these cases clinical history for classic migraine was quite atypical. The authors concluded that persistent and nonprogressive neurological sequelae such as homonymous hemianopsia and hemiparesis are caused by cerebral infarction, and that only progressive neurological deficits such as focal epilepsy, focal neurological findings and papilledema are indications for angiography in patients with migraine.[9]

Of 200 patients with the clinical diagnosis of migraine who underwent CT, two clinically unsuspected lesions were detected. In these cases, careful visual field examination showed homonymous hemianopsia; EEG and isotope scan demonstrated localized abnormalities. CT findings were consistent with angioma and glioma located in the occipital cortex; this was confirmed by surgical findings. In four other patients with the clinical diagnosis of complicated migraine who developed focal neurological deficit (homonymous hemianopsia, hemisensory deficit or hemiparesis), CT findings were consistent with vascular ischemia or infarction (Fig. 15–1). Abnormal CT patterns included the following: (1) isodense occipital gyral enhancing lesion without mass effect that resolved within 10 days; (2) hypodense sharply marginated nonenhancing unilateral occipital lesion and (3) hypodense nonenhancing bioccipital lesion. In our experience, abnormal CT findings were seen only in patients with complicated migraine who had neurological deficit during an acute migraine syndrome. The incidence of CT findings did not correlate with the frequency of migraine episodes or duration of attacks. The incidence of generalized cerebral atrophy in patients with migraine did not differ from that in normal controls. In other studies, one third to one half of migraine patients showed CT abnormalities. Findings included: (1) focal hypodense regions that do not enhance or cause mass effect; these spontaneously resolved within several weeks and (2) diffuse or focal ventricular and cortical sulcal space enlargement. It is postulated that atrophic changes represent the cumulative pathological effect of migraine episodes; however, comparison with age-matched controls was not attempted.[10, 11]

Basilar Artery Migraine. Initial symptomatology includes bilateral visual aberrations (bright flashing lights, visual dimming), gait ataxia, dysarthria, diplopia, vertigo and facial or tongue paresthesia. This is followed by severe throbbing headache, maximal in the occipital region and accompanied by nausea and vomiting. Consciousness may be impaired because of brain stem ischemia.[12] Diagnosis is established by these clinical criteria: (1) normal interictal neurological findings, (2) family history of migraine, (3) rapid clearing of neurological disorder and (4) young age of the patient. Ruptured aneurysm and angioma may simulate this disorder; these conditions are excluded by normal CSF examination. In basilar artery migraine, CT is usually normal, but we have seen two patients with hypodense nonenhancing occipital lesions; these resolved within several days after the disappearance of the neurological abnormalities and headache.

Ophthalmoplegic Migraine. This migraine variant is associated with impaired ocular motility and abnormal pupillary reactivity. The disorder usually occurs in patients younger than 20 years old who frequently have a negative family history of migraine. Patients initially develop unilateral pulsatile headache. Ophthalmoplegia, most frequently involving all branches of the oculomotor nerve, develops later. It is located ipsilateral to the headache. Headache disappears within several days; however, oculomotor paresis may not resolve for several weeks. Diagnostic studies are necessary to exclude posterior communicating–internal carotid artery aneurysm, pituitary apoplexy and Tolosa-Hunt syndrome. In all cases of ophthalmoplegic migraine, CT has been negative. There was no evidence of asymmetrical cavernous sinus enhancement. This latter finding is useful in excluding cavernous sinus lesion.

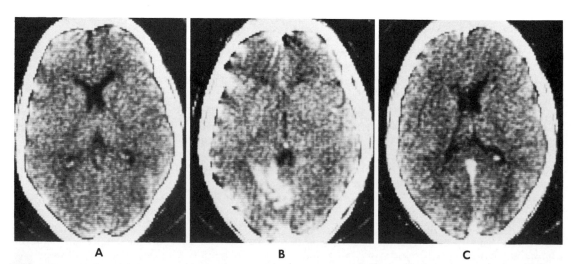

A	B	C

Figure 15–1. A 19-year-old saw flashing lights on the right side. This was followed by severe left temporal headache. The finding was right homonymous hemianopsia. EEG showed left hemispheric delta activity. *CT findings:* left occipital isodense (A) gyral enhancing lesion (B). Angiogram was normal. One month later he was neurologically normal. EEG and CT were also normal (C).

Raeder's Syndrome (Paratrigeminal Syndrome). This consists of two types—migrainous and symptomatic.[13, 14] In the migrainous type, patients are afflicted by episodes of unilateral pulsatile supraorbital pain, sometimes accompanied by palpebral or periorbital paresthesias. There is an accompanying oculosympathetic paresis that consists of ptosis and miosis with normal facial sweating. This is caused by involvement of sympathetic fibers distal to the bifurcation of the carotid artery at the base of the middle fossa. This disorder most usually occurs in males and initial symptoms may occur in middle-aged or older patients. These patients usually have had long-standing headache with intermittent attacks. These may recur at regular intervals every several months, each lasting several days to weeks, but the course is usually self-limited. There have been reports of this syndrome being caused by carotid aneurysm; however, this is quite rare and carotid angiography is of questionable value in patients with these clinical features. CT has been uniformly negative in these patients, even with careful attention to the basal skull and parasellar region.

In other patients with Raeder's syndrome, the onset of supraorbital pain is sudden and the pain progressively worsens. There is trigeminal nerve involvement that is manifested by facial paresthesias, decreased corneal reflex, tic-like bursts of pain and weakness of jaw muscles. In addition to oculosympathetic paresis and facial pain, these patients sometimes have evidence of parasellar (abducens, trochlear, oculomotor) cranial nerve involvement. The causes of this symptomatic type of Raeder's syndrome include supraclinoid carotid aneurysm, ectatic carotid artery (Fig. 15–2), extra-axial middle fossa tumors (metastases, pituitary adenoma), and trauma to the skull base involving the apex of the petrous bone. Diagnostic studies should include: (1) skull roentgenogram, (2) conventional tomography of sella and skull base, (2) carotid angiogram and (3) CT scan with special attention to the middle fossa floor and parasellar region.

Trigeminal Neuralgia (Tic Douloureux). This disorder is characterized by brief and sometimes repetitive bursts of severe pain located within single or multiple divisions of the trigeminal nerve. The pain occurs most commonly in the mandibular division (70 percent); less commonly, in the maxillary or ophthalamic branch. The pain begins in one region and may spread to a larger area, sometimes the entire face. There is usually a trigger point that precipitates the pain.

In rare instances tic douloureux is symptomatic of an underlying lesion, and there are usually associated neurological abnormalities such as decreased facial sensation, abnormal corneal reflex and abducens or facial nerve paresis. Causes of symptomatic tic douloureux include: (1) multiple sclerosis; (2) posterior fossa tumors such as trigeminal or acoustic neuromas, meningiomas and epidermoid cysts; (3) vascular malformations such as angiomas, posterior fossa berry aneurysms and vertebral-basilar ectatic aneurysms and (4) middle fossa extra-axial or tentorial lesions. In rare instances small tumors (neuromas and meningiomas) may cause tic douloureux, but neurological examination shows no abnormalities.[15]

It is important to define the clinical features of the facial pain, because other disorders may simulate tic douloureux. Atypical trigeminal

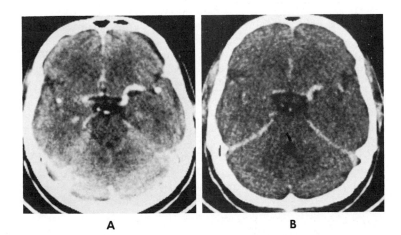

Figure 15–2. A 54-year-old man had three clusters of right-sided supraorbital pain with accompanying subjective paresthesias. He had decreased sensation in the ophthalmic division of the trigeminal nerve. *CT findings:* right-sided parasellar curvilinear enhancing structure consistent with carotid aneurysm (A,B). Angiogram showed ectatic carotid artery.

A

B

neuralgia is characterized by more constant and deep aching pain. It is located in all divisions of the trigeminal nerve. It may be caused by lesions involving the gasserian ganglion or supratentorial region. Differentiation of atypical trigeminal neuralgia from tic douloureux is important because diagnostic investigations and treatment are different.

In patients with trigeminal neuralgia who have abnormal neurological findings, neurodiagnostic evaluation is performed to investigate posterior fossa lesions. This includes: (1) skull x-rays with Towne and Stenver views, (2) base of skull tomograms, (3) CT with thin tissue sections to include the petrous apex and (4) angiogram to detect posterior fossa vascular malformation. It is possible for some tumors that cause tic douloureux to *not* be detected on initial studies. If the pain symptoms do not respond to medical management, diagnostic reassessment may be indicated several months later, especially if surgical treatment of face pain is considered.

Cluster Headache. These consist of unilateral supraorbital headaches of deep-aching quality that reach maximal severity very rapidly. These headaches frequently awaken the patient. Associated symptoms include lacrimation and conjunctival and facial reddening. The attack lasts several hours, and these headaches occur in clusters, each of which lasts several weeks. Males are affected most commonly. The attacks usually begin when patients are in their thirties. Because headaches usually remain lateralized to one side, these patients frequently are referred for neurodiagnostic evaluation; however, it is quite unusual to demonstrate lesions such as carotid aneurysm, angioma and neoplasm. Because cluster headaches are believed to be caused by abnormal vascular reaction in the carotid artery, it is possible that CT and angiography may show such a lesion; however, there are no examples of aneurysm simulating cluster headache. We have seen one patient with classic cluster headache; CT showed subfrontal meningioma. Symptoms were unchanged following surgical removal of this apparently clinically unrelated lesion.

Temporal Arteritis. The headache is usually unilateral or bilateral temporal-parietal in location. It has an aching quality and there is tenderness over the scalp in the temporal region. The temporal artery is thickened; it is easily palpable and tender. This condition develops most commonly in older patients.

Headache usually precedes visual deterioration. This visual complication develops rapidly and may be irreversible. Ophthalmoplegia results from cranial nerve ischemia. Diagnosis is established by these criteria: First, markedly elevated erythrocyte sedimentation rate and second, temporal artery biopsy findings of giant cell granulomatous arteritis. Headache may be successfully treated with corticosteroids, but visual loss is usually irreversible.[16]

In patients who present with headache and unilateral visual symptoms, an occult prechiasmal optic nerve lesion may simulate temporal arteritis. We have seen two patients who were diagnosed as having temporal arteritis *without* biopsy confirmation whose clinical features (headache, visual loss) responded to corticosteroid medication. Headache and vision deterioration recurred several months later and CT demonstrated prechiasmal lesion. To demonstrate these lesions, careful thin sections through the orbital apex and parasellar region are indicated.

Tolosa-Hunt Syndrome. Initial symptoms are deep aching and constant orbital pain. It may be severe and awaken the patient from sleep. The pain may be accompanied by diplopia and facial paresthesias. Neurological findings include: (1) ophthalmoplegias, (2) pupillary abnormalities (most commonly dilated and poorly reactive) and (3) normal visual acuity and normal funduscopic examination. This disorder represents an inflammatory condition involving the superior orbital fissure or cavernous sinus. Symptoms respond to corticosteroids; however, the condition may recur. Pathological confirmation of the diagnosis is rarely possible; diagnostic evaluation is necessary. This includes: (1) skull x-ray with superior orbital fissure views and paranasal sinus views, (2) hypocycloidal sella tomography, (3) CT scan with thin sections of the orbit and parasellar regions, (4) carotid angiogram and (5) orbital venography.[17] Angiography may show narrowing of the intracavernous carotid artery.[18] CT has been negative in the Tolosa-Hunt syndrome. We have seen two cases in which CT showed parasellar abnormalities; however, biopsy showed other lesions (pituitary adenoma, meningioma). It should be emphasized that in these cases, clinical symptoms dramatically improved with corticosteroids; they subsequently exacerbated as the dose was tapered to suggest falsely inflammatory Tolosa-Hunt syndrome (Fig. 15–3).

Neoplasms as Cause of Headache. In pa-

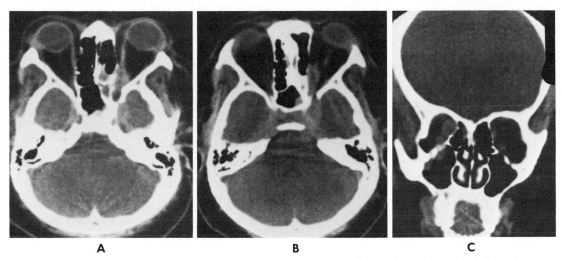

Figure 15–3. This 30-year-old woman experienced multiple recurrent bilateral episodes of painful ophthalmoplegia. These responded dramatically to corticosteroids. During this episode she developed vision loss in her right eye. She had Marcus-Gunn pupil with superior and medial rectus paresis. Sella tomograms were normal. CT findings: right posterior-inferior (A) and medial (B) enhancing orbital mass extending into the cavernous sinus (C). Biopsy showed pituitary adenoma.

tients with intracranial tumors, headache may be an early and prominent symptom; however, neurological examination shows abnormalities, and other studies (skull x-ray, EEG and isotope scan) are usually also positive. There was no difference between a rapidly growing neoplasm and a slowly growing one in respect to headache frequency. The incidence of headache with different neoplasms was comparable—meningioma (46 percent), pituitary adenoma (51 percent), glioblastoma (57 percent) and metastases (65 percent). The sudden onset of headache suggests hemorrhage into the neoplasm, e.g., pituitary adenoma or melanoma, or ventricular obstruction, as with colloid cyst.[19] Headache caused by neoplasm may be intermittent; there may be remissions rather than progressive worsening. In certain cases in which headache is the only neurological abnormality, the patient has sought medical help because of concern about the possibility of an underlying brain tumor. In this situation, performance of CT may detect incidental lesions and lead to therapeutic intervention for an unrelated finding. Small meningiomas may represent incidental necropsy findings.[20] Of 300 asymptomatic neoplasms detected at necropsy, one hundred were meningiomas—parasagittal (31 percent), convexity (25 percent), sphenoid ridge (10 percent), parasellar (13 percent), posterior fossa (9 percent) and olfactory or basal-frontal (7 percent). These tumors were sharply circumscribed and

encapsulated. They varied in size—less than 1 cm (61 percent), less than 2 cm (22 percent) and greater than 2 cm (17 percent). Routine necropsy studies of asymptomatic patients have shown that one third had pituitary adenomas. These are usually small, but some extend upward above the pituitary fossa. Before CT came into use, diagnosis of asymptomatic pituitary adenoma was initially suggested by the finding of abnormal sella.[21] This frequently occurred when skull x-ray was obtained, for example, following head injury.[22] With CT we have detected four pituitary adenomas in patients with headache without endocrine or visual findings.

REFERENCES

1. Carrera GF, Gerson DE, Schnur J: Computed tomography of the brain in patients with headache or temporal lobe epilepsy: findings and cost effectiveness. J Comput Assist Tomogr 1:200, 1977
2. Stein HJ: Is headache going to the CATS? Headache 18:5, 1978
3. Weisberg LA: Incidental CT findings. J Neurol Neurosurg Psychiatr 45:715, 1982
4. Hockaday JM, Whitty CWM: Factors determining the EEG in migraine. Brain 92:769, 1969
5. Hughes JR: EEG in headache. Headache 11:162, 1972
6. Dukes HT, Vieth RG: Cerebral angiography during migraine prodrome and headache. Neurology 14:636, 1964
7. Dorfman LJ, Marshall WH, Enzmann DR: Cerebral

infarction in migraine: clinical and radiologic correlations. Neurology 29:317, 1979

8. Troost BT, Newton TH: Occipital lobe arteriovenous malformations: clinical and radiological features in 26 cases with comments on differentiation from migraine. Arch Ophthalmol 93:250, 1975

9. Pearce JMS, Foster JB: An investigation of complicated migraine. Neurology 15:333, 1965

10. Hungerford GD, duBoulay GH: CT in patients with severe migraine. J Neurol Neurosurg Psychiatr 39:990, 1976

11. Mathew NT, Meyer JS: Abnormal CT scans in migraine. Headache 16:272, 1976

12. Bickerstaff ER: Basilar artery migraine. Lancet 1:15, 1961

13. Law WR, Nelson ER: Internal carotid aneurysm as a cause of Raeder's paratrigeminal syndrome. Neurology 18:43, 1968

14. Mokri B: Raeder's paratrigeminal syndrome. Arch Neurol 39:395, 1982

15. Dandy WE: Concerning the cause of trigeminal neuralgia. Am J Surg 24:447, 1934

16. Hamilton CR, Shelley WM, Tumulty PA: Giant cell arteritis: including temporal arteritis and polymyalgia rheumatica. Medicine 50:1, 1979

17. Freeman NR, Shraberg D: Alternating painful ophthalmoplegia. South Med J 73:1398, 1980

18. Sondheimer FK, Knapp J: Angiographic findings in the Tolosa-Hunt syndrome; painful ophthalmoplegia. Radiology 106:105, 1973

19. Heyck H: Examination and differential diagnosis of headache. *In* PJ Vinken, GW Bruyn (eds). Handbook of Neurology. Vol 5. Amsterdam, North Holland Publishing Co., 1968, pp. 25–36

20. Wood MW, White RJ, Kernohan JW: One hundred intracranial meningiomas found incidentally at necropsy. J Neuropathol Exp Neurol 16:337, 1957

21. Weisberg LA: Asymptomatic enlargement of the sella turcica. Arch Neurol 33:483, 1975

22. Chernow B, Buck DR, Early CB: Rapid shrinkage of a prolactin-secreting pituitary adenoma with bromocriptine: CT documentation. Am J Neuroradiol 3:442, 1982

Chapter 16

SEIZURE DISORDERS AND ELECTROENCEPHALO-GRAPHIC PATTERNS

The purpose of this chapter is threefold. First, we present an analysis of CT findings in our patients with syncope and seizures and compare these results with those reported in other studies. Second, in patients with poorly controlled seizures we have attempted to determine if multiple or prolonged episodes were associated with morphological CT abnormalities. Third, there are certain EEG patterns such as bifrontal monorhythmic delta and focal delta that have been associated with focal pathological processes. Other EEG patterns such as bitemporal or generalized slowing have been of less certain clinical significance. We have correlated these EEG patterns with CT and pathological findings.

One hundred patients were referred for CT because of "possible epileptic disorder," but clinical features were consistent with syncope. Neurological examination was normal. EEG was normal or showed slight diffuse slowing; none showed bursts of spike discharges or focal abnormalities. Three focal lesions were detected by CT. One represented parietal meningioma. Neurological examination and other neurodiagnostic studies were normal. Following surgical removal, syncopal episodes persisted. Ten months later, focal seizures developed. These were presumed to be caused by cortical gliotic scar because CT showed no recurrent neoplasm. One patient with postural syncope had skull radiographic evidence of enlarged sella turcica and CT findings consistent with pituitary adenoma. The syncopal episodes were believed to result from adrenal insufficiency. In the other patient unilateral throbbing headache preceded syncope. Several interictal EEG patterns were normal; however, immediately following one episode EEG showed focal spike and slow wave pattern. Isotope scan showed no abnormal uptake. CT showed hypodense nonenhancing occipital lesion without mass effect. This was believed caused by migraine with ischemic changes rather than angioma; this diagnosis was confirmed by angiographic findings. From this we conclude that CT is not a high-yield diagnostic study in patients with syncope unless other clinical features such as focal EEG pattern or abnormal skull x-ray are present that suggest a neurological disorder.

Fifty consecutive patients had sudden episodic loss of consciousness. In these patients, there were no witnesses to the episode and there were some atypical features for syncope such as absence of presyncopal symptoms, urinary incontinence, tonic posturing and non-rhythmical myoclonic jerking. CT was performed because EEG was abnormal. These were of three types: first, generalized single spikes or polyspikes (30 percent), second, generalized slowing (50 percent) and third, bitemporal slow wave activity (20 percent). No patient had abnormalities on neurological examination. In patients with bilateral symmetrical spikes or diffuse slow wave activity, CT was normal. Ten patients had bitemporal slow wave activity; isotope scan was normal. These patients had CT findings consistent with middle cerebral artery ischemia or infarction. Focal cerebrovascular ischemia caused by carotid artery occlusive disease may result in syncope; however, this would be an unlikely occurrence because of the paucity of focal neurological deficit in these patients. In six cases CT showed isodense enhancing lesions.

The syncopal attacks ceased within two months and CT showed no residual abnormalities. In four other patients CT showed hypodense nonenhancing lesions. The attacks persisted in these patients and CT lesion did not change. From this we conclude that focal pathological lesions other than vascular ischemia or infarction are unlikely to be defined by CT unless there are focal neurological or EEG findings. It was indeed surprising that these patients with CT evidence of nonhemorrhagic cerebrovascular disease had normal neurological examination.

In patients with electroencephalographic and clinical evidence of epilepsy, an attempt was made to classify seizure disorders utilizing International League Against Epilepsy criteria and to correlate these with CT findings.[1, 2] Primary generalized epilepsy (PGE) refers to two common clinical patterns. In one type, patients suddenly lose consciousness without prior aura. The patient exhibits symmetrical tonic-clonic activity, usually with tongue biting and incontinence. Following the episode, patients may be disoriented but focal neurological deficit is not present (major motor). EEG shows symmetrical bursts of single or polyspikes sometimes with interspersed slowing; however, in 20 percent of cases no abnormalities are seen. In the second type, patients have brief episodes of unawareness without abnormal motor activity (absence attacks). Following this attack, the patient is alert and resumes previous activities. EEG shows a characteristic symmetrical three cycles per second spike and wave discharge; however, asymmetrical or atypical EEG variants may be seen. Unless EEG shows a spike wave pattern slower than 2.5 cps or there is marked hemispheric asymmetry, an underlying focal pathological lesion is unlikely.[3, 4] Patients with PGE usually are symptomatic before age 20. Their condition frequently has a genetic origin rather than being caused by an underlying pathological lesion of focal or diffuse type.

Because PGE represents a generalized cerebral electrophysiological disturbance, diagnostic yield from noninvasive diagnostic studies (skull x-ray, isotope scan, echoencephalogram) and invasive ones (CSF examination, air studies, angiogram) has been quite low. Gastaut reported that CT showed abnormalities in 10 percent of patients with PGE; other studies have shown abnormalities ranging from zero to 10 percent.[5] The wide range of abnormalities reported may relate to factors such as source of clinical material and adequacy of seizure classification. There are rare reports of supratentorial tumors detected in patients with absence attacks; however, it is likely that clinical diagnosis actually was partial complex (psychomotor) seizures and EEG did not show symmetrical spike-wave pattern. In those patients with true absence attacks and CT findings of supratentorial tumor, seizures were not modified by tumor resection. In 50 patients with absence attacks and EEG findings of symmetrical 3 cps spike wave pattern, plain and enhanced CT showed no abnormalities. If EEG pattern showed clear-cut atypical features such as slowing (less than 2.5 cps spike wave) or focal spike wave activity, CT showed abnormalities in 25 percent of patients (see the discussion of infantile spasms).

We have evaluated one hundred patients with PGE of the major motor type. All patients were younger than 25; neurological examination was normal. EEG showed symmetrical single or polyspike activity. Only 2 percent of patients had focal lesion detected by CT. These were well-delineated on noncontrast scan. In one patient with epidermoid cyst, CT had been performed because of poor seizure control despite the patient's having adequate anticonvulsant blood levels (Fig. 16–1). In the other patient, initial clinical and EEG findings were consistent with PGE; however, CT was

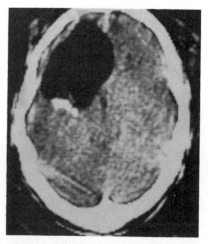

Figure 16–1. A 33-year-old man had primary generalized seizure. Examination, EEG and isotope scan were normal. Despite adequate anticonvulsant levels, seizures increased in frequency. Skull x-ray showed left frontal calcification. *CT findings:* hypodense lesion (with negative values representing fat) and interspersed calcification in frontal lesion. *Operative finding:* dermoid cyst.

not initially performed. The patient had two seizures during a six-month interval despite adequate anticonvulsant levels, and the pattern of the seizures changed in that the attack was now preceded by an aura. Because of seizure recurrence and change in seizure pattern, reassessment was initiated and EEG showed focal slow wave activity. CT scan was consistent with malignant glioma; this was confirmed by surgical biopsy.

In patients with PGE, we attempted to correlate seizure control with abnormal CT findings. We compared those patients who had two or more seizures per month and motor activity that persisted for more than 10 minutes during each episode with those who had infrequent attacks—that is, one or two attacks per year and short-duration seizures. There was no difference in the incidence of focal lesions or generalized cerebral atrophy demonstrated by CT in these patients. However, patients who had episodes of status epilepticus had CT evidence of mild to moderate diffuse cerebral atrophy. Those patients with seizures that had been poorly controlled who had taken phenytoin for longer than five years showed CT evidence of cerebellar atrophy; however, these patients had no clinical evidence of gait ataxia. These CT findings were not seen in patients who had taken other types of anticonvulsants and had good seizure control; however, the CT finding of cerebellar atrophy was also seen in some patients without seizures who had never taken phenytoin and had no abnormal neurological findings. It is not known whether cerebellar atrophy is related to phenytoin or hypoxia resulting from frequent seizures.

The partial (focal) epilepsies are of two types. Simple partial seizures consist of episodes that begin with focal neurological symptoms with abnormal motor, sensory, auditory, visual and language dysfunction. Consciousness is initially preserved; however, subsequent impairment may develop (secondary generalization). Complex partial seizures consist of attacks in which there is initial loss of awareness or consciousness. There may be accompanying abnormal motor activity consisting of automatic stereotyped movements. The partial epilepsies are usually acquired disorders; therefore, the reported incidence of underlying pathological lesions is quite high. The highest incidence of focal pathological lesions has been reported in patients having partial seizures with secondary generalization. In patients with partial epilepsies, EEG usually shows focal spike or slow wave activity. Focal EEG abnormalities are more likely detected with superficial lesions, whereas EEG abnormalities may not be detected with deep and medial temporal lesions unless special recording electrodes (nasopharyngeal) are utilized. If partial seizures develop in patients older than 20, underlying pathological lesions must be strongly suspected. In selected cases of children and adolescents, partial seizures may be benign without evidence of underlying lesion. These partial seizures that are idiopathic do not usually secondarily generalize. EEG usually shows focal spike focus, and other neurodiagnostic studies are negative.

If partial seizures occur after age 20, neurodiagnostic studies are necessary. The common etiologies depend upon age of onset: (1) between age 20 to 35, head trauma and neoplasm are most common; (2) between 35 and 55, vascular disorders and neoplasms are most common and (3) after age 55, degenerative disorders are most likely to occur.[6] The presence of focal slow wave is more frequently associated with structural lesion than is spike focus alone.[7] Sixty percent of patients with interictal neurological deficit who had partial seizures were found to have an underlying neoplasm.[8] Before the advent of CT, it was suggested that patients with partial seizures should undergo angiography and air studies because of the probability of detecting an underlying pathological lesion. Despite complete neuroradiographic studies, 25 to 40 percent of adult patients with partial seizures have no detectable abnormalities. The incidence of negative studies in patients with simple partial seizures is higher in children than adults.

CT provides a new approach to patients with partial seizures. Bogdanoff and colleagues reported CT findings in 50 patients who had focal seizures based on clinical or EEG findings; CT abnormalities were found in 60 percent.[9] Two patients had neoplasms (4 percent); however, certain lesions (focal or generalized atrophy, hydrocephalus, cerebellar hypoplasia) were previously detected only by air studies. Of eight patients with interictal neurological deficit, six had focal CT abnormalities. If EEG showed focal spike focus, 15 percent had CT abnormalities; 66 percent of patients had CT abnormalities if EEG showed focal slow wave activity.

We have investigated one hundred consecutive patients with simple partial seizures. Sixty percent of patients had no interictal neurological deficit. EEG showed these patterns: (1) focal slow wave pattern (15 percent), (2) focal slow wave with interspersed spikes (33 percent), (3) focal spike (35 percent) and (4) focal spikes with occasional interspersed slow waves (17 percent). CT showed evidence of focal lesion in all cases if there was interictal neurological deficit and EEG showed focal slow wave activity. CT showed focal abnormality in only 8 percent of cases if neurological examination was normal and EEG showed focal spike discharges only. In these patients with simple partial seizures, 68 percent had CT abnormalities. This included neoplasms (18 percent), cerebral infarction (15 percent), porencephalic cyst (9 percent), subarachnoid cyst (5 percent), focal atrophy (11 percent), diffuse atrophy (5 percent) and angioma (5 percent). In two cases, initial CT showed no abnormality; however repeat scan showed pa-

rietal metastases (three weeks later) and malignant glioma (four months later). In both cases, initial EEG showed focal slowing; however, neurological examination was normal. In patients with partial epilepsies, all neoplasms and cysts were visualized on the plain scan. Ten percent of patients had normal plain scan, and the lesion was detected only on enhanced scan. These isodense enhancing lesions represented cerebral infarction.

Five patients presented with partial simple seizure; they were neurologically normal in the interictal period. EEG showed extensive focal delta activity without spikes. Because these patients had partial seizures and focal slow wave activity, neoplasm was considered the most likely underlying lesion. CT showed hypodense or isodense parietal gyral enhancing lesion without mass effect. Angiogram showed middle cerebral artery branch occlusion. Follow-up CT showed diminution or disappearance of enhancement pattern; this spontaneous resolution was consistent with

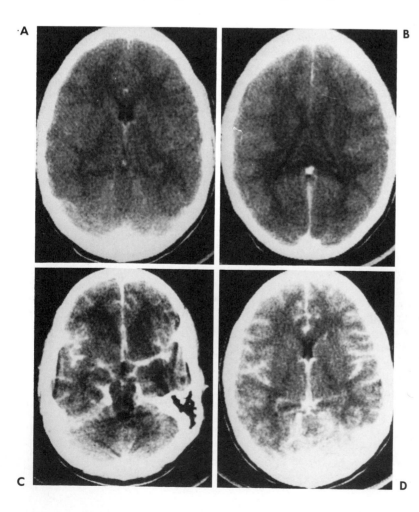

Figure 16–2. An 18-year-old woman developed multiple frequent partial complex seizures and remained confused. EEG showed bitemporal spikes; CSF showed sterile pleocytosis. *CT findings:* no abnormal density (A) or enhancement pattern (B). Following three days of continued seizures, she remained obtunded. *CT findings:* dense symmetrical bilateral (C) hemispheric enhancement (D). She died following cardiopulmonary arrest. Necropsy showed hypoxic-ischemic brain damage but no evidence of herpes encephalitis.

Figure 16–3. This 35-year-old developed episodes of déjà vu and auditory hallucinations. Examination was normal. EEG showed left temporal delta pattern with interspersed spike discharges. *CT findings:* hypodense irregularly marginated (*A*) (reader's right) temporal nonenhancing lesion with prominent mass effect (*B*). Angiogram showed avascular mass. Four years later he had infrequent partial complex seizures and some word-finding aphasic deficit. This is presumed to represent low-grade glioma.

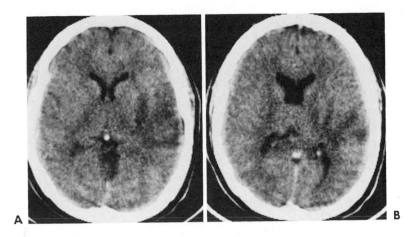

ischemic process. These cases represent exceptions to a previously useful clinical rule that focal extensive slow wave activity occurring in patients with only mild neurological deficit is caused by mass lesion, e.g. neoplasm, abscess, angioma. Two of these five patients with cerebral infarction had positive isotope scan within 72 hours after the seizure. This pattern is not consistent with vascular infarction in which isotope scan becomes positive in the second week; however, positive isotope scan has been reported immediately following seizure and this is caused by vascular hyperperfusion (Fig. 16–2). We have seen CT evidence of vascular enhancement as well as cerebral hemispheric gyral enhancement following generalized and partial seizures; this is believed to represent hyperperfusion.[10, 11]

In patients with complex partial (temporal lobe, psychomotor) seizures, neurodiagnostic studies have demonstrated structural lesions in 25 to 35 percent of cases.[12, 14] The majority of tumors are located in the temporal lobe, but lesions may be in other locations. Most common are gliomas (Fig. 16–3); however, others were meningiomas, angiomas, cysts, infectious-inflammatory disorders (Fig. 16–4) and hamartomas (Fig. 16–5). Currie et al. described abnormal angiographic and pneumographic temporal lobe findings in one third of nontumorous cases.[14] Perinatal vascular ischemic vascular damage involving the posterior cerebral arteries may cause tissue damage involving the occipital lobe, parahippocampal gyrus and inferior and mesial temporal cortex. This tissue injury is expressed electrically as spike or slow waves and clinically as partial complex seizures.[15, 16] Air studies have shown

Figure 16–4. A 30-year-old had had viral encephalitis 10 years previously. He developed partial complex seizures; EEG showed unilateral posterior temporal spike discharge. *CT findings:* unilateral posterior temporal calcified regions (*A*) seen on coronal (*B*) and sagittal (*C*) reformated projections.

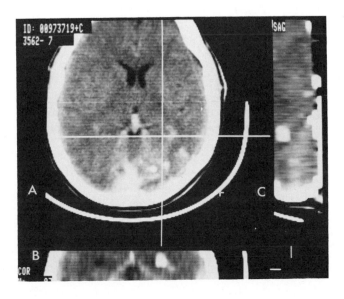

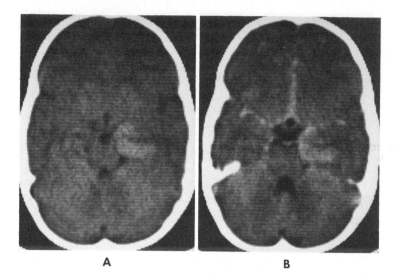

A   B

Figure 16–5. A 7-year-old developed partial complex seizures. Examination was normal. EEG showed right temporal spike focus. Angiogram showed no mass effect. *CT findings:* comma-shaped (A) medial temporal hyperdense lesion that showed slight enhancement (B). Because of persistent seizures, temporal lobectomy was performed and showed hamartoma.

localized dilatation of the temporal horn caused by uncal and hippocampal tissue damage from mesial temporal sclerosis.

We have investigated one hundred patients with partial complex seizures. Forty percent had abnormal CT findings; 35 percent had focal and 5 percent had diffuse lesions. Of those with CT evidence of neoplasm, 75 percent of patients had neurological deficit. Twenty percent of patients with partial complex seizures and localized temporal EEG abnormalities had a focal CT finding (neoplasm, cyst, angioma) and in 3 percent these were located external to temporal lobe. Porencephalic cysts and focal hemispheric atrophy were the next most common CT abnormalities. In several of these cases isotope scan showed decreased perfusion in the abnormal hemisphere on flow study. CT was most likely to be abnormal if EEG showed focal slowing and least likely to be abnormal if there were focal spikes. There was one CT finding that correlated with focal spike discharge. This consisted of unilateral temporal horn dilatation without evidence of abnormal density pattern (Fig. 16–6). It is possible that this represents mesial temporal sclerosis; however, we have no biopsy confirmation in these cases. The sensitivity of CT for demonstrating temporal horn dilatation has improved with newer scanning technology. Air studies sometimes demonstrated temporal horn dilatation that was not confirmed by early model CT scanners; however, CT is now quite sensitive in detecting temporal horn dilatation. Our findings are consistent with those reported by other studies of patients with partial complex seizures.[17, 18] Gastaut reported that in patients

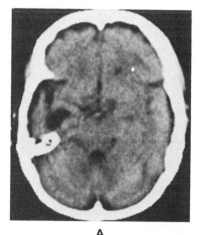

A

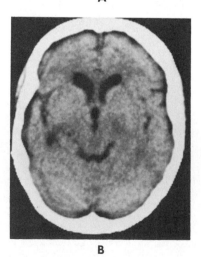

B

Figure 16–6. A 22-year-old developed partial complex seizures. EEG showed left temporal spike focus. *CT findings:* marked enlargement of the left temporal horn (A) with slight enlargement of other regions of the lateral ventricle (B) but no abnormal tissue density.

with partial complex seizures, CT showed abnormalities (focal, 30 percent; diffuse, 20 percent) in 50 percent. This included nine patients who had neurological findings (mental retardation, hemiplegia, homonymous hemianopsia) in addition to seizures. In these latter cases, CT showed sharply marginated hypodense temporal-occipital lesions that represented porencephalic cysts. These were believed to result from posterior cerebral artery infarction, and these lesions were consistent with angiographic and pneumographic findings. Mesial temporal sclerosis is found in 75 percent of pathological specimens in patients with partial complex seizures. This is usually represented by localized temporal atrophy with temporal horn dilatation. Jabbari and coworkers had reported one case of arcuate temporal calcification representing mesial temporal sclerosis.[16]

Infantile Spasms

This occurs in children who frequently have prior history of perinatal hypoxic-ischemic brain damage (Fig. 16–7). Most children have poor neurological development prior to onset of seizures; however, certain patients are entirely normal before seizures develop. EEG shows characteristic hypsarrhythmia pattern. In those children who were neurologically normal prior to onset of spasms, careful investigation for metabolic disorders and neurocutaneous disorders should be undertaken. Tu-berous sclerosis is the most common associated disorder. CT may detect subependymal hyperdense tubers before cutaneous manifestations or intracranial calcification develop. CT is important to define the presence, type and severity of the underlying lesion; however, seizure control was not directly correlated with normal CT.

Lennox-Gastaut Syndrome

This consists of mixed minor motor seizures associated with slow spike and wave pattern, less than 2.5 cycles per second spike—this EEG pattern may be symmetrical or asymmetrical. These children show developmental delay and are usually mentally retarded. This represents a predominantly generalized paroxysmal disorder with strong suggestive evidence of underlying pathological lesion. Some children with infantile spasms later develop this clinical and EEG pattern. Of 42 patients studied by Gastaut, 60 percent showed CT abnormalities. Most frequent was diffuse or focal atrophy; however, several patients had focal lesions, including one parietal-occipital neoplasm. This is most unusual because it is believed that a diffuse pathological process is the underlying disorder. Of 38 patients studied by Zimmerman et al., 18 had abnormal CT findings. The most frequent finding was generalized cerebral atrophy. There were two patients with CT findings of cerebellar atrophy. This may reflect the effect of hypoxic

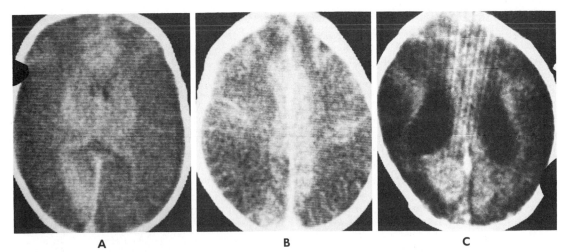

A   **B**   **C**

Figure 16–7. A neonate suffered hypoxic-ischemic birth damage. She had poor neurological development. EEG was diffusely slow with prominent burst suppression pattern. *CT findings:* bilateral hypodense symmetrical hemispheric lesions (*A*) with normal-sized ventricles (*B*). Two months later, EEG showed hypsarrhythmia and the patient had infantile spasms. *CT findings:* hypodense bilateral hemispheric lesions (*C*) and marked ventricular and subarachnoid space enlargement.

brain damage or represent the role of the cerebellum in causing the seizure disorder. There was some suggestive evidence that structural brain changes progressively worsen, because all patients older than 20 had abnormal CT findings.[19]

EEG Abnormalities

Focal Slow Wave Pattern. Joynt and coworkers investigated the clinical significance of focal polymorphic delta activity; two thirds of patients had vascular disease and neoplasm.[20] Seventy percent of patients with focal delta activity had abnormal neurological signs. In 20 percent of patients who were neurologically normal, focal delta activity was presumed caused by epilepsy; however, in 10 percent, no etiology was defined. Although adequate follow-up was not obtained in these 10 percent, it was postulated that focal delta activity represented an early sign of neurological dysfunction that was not demonstrated by clinical examination or other diagnostic studies.

In 50 consecutive patients who had neurological signs with unilateral temporal delta pattern, CT showed neoplasm (40 percent), vascular lesions (20 percent), generalized cerebral atrophy (16 percent) and hydrocephalus (4 percent). Twenty percent of patients showed no abnormality. In these latter patterns, clinical evidence of epilepsy was demonstrated in one half; however, no neurological disorder was subsequently detected in the other patients with follow-up extending up to four years. It is possible that some of these represented ischemic stroke that is not always detected by CT; however, none had clinical findings consistent with stroke or transient ischemic attacks. In 20 other cases, unilateral delta pattern was demonstrated in patients without abnormal neurological findings. Skull x-ray, isotope scan and CSF examination were normal. CT was normal in 14 cases. Three patients had CT findings of generalized atrophic process. Follow-up clinical studies showed that they had clinical evidence of dementia of Alzheimer type within one year. Three other patients had CT evidence of cerebral infarction. No asymptomatic patient had a neoplasm.

Our findings in patients with focal delta activity are similar to other studies. Brenner and Gilmore reported CT abnormalities in 68 percent of patients with polymorphic focal delta activity. These included: ischemic stroke (32 percent), hemorrhagic stroke (6 percent), seizures (21 percent), neoplasm (13 percent), trauma without hematoma (13 percent) and trauma with hematoma (11 percent). Of patients with focal neurological signs, 79 percent had a focal lesion; and of patients without focal signs, 62 percent had a focal lesion. Of patients with focal delta activity and normal neurological examination, 35 percent had a focal lesion. If the patient with focal delta activity has normal CT, the diagnosis of epilepsy, concussion or ischemic stroke is most likely.[21] In another study, patients were evaluated who had neurodiagnostic assessment for several neurological disorders (seizure, headache, dementia or transient ischemic attacks) but had no focal signs. It was found that all patients with a focal CT lesion also had focal EEG activity. Of patients who had focal EEG slow wave activity, 20 percent had CT evidence of focal lesion; however, of those patients with diffuse EEG 3 percent had a focal CT lesion.[22]

Monorhythmic Frontal Delta (MRFD) Activity. This pattern is believed to be an indicator of increased intracranial pressure usually caused by ventricular obstruction; however, it has been reported in other conditions such as epilepsy, concussion-contusion, degenerative disorders and toxic or metabolic disturbances.[23] Gliomas are the most likely neoplasm to cause this electrical pattern. Most commonly they are deep medial-frontal, but they may be posterior fossa in location. The exact site of origin of this rhythmic pattern is not known. Regions that have been implicated include the upper midbrain or diencephalon and the dorsal-medial and intralaminar thalamic nuclei. In one hundred cases of patients with these findings reported by Cordeau, final diagnoses included tumors (42 percent), degenerative disorders (8 percent), vascular disorders (7 percent), meningitis (3 percent), head injury (2 percent) and aqueductal stenosis (1 percent). Twenty-five percent of patients had clinical epilepsy. Ten percent had "psychiatric disturbances" for which they had prefrontal leucotomy performed. Vascular lesions represented only 2 percent (cerebral infarction and intracerebral hematoma).

We have studied 27 patients with electrical evidence of MRFD activity. Twelve patients presented with clinical evidence of intracranial hypertension; CT showed obstructive hydrocephalus caused by deep midline (9) or posterior fossa (3) tumor. Twelve other patients were disoriented but without focal deficit or papilledema; CT was normal and subsequent laboratory investigations demonstrated toxic-metabolic encephalopathy. Three patients had this pattern immediately following head trauma but had no clinical evidence of intracranial hypertension (although adequate intracranial pressure monitoring was not utilized); CT showed no evidence of cerebral edema or acute brain swelling. Clinical recovery was noted. The patient was neurologically asymptomatic three days later and EEG no longer showed MRFD activity.

Diffuse Slow Wave Pattern. In senescence the frequency of the background basic alpha rhythm is decreased; the amount of the theta and delta activity is increased. This is most common in the temporal regions.[24] It is believed that diffuse slowing correlates with intellectual deterioration. Stefoski and Bergen studied 35 patients with clinical dementia who were older than 59 and attempted to correlate ventricular size with EEG slowing.[25] Twenty-three percent of demented patients had normal background rhythm, 40 percent had mild generalized slowing and 37 percent had severe generalized slowing. There was no correlation between degree of EEG slowing and amount of ventricular and subarachnoid size enlargement. We have found that almost all patients with clinical dementia who were no longer capable of living independently or of handling their own finances had moderate to severe CT evidence of diffuse atrophy. This was accompanied by moderate diffuse slowing of EEG pattern.

Fifty patients without clinical evidence of dementia or seizures had EEG evidence of diffuse slowing. Twenty-eight patients had CT evidence of moderate ventricular and sulcal space enlargement as compared with controls. Follow-up of these patients has demonstrated that clinical dementia developed in 22 patients within 3 years. It is inferred from these studies that EEG and CT abnormalities may precede clinical intellectual deterioration. In 22 other patients with diffuse slowing, CT was entirely normal. Follow-up of these patients has shown no subsequent development of neurological or CT abnormalities within a three-year interval.

REFERENCES

1. Gastaut H, Gastaut JL: Computerized transverse axial tomography in epilepsy. Epilepsia 17:35, 1976
2. Gastaut H: Conclusions: computerized transverse axial tomography in epilepsy. Epilepsia 17:337, 1976
3. Stevens JR: Focal abnormality in petit mal: intracranial recordings and pathological findings. Neurology 20:1069, 1970
4. O'Brien JL: EEG abnormalities in addition to bilaterally synchronous three per second spike and wave in petit mal. Electroencephalog Clin Neurophysiol 11:747, 1959
5. Yang PJ, Berger PE, Cohen ME: Computerized tomography in childhood seizure disorders. Neurology 29:1084, 1979
6. Peafield W, Jasper HH: Epilepsy and functional anatomy of the brain. Little Brown and Co., Boston, 1954, pp. 50–65
7. Wallace JC: Radionuclide brain scanning in investigation of late onset seizures. Lancet 2:1467, 1974
8. Sumi SM, Teasdall RD: Focal seizures. Neurology 13:582, 1963
9. Bogdanoff BM, Stafford CR, Green L: Computerized transaxial tomography in the evaluation of patients with focal epilepsy. Neurology 25:1013, 1975
10. Prensky AL, Swisher CN, DeVivo DC: Positive brain scans in children with idiopathic focal epileptic seizures. Neurology 23:798, 1973
11. Yarnell PR, Burdick D, Sanders B: Focal seizures early veins, and increased flow. Neurology 24:512, 1974
12. Falconer MA, Serafetinides EA, Corsellis JA: Etiology and pathogenesis of temporal lobe epilepsy. Arch Neurol 10:233, 1964
13. Newcombe RL, Shah SH: Radiological abnormalities in temporal lobe epilepsy with clinicopathological correlations. J Neurol Neurosurg Psychiatr 38:279, 1975
14. Currie S, Heathfield WG, Henson RA: Clinical course and prognosis of temporal lobe epilepsy. Brain 94:173, 1971
15. Remillard GM, Ethier R, Andermann F: Temporal lobe epilepsy and perinatal occlusion of posterior cerebral artery. Neurology 24:1001, 1974
16. Jabbari B, DiChiro G, McCarthy JP: Mesial temporal sclerosis detected by computed tomography. J Comput Assist Tomogr 3:527, 1979
17. Jabbari B, Huott AD, DiChiro G: Surgically correctable lesions detected by CT in 143 patients with chronic epilepsy. Surg Neurol 10:319, 1978
18. McGahan JP, Dublin AB, Hill RP: The evaluation of seizure disorders by computerized tomography. J Neurosurg 50:328, 1979
19. Zimmerman FJ, Niedermeyer F, Hodges FJ: Lennox-Gastaut syndrome and computerized tomography findings. Epilepsia 18:463, 1977
20. Joynt RJ, Cape CA, Knott JR: Significance of focal delta activity in adult encephalogram. Arch Neurol 12:631, 1965
21. Brenner RP, Gilmore PC: Correlation of EEG, computerized tomography and clinical findings. Arch Neurol 38:37, 1981
22. Rosenberg CE, Anderson DC, Mahowald MW: Computed tomography and EEG in patients without focal neurologic findings. Arch Neurol 39:291, 1982
23. Cordeau JP: Monorhythmic frontal delta activity in the human EEG. Electroencephalog Clin Neurophysiol 11:733, 1959
24. Obrist WD: EEG of normal aged adults. Electroencephalog Clin Neurophysiol 6:235, 1954
25. Stefoski D, Bergen D: Correlation between diffuse EEG abnormalities and cerebral atrophy in senile dementia. J Neurol Neurosurg Psychiatr 39:751, 1976

Chapter 17

INTRACRANIAL CALCIFICATION AND BONE ABNORMALITIES

Intracranial mineral deposition is frequently found at necropsy examination. This occurs in brain parenchyma, blood vessels, dural structures and choroid plexus. Histochemical studies have shown that the basophilic vascular granular deposits contain calcium, iron and copper.[1] Of these, only calcium is sufficiently radiopaque to be detected radiographically. For example, iron deposits may occur in the basal ganglia in Hallevorden-Spatz disease and infantile neuroaxonal dystrophy, and copper is deposited in the basal ganglia in Wilson's disease. However, in these conditions radiopaque regions are not detected by radiographic studies, including CT.

Intracranial calcification may be caused by pathological processes (Table 17–1) or develop spontaneously. Radiographic evidence of intracranial calcification is uncommon in children; this increases in frequency with age. It is possible that this represents a degenerative or "aging" process or it may possibly reflect the effects of hormonal changes. Siderocalcific deposits are detected most frequently in the pineal gland, globus pallidus, putamen, caudate, thalamus, dentate nucleus of the cerebellum, cerebral cortex and choroid plexus. Phantom model studies have shown that CT is 5 to 15 times more sensitive than plain shadow radiography for detection of intracranial calcification.[2]

Pineal gland calcification is detected in 55 to 80 percent of plain skull radiographs in patients older than 20 years.[3, 4] It may measure up to 15 mm in size. It is most sensitively detected on lateral radiographic projections, but its midline position is most readily and accurately assessed on coronal (anteroposterior) projections. In some cases the pineal is obscured by the thick midline occiput in Towne's view or the frontal sinus in frontal projection. If frontal tomograms are utilized, the pineal is visualized in 40 percent of cases in which it is not detected by routine views.[4]

In routine CT scans (10-mm tissue section), the pineal is visualized in 75 percent of patients over age 20 to 96 percent of patients over age 40. The demonstration of pineal calcification is enhanced if thinner tissue sections are utilized because partial volume averaging is diminished. From a review of normal young subjects, pineal calcification was reported to occur in these frequencies: birth to 4 years (0 percent), 5 to 8 years (3 percent), 9 to 12 years (12.7 percent), 13 to 16 years (18.9 percent) and 17 to 20 years (43.3 percent).[5] Because the hyperdense pineal gland is surrounded by hypodense CSF in the diamond-shaped quadrigeminal cistern–third ventricular region, it may be visualized even if it is only faintly calcified. In patients with funduscopic evidence of papilledema caused by increased intracranial pressure, the pineal was visualized less frequently by skull radiography but there were no significant differences in detection by CT. The lower evidence of visualization by skull x-ray is the result of pineal body demineralization by intracranial hypertension. This renders the pineal invisible by conventional skull roentgenogram. However, there was no difference in frequency with which the pineal gland was visualized by CT in normal subjects and those with increased intracranial pressure. This indicates that although demineralization had occurred, this did not decrease the contrast resolution of the pineal by CT.

Because of the small size of Polaroid picture

294

TABLE 17–1. Etiologies of Basal Ganglionic Calcification

Metabolic-endocrine
Hypoparathyroidism
Pseudohypoparathyroidism
Pseudopseudohypoparathyroidism

Congenital
Cerebral vascular ferrocalcinosis (Fahr disease)
Cockayne syndrome
Tuberous sclerosis
Oculocraniosomatic disease (Kearns-Sayre syndrome)

Infectious-inflammatory
Cysticercosis
Postviral encephalitis
Toxoplasmosis
Cytomegalic inclusion disease
Granuloma (tuberculous)

Toxic
Carbon monoxide
Radiation therapy
Methotrexate
Lead encephalopathy

Vascular
Angioma
Aneurysms

Neoplastic
Glioma

devised a technique to magnify the scan image. The calvarial diameter measurement and pineal distance from the inner table are determined. These are expressed as a percentage of pineal shift normalized to calvarial diameter. The diameter ranges from 31 to 37 millimeters; pineal displacement that measures 0.9 millimeters represents a 2.6 percent shift. Ninety-nine percent of normal subjects show less shift. In several cases skull roentgenogram was interpreted as showing pineal shift. Subsequent CT scan showed that multiple intracranial calcifications were present, including those in the tentorium and perimesencephalic cistern. CT identified the midline pineal position as well as the characteristic shape and location of tentorial calcification (Fig. 17–1).

The size of the calcified pineal did not always correlate with occurrence of pineal tumor; however, all pineal calcifications with a diameter greater than 20 mm were pathological. Multilobulation of the pineal was another pathological feature. The pineal usually appeared homogeneously calcified; however, in several cases the central portion was hypodense (Fig. 17–2). Because there was no evidence of mass effect or enhancement, no further diagnostic studies were performed.

Other intracranial structures that are sometimes visualized on plain skull x-ray because of calcification include the choroid plexus, habenular, basal ganglia, dentate and falx cerebri. Choroid plexus is visualized on 67 percent of CT studies in normal subjects older than 45, and in 30 percent of those who are 20 to 44 years old. This is most common in the glomus of the atrial portion of the lateral ventricle. In one third of these cases, choroid plexus calcification appeared asymmetrical;

or multiformat x-ray, it is sometimes difficult to make an accurate assessment of the pineal position by CT. Significant shift of the pineal is shown by CT without difficulty; however, evidence of a small degree of shift may be equivocal by CT measurement. A slight degree of head rotation may influence the measurement of the pineal position. Hahn et al.

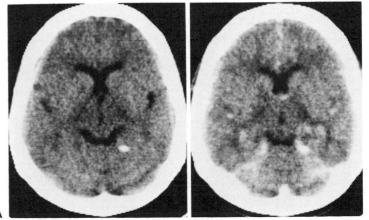

Figure 17–1. A 40-year-old had chronic headaches. Skull x-ray showed midline pineal shift; however, CT showed that this represented tentorial calcification (*A,B*) and not shifted pineal.

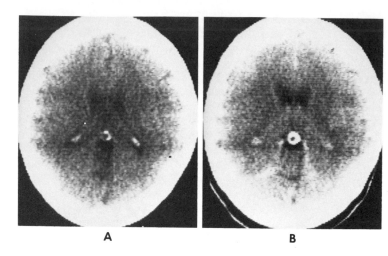

A   B

Figure 17–2. This 62-year-old woman had light-headedness and normal neurological examinaton. *CT findings:* calcified lesion *(A)* with dense peripheral enhancement and a hypodense central region *(B)* located in the quadrigeminal cistern. There is no mass effect or hydrocephalus.

however, unless there are other signs of mass effect, this is not a significant diagnostic finding. The falx cerebri appears calcified in 42 percent of adult patients. This is an age-dependent phenomenon and is most common in patients older than 60 years. Calcification is more commonly present in the anterior than the posterior portion. The falx most commonly appears as a linear hyperdense band; however, rarely it appears as a thick plaque or globular mass. In pediatric patients the presence of hyperdense falx may be caused by subarachnoid hemorrhage and the falx is infrequently visualized in normal subjects; however, in adults it is quite difficult to differentiate hemorrhage in this region from normal calcified falx. The linear falx usually enhances on postcontrast scan. The finding of a hyperdense thickened calcified falx is suggestive of meningioma; however, lack of enhancement in the contiguous frontal region makes a diagnosis of meningioma unlikely (Fig. 17–3). Cerebellar dentate calcifications are usually bilateral, and these are seen in 0.1 percent of normal subjects (Fig. 17–4). The habenular calcification is usually not visualized as a distinct region on CT as it is seen with plain skull roentgenogram.

Basal ganglionic calcification was seen in 0.8 percent of CT scans. This percentage is slightly higher than those reported in other series.[6, 7] These lesions are usually bilateral and symmetrical. The calcified regions appeared asymmetrical in 20 percent of cases. In 6 percent of patients, basal ganglionic calcification appeared unilateral. Serial CT scans will be necessary to determine if unilateral calcification evolves to a bilateral process. If a hyperdense ganglionic lesion is unilateral, it

may be difficult to differentiate calcification from hemorrhage. This problem is further compounded if the calcified lesion is small and attenuation values overlap those of hemorrhage. Ganglionic hematomas extend across the internal capsule and have irregular margination, whereas ganglionic calcifications are usually confined and outline gray matter subcortical masses. The initial pathological process is deposition of colloid material in and around blood vessel walls; this colloid material subsequently calcifies.

Basal ganglionic calcification is most commonly seen in the globus pallidus; but this may also involve the putamen or caudate. They may be associated with dentate nucleus and cerebral cortex calcification. The etiolo-

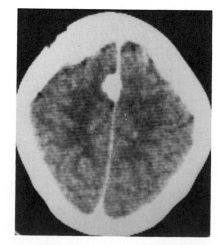

Figure 17–3. A 47-year-old with malignant melanoma developed headache. Examination, EEG and isotope scan were negative. *CT finding:* localized hyperdense calcified nonenhancing falx and not representing a neoplasm.

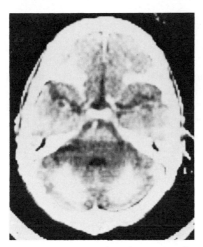

Figure 17–4. A 50-year-old had no neurological abnormalities. *CT findings:* bilateral dentate cerebellar calcification with normal fourth ventricle.

gies of ganglionic calcifications are listed in Table 17–1. Disturbances of calcium metabolism have been detected in 40 to 66 percent of cases (Fig. 17–5). In 20 percent of cases, this is believed to be an age-related phenomenon. This physiological calcification is uncommon before age 60 (Fig. 17–6). All patients under age 40 with CT evidence of ganglionic calcification should be completely investigated for the conditions listed in Table 17–1. In addition, patients with *widespread* intracranial calcification should be thoroughly studied, irrespective of age.

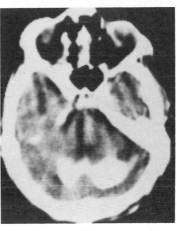

A

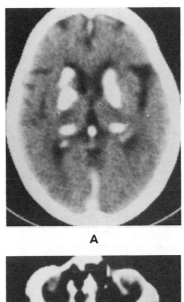

B

Figure 17–6. A 60-year-old woman had dementia but no parkinsonian features. Skull x-ray showed bilateral basal ganglionic calcification. *CT findings:* bilateral basal ganglionic, thalamic *(A)* and cerebellar calcification *(B)*.

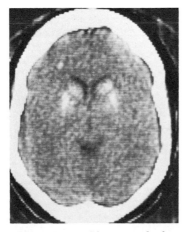

Figure 17–5. A 25-year-old woman had generalized seizures that were poorly controlled with anticonvulsants. Skull x-ray showed no calcification. Laboratory studies showed marked hypocalcemia. *CT findings:* bilateral frontal caudate and globus pallidus calcification.

There are some patients with CT evidence of globus pallidus calcification who have clinical signs of extrapyramidal syndrome. There have been reports of patients with the diagnosis of parkinsonism who show poor response to levodopa therapy; in some of these, CT showed bilateral basal ganglionic calcification. In those patients with abnormal calcium and phosphorus metabolism causing basal ganglionic calcification, skull x-ray usually also showed the lesions. In patients with other conditions such as toxoplasmosis and tuberous sclerosis causing basal ganglionic calcification, calcified lesions are more widespread, involving cerebral hemispheres and cerebellum.

CONDITIONS CAUSING INTRACRANIAL CALCIFICATION

Tuberous Sclerosis. Intracranial calcification is the most common radiographic abnormality in this disorder. It has been detected in 40 to 50 percent of cases; however, it becomes more dense with increasing age. The calcified lesions appear as multiple dense round lesions located periventricularly, and in some cases they are also seen in the cerebral cortex, basal ganglia and cerebellum. These lesions are believed to represent foci of cortical gliosis that contain abnormal neuronal and glial elements and subsequently calcify. The calcified periventricular lesions of tuberous sclerosis may be seen before cutaneous manifestations develop.[8]

Infectious-Inflammatory. Many varied disorders such as cytomegalic inclusion body disease (CID), toxoplasmosis, cysticercosis and tuberculosis are associated with intracranial calcification. Toxoplasmosis and CID show multiple periventricular lesions. These may progress such that they delineate the entire ventricular surface. Cysticercosis causes single or multiple cerebral cortical calcified lesions. These are usually not identified by plain skull x-ray. The calcification may be seen in the cyst wall and the scolex to create a characteristic appearance. Tuberculous granulomas may calcify and appear as single or multiple, most commonly located in the cerebral cortex.

Vascular. Giant (berry) aneurysms that are partially or completely thrombosed frequently show evidence of calcification in the peripheral wall or thrombosed portion. Calcium is deposited in fibrous tissue that has replaced the normal muscular and elastic component of vessel wall. The calcified lesion may be curvilinear or ring-shaped or may appear as dense and egg-shaped. Ectatic fusiform aneurysms are tortuous in shape; calcified lesions may have a serpentine S-shaped configuration. Arteriovenous malformations show evidence of calcification in one quarter of cases. The calcified portion of angiomas may be curvilinear, dense globular, ring-like or punctate in appearance. Thrombosed (occult) angiomas show calcified components in almost all cases. In Sturge-Weber syndrome (capillary-venous malformation) there may be characteristic calcified lesions that resemble railway tracks. The calcification is located in the atrophic and gliotic occipital gyri rather than within the walls of the vessel malformation. There have been occasional reports of spontaneous parenchymal hematomas (cerebral, hemisphere, cerebellum) that have subsequently calcified.[9] It is most likely that these have resulted from underlying angioma or aneurysm; however, in some cases the hematoma appeared to have no underlying etiology.

Neoplasms. Calcification is most frequent in slow-growing and less malignant neoplasms.[10] The incidence of histological and radiographic calcification is highest in meningiomas, craniopharyngiomas, oligodendrogliomas, ependymomas and low-grade (Grades I and II) astrocytomas. Because of their malignant potential and rapid growth rate, glioblastoma multiforme and metastases are unlikely to show evidence of calcification. The malignant neoplasms also contain foci of hemorrhage and necrotic portions that have the potential to undergo calcification, but they rarely show radiographic calcification.[11] Plain skull radiography has shown that 25 percent of low-grade (Grades I and II) astrocytomas calcify. This has been consistent with CT findings. Glioblastomas show plain skull radiographic calcification in less than 1 percent; however, we have seen CT foci of calcification in 5 percent. Although medulloblastomas rarely show radiographic calcification, we have seen this finding in 10 percent diagnosed with CT. Oligodendrogliomas are the most common glioma to show radiographic calcification; this is consistent with CT findings.

Meningiomas frequently show histological evidence of psammomatous body calcification. These dispersed areas of calcification are not always detected on x-rays, but 60 percent showed hyperdense speckled portions consistent with psammoma bodies with CT. In 4 percent, meningiomas appear densely calcified (Fig. 17–7). Lateral ventricular calcified masses usually represent meningioma or choroid plexus papilloma. Intrasellar calcification is usually caused by pituitary adenoma or craniopharyngioma. Suprasellar calcifications may be caused by multiple tumor types, including craniopharyngioma, pituitary adenoma, meningioma, teratoma, chordoma, hypothalamic glioma and aneurysm. Lipomas of the corpus callosum appear as curvilinear calcified lesions with a central hypodense component. Atypical teratomas and pinealomas may appear as calcified lesions in the pineal–third ventricular or suprasellar–anterior third ventricular region. Dermoid and epidermoid tumors may calcify. They may appear as dense nodular or curvilinear calcified lesions.

Figure 17–7. A 67-year-old had headache and normal neurological examination. Skull x-ray showed parietal hyperostosis. *CT findings:* posterior parietal densely calcified homogeneous lesion *(A)* that appears more heterogeneous with bone settings *(B).*

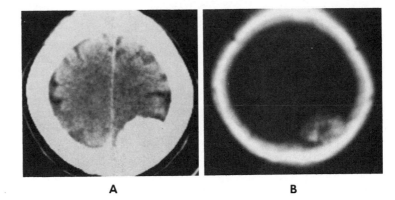

A   B

BONE ABNORMALITIES

Fibrous Dysplasia. This is a condition affecting children and adolescents.[12] The skull may be the only involved area (monostotic); however, in the other form, skull and multiple long bones are involved (polyostotic). If the skull is involved, there is thickening of the bones comprising the orbit and the anterior and middle fossa floor. There may be foraminal encroachment with resultant cranial nerve dysfunction, as in visual loss caused by optic nerve compression within the optic canal. When the sphenoid bone is the only bone that appears thickened, differentiation of fibrous dysplasia from meningioma may be difficult. Radiographic findings of fibrous dysplasia include dense bone sclerosis and lucent lesions within diploic spaces caused by cystic spaces filled with poorly calcified bone. Isotope scan may show localized uptake caused by increased bone turnover in this condition. There is pathological evidence of replacement of bone by actively proliferating fibroblasts. CT may show localized bone thickening with interspersed hypodense regions and there may be abnormal enhancement. In rare instances, certain neurodiagnostic studies including plain skull x-ray, isotope scan and CT may suggest meningioma; however, angiography shows no tumor stain in fibrous dysplasia.

Paget's Disease. This is a disorder that commonly affects patients in middle life. There is bone overgrowth leading to skull enlargement. Clinical symptoms include: (1) basilar invagination caused by involvement of the skull base, (2) visual loss from optic nerve compression and (3) deafness resulting from temporal bone involvement. Initial pathological bone changes are osteolytic; skull x-ray shows sharply circumscribed demineralized osteoporotic areas.

In the next phase bone destruction and bone formation occur simultaneously. Skull x-ray shows calvarial thickening with frontal bossing. Sclerotic areas are seen and coalesce into a "cotton-wool" appearance. CT shows skull bone to be thickened and to contain interspersed multiple honeycombed lucent regions (Fig. 17–8).

Hyperostosis Frontalis Interna. This disorder consists of thickening of the inner table of the frontal bone that tapers down toward the midline. The outer table is spared and there is no attachment to the falx (Fig. 17–9). The thickened bone may project into the anterior fossa. The condition is usually bilateral but may be unilateral. Isotope scan is negative. CT shows thickened frontal bone that may be lobulated and project into the anterior fossa. There is no contrast enhancement.

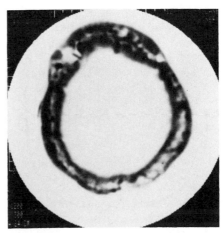

Figure 17–8. In this elderly woman with Paget's disease, CT findings taken with bone settings were marked bone thickening with interspersed sclerotic and lucent regions.

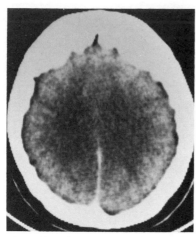

Figure 17–9. A young woman with dizziness and marked frontal bone thickening on skull x-ray had CT findings of marked lobulated thickening of frontal bone that tapered toward the midline. This represented hyperostosis frontalis interna.

Arachnoid Granulations. These may project into venous sinuses or cerebral veins along the cerebral hemispheres; these are most common in relationship to the superior sagittal sinus. They are usually located in the posterior frontal-anterior parietal region and are paramedian in position; however, they may be seen in other locations (occipital) in relation to the torcular herophili. Skull x-ray shows lucent lesions. These may protrude through

the inner table or rarely through the outer table. They usually are multiple but may be solitary. Solitary arachnoid granulations eroding through the inner table may simulate superficial intracranial tumor. CT shows hypodense lesions eroding through the inner table. It is possible that these arachnoid granulations would show dense contrast enhancement; however, we have not had the opportunity to test this hypothesis.

Encephaloceles. In this condition both brain and CSF protrude through abnormal foramina in the bony calvarium. If the protruding tissue consists only of meninges (meningocele), the density of the material is that of CSF. These are usually midline lesions, and the majority occur in the occipital region. CT shows bony defect and brain tissue that herniates through it. Regional encephaloceles that contain CSF only may show communication with the quadrigeminal cistern and posterior third ventricle. Meningoencephaloceles may be associated with other congenital abnormalities. Pseudomeningomyeloceles may develop as a surgical complication (Fig. 17–10).

BENIGN TUMORS OF THE SKULL

Osteoma. These may originate from the outer table and project externally as skull masses or they may arise from the inner table and project into the cranial visit. These represent the most common benign tumors involving the skull. Sites of predilection include the calvarium or paranasal sinuses (frontal, ethmoidal). Skull x-ray shows a dense sclerotic sharply marginated lesion without involvement of diploic spaces. CT shows a homogeneous hyperdense nonenhancing mass that has the same density as bone. These may simulate the CT appearance of meningioma. Osteomas are usually small, whereas calcified meningiomas are usually larger lesions. CT may detect sinus, orbital and intracranial extension of the osteoma.

Hemangioma. Those involving the calvarium originate within and expand the diploic spaces. Skull x-ray shows a lucent lesion with sharply marginated borders without sclerosis. CT shows a hypodense lesion that expands into the diploic spaces; however, it is the skull radiographic findings that are characteristic of this lesion.

Eosinophilic Granuloma. This represents

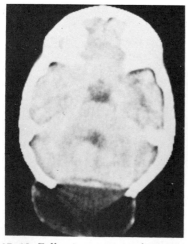

Figure 17–10. Following posterior fossa craniotomy, this girl developed swelling at the operative site. CT findings: marked bulging containing CSF and brain parenchyma density material caused by pseudomeningomyocele.

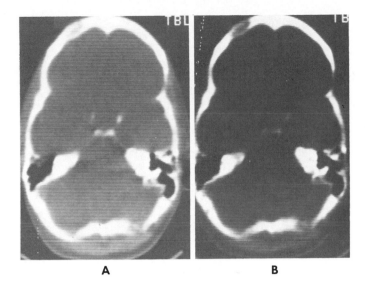

Figure 17–11. A 22-year-old woman noticed a lump in the left frontal region. Skull x-ray showed a sclerotic lesion; isotope scan was positive. *CT findings:* left frontal hypodense lesion *(A)* within diploic spaces of frontal bone *(B).* Biopsy showed an eosinophilic granuloma.

A   B

one manifestation of inflammatory histiocytosis.[13] It occurs most commonly in adolescents and young adults and usually involves frontal bone. Skull x-ray shows irregularly marginated lucent lesions without surrounding sclerosis. The edges may be beveled because of the greater degree of outer table bone erosion. Solitary lesions are more common than multiple lesions (Fig. 17–11). There may be a central sclerotic region (button sequestrum). CT findings include: (1) a hypodense lesion within the diploic space of frontal bone, (2) central hyperdense region and (3) overlying soft-tissue mass.

Epidermoid Cyst. These may cause bone destruction because of pressure erosion. Skull x-ray shows a sharply marginated hypodense lesion with surrounding sclerotic border. CT shows thinning of bone with a homogeneous hypodense region and medial hyperdense rim. The underlying brain appears normal.[14]

MALIGNANT TUMORS OF THE SKULL

Metastatic Carcinoma. These most commonly originate from breast, lung and prostate. They may be osteolytic with a hypodense region or osteoblastic with sclerotic regions. The base of skull lesions caused by direct extension from the paranasal sinus or nasopharynx is best delineated by hypocycloidal tomography (see discussion under metastatic disease).

Neuroblastoma. This tumor of childhood metastasizes to the skull. There may be multiple areas of bone destruction possibly involving the calvarium or orbital region. Tumor deposits may occur between the dura and inner table.

Chondrosarcoma. These are rare tumors that occur in the parasellar, cerebellopontine angle and convexity regions.[15] Skull x-rays usually show speckled or ring-like calcification and osteolytic bone lesions. CT shows a soft-tissue mass with interspersed calcification. The noncalcified portion enhances in a heterogeneous pattern. Differentiation from chordoma or meningioma is not usually possible.

REGIONS OF SPECIAL INTEREST

Paranasal Sinuses. Diagnostic assessment includes the following: (1) conventional radiography (Waters, Caldwell, lateral, basal projections) and (2) pluridirectional tomography and (3) computed tomography.[16] Pluridirectional tomography is slightly more sensitive in detecting bone abnormalities than CT; however, CT better delineates soft-tissue lesions and extension into contiguous regions such as the orbit and cranium. Complete CT examination of the paranasal sinuses includes axial and coronal projections. To obtain adequate bone detail, high spatial resolution is necessary. This is obtained by thin tissue sections (1.0 to 3.0 mm), fine matrix size (256 × 256, 512 × 512) and small pixel size (less than 1.0 × 1.0

mm). This technique will detect small bone abnormalities; however, for detection of soft-tissue lesions, 4 mm sections are adequate. It has been reported that direct coronal images are superior to the computer-generated reformated images; however, we have found reformated images to be of equal value, especially since we obtain 2 mm axial sections from which reformated images are based. This reformated technique avoids image-degrading artifacts that frequently emanate from such high-density objects as dental fillings and also avoids limitation in patient positioning because of inability to hyperextend the patient's neck. As has been the experience with orbit CT, contrast medium–enhanced scans do not provide supplemental information except in rare cases, as in angiofibroma or vascular malformation or if intracranial extension is suspected. If there is bone erosion extending toward the intracranial cavity, contrast medium–enhanced study should be utilized.

CT is the most useful diagnostic procedure in patients with sinusitis, sinus or facial bone fracture or if intracranial extension of sinus infection is suspected. Neoplasms of the paranasal sinuses show extensive bone destruction, soft-tissue masses and evidence of orbital and infratemporal extension. Mucoceles and cysts may expand the sinus and cause bone erosion, and these are well-delineated by CT.

Temporal Bone. By certain modifications in technique, spatial resolution of the petrous temporal bone may be better than 0.6 mm. This involves improvements in high resolution technology of both hardware and software capabilities. It is therefore possible that the detailed anatomy of middle ear structures and the internal acoustic canal are clearly visualized. It should be emphasized that this is possible only in an area of inherent high contrast, such as the petrous temporal bone, and with these specific technical modifications. For a detailed discussion of the anatomy and pathology of this region, the reader is referred to other sources.[17]

REFERENCES

1. Wagner JA, Slager UT: Incidence and composition of radiopaque deposits in basal ganglia of brain. Am J Roentgenol 74:232, 1955
2. Norman D, Diamond C, Boyd D: Relative detectability of intracranial calcifications on computed tomography and skull radiography. J Comput Assist Tomogr 2:61, 1978
3. Hahn FJY, Rim K, Schapiro RL: The normal range and position of the pineal gland on computed tomography. Radiology 119:599, 1976
4. Goree JA, Wallace KK, Bean RL: The pineal tomogram: visualization of the faintly calcified pineal gland. Am J Roentgenol 89:1209, 1963
5. Zimmerman RA, Bilaniuk LT: Age-related incidence of pineal calcification detected by computed tomography. Radiology 142:659, 1982
6. Koller WC, Cochran JW, Klawans HL: Calcifications of the basal ganglia: computerized tomography and clinical correlation. Neurology 29:328, 1979
7. Cohen OR, Duchesneau PM, Weinstein MA: Calcification of the basal ganglia as visualized by computed tomography. Radiology 134:97, 1980
8. Schafer JA, Berg BD, Norman D: Cerebellar calcification in tuberous sclerosis. Arch Neurol 32:642, 1975
9. Kawakami Y, Nakao Y, Tabuchi K: Bilateral intracerebellar calcification associated with cerebellar hematoma. J Neurosurg 49:744, 1978.
10. Gouliamos AD, Jimenez JP, Goree JA: Computed tomography and skull radiography in the diagnosis of calcified brain tumor. Am J Roentgenol 130:761, 1978
11. Dohrmann GJ, Geehr RB, Robinson F: Small hemorrhages versus small calcification in brain tumors: difficulty in differentiation by computed tomography. Surg Neurol 10:309, 1978
12. Olmsted W: Some skeletogenic lesions with common calvarial manifestations. Radiol Clin North Am 19:703, 1981
13. Mitnick JS, Pinto RS: Computed tomography in the diagnosis of eosinophilic granuloma. J Comput Assist Tomogr 4:791, 1980
14. Garcia J, Lagier R, Hoessly M: Computed tomography-pathology correlation in skull epidermoid cyst. J Comput Assist Tomogr 6:818, 1982
15. Grossman RI, Davis KR: Cranial computed tomographic appearance of chondrosarcoma of the base of skull. Radiology 141:403, 1981
16. Bilaniuk LT, Zimmerman RA: Computed tomography of the paranasal sinuses. Radiol Clin North Am 20:51, 1982
17. Taylor S: The petrous temporal bone (including the cerebellopontine angle). Radiol Clin North Am 20:67, 1982.

Chapter 18

PEDIATRIC CONDITIONS

Interpretation of CT in neonates, infants and young children requires understanding of maturational brain growth changes. These are most rapid within the first six months of life but continue at slower rates probably into the second decade. These changes include: (1) increased size, (2) increased dry weight, (3) decreased water content, (4) increased lipid and protein content, (5) decreased lateral (frontal horn, bodies) and third ventricular size and (6) decreased CSF-filled space (subdural, subarachnoid).[1,2] There are detectable differences in gray and white matter CT attenuation values; these are most marked in premature infants. This visually detectable difference lessens with age (Fig. 18–1). Gray matter attenuation values show minimal change after birth. However, white matter attenuation values increase because of reduced water content and rapid myelination. Cerebral hemisphere myelination is poorly formed at term. Rapid myelination occurs for several years and probably continues at a slower rate up to the second decade. In premature infants, CT shows symmetrical periventricular hypodense regions. These are more prominent in the frontal than in the parietal and occipital regions. The periventricular hypodensities markedly decrease within six months. It is important to be careful to distinguish this normal pattern from that resulting from perinatal hypoxic-ischemic brain injury.

There is doubling of dry brain weight within 6 months; the brain is 80 percent of full adult weight within 2 years. CSF spaces appear enlarged in neonates and infants. Those in the frontal region may measure up to 8 mm for 12 months. Other measurements in normal subjects up to 12 months include: sylvian cistern, 10 mm; interhemispheric fissure, 6 mm; third ventricular width, 6 mm and fourth ventricular height, 15 mm. The Evans ratio (maximum distance between the internal laminae at the same level divided by the maximum frontal horn distance) is .22 to .32—this does not change with age. We identify no more than two or three cerebral sulci in supraventricular sections of normal children.[3] After 12 months, these CSF spaces decrease in size; therefore, diagnosis of brain atrophy before this time should be made with caution. CSF protein content is high at term (maximum of 90 mg percent); CSF appears more radiodense, acting to blur the ventricular-brain interphase. This interferes with ventricular size measurements. CSF protein content decreases by 50 percent within 2 months.

In the diagnostic assessment of children in two areas unique to pediatric practice, CT has modified our clinical approach. CT has been most helpful in evaluating children with enlarged head size.[4] It is also important in assessing children with developmental delay, especially when accompanied by the following: dysmorphic features (abnormal appearance caused by congenital malformations); skin lesions (neurocutaneous disorders); seizures, especially infantile spasms and minor motor attacks caused by congenital anomalies or metabolic disorders; and small head (microcephaly).

CLINICAL PROBLEMS OF CHILDHOOD

Macrocrania (Megalocephaly)

This is defined as head circumference above the 97th percentile.[5] The condition may result from abnormalities in one or more intracranial compartments. The calvarium may be thickened as a result of anemia, rickets or osteopetrosis. The subdural region may be affected by effusion, hygroma, hematoma or empyema, and the ventricles by obstructive intraventric-

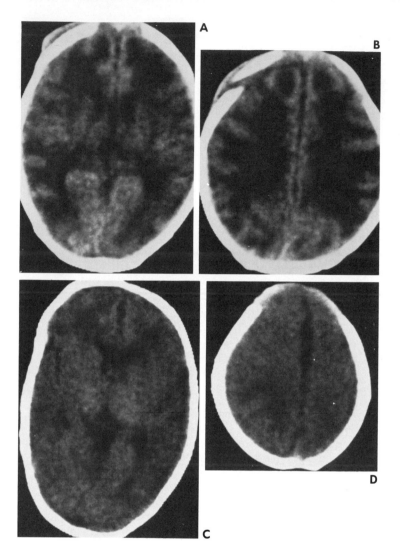

Figure 18–1. This 2-week-old neonate was born 4 weeks prematurely. She had poor suck reflex and was hypotonic. *CT findings:* symmetrical cerebral hemispheric hypodense regions with enlarged sulci and ventricles (*A,B*). Two months later her neurological development was normal. *CT findings:* normal density pattern in both hemispheres with normal-sized ventricles (*C,D*).

ular or extraventricular hydrocephalus. Cerebral edema may result from toxic or metabolic causes, venous occlusion or neoplasm. "Large brain" (megalencephaly) may be caused by familial conditions, neurocutaneous syndromes or metabolic conditions (aminoaciduria, leukodystrophy, mucopolysaccaridosis, gangliosidosis). To delineate the etiology of macrocrania, four baseline parameters should be analyzed (Table 18–1). These are rate of head circumference growth and shape of the head, developmental history and neurological examination, family history of enlarged head size, and CT findings.

Benign Megalencephaly

Children with large heads may be neurologically normal and have no evidence of developmental delay. Serial measurements show gradual and proportional enlargement of head size, and head shape is normal. Skull roentgenogram may be normal or may show suture diastasis. CT is performed to exclude occult hydrocephalus. If cerebroventricular indexes (bifrontal or bicaudate distance divided by brain diameter at a similar level) are calculated, ventricular size is normal; however, if absolute ventricular size is measured, the ventricles may be slightly dilated compared with those of children with normal-sized heads. The failure to calculate this ratio may account for results in some studies in which normal ventricles are reported and others in which enlarged ones are reported. The bifrontal ratio should not exceed 40 percent and the bicaudate ratio should be less than 23 percent. The characteristic feature of benign megalencephaly is the positive family history. At least one

TABLE 18–1. **Common Causes of Macrocephaly**

Birth to 6 Months
A. Hydrocephalus
    1. Congenital–spina bifida cystica, Arnold-Chiari malformation, aqueductal stenosis, holoprosencephaly
    2. Mass lesions–vein of Galen aneurysm, cysts, neoplasm
    3. Intrauterine infections–toxoplasmosis, cytomegalic inclusion disease, syphilis, rubella
    4. Perinatal infections–bacterial, tuberculous
B. Hydranencephaly
C. Subdural effusion

6 Months to 2 Years
A. Hydrocephalus
    1. Mass lesions–cysts, neoplasm, abscess
    2. Infectious–postmeningitic
    3. Dysraphism–Dandy-Walker syndrome, Arnold-Chiari malformation
    4. Posthemorrhagic–trauma, vascular malformation
B. Subdural effusion
C. Increased intracranial pressure syndrome
D. Megalencephaly
    1. Metabolic–leukodystrophy, lipidosis (Tay-Sachs)
    2. Neurocutaneous syndrome–tuberous sclerosis, Sturge-Weber syndrome, von Recklinghausen's disease
E. Primary megalencephaly

After 2 Years
A. Hydrocephalus
    1. Mass lesions–neoplasms, angioma
    2. Dysraphism–aqueductal stenosis, Arnold-Chiari malformation
    3. Postinfectious–bacterial, tuberculosis
    4. Hemorrhagic–trauma, angioma
B. Megalencephaly
C. Pseudotumor cerebri
D. Cerebral edema of multiple diverse causes

parent and frequently one or more siblings have large head size. In these children other diagnostic studies such as serial CT scan and cisternogram (metrizamide, radionuclide) are not necessary. Follow-up of these patients has confirmed the benign nature of this condition if the child has a normal cerebroventricular ratio, positive family history, and is neurologically normal even if the ventricles are mildly enlarged.[6]

External Hydrocephalus

Other children with macrocrania have no family history of enlarged head size. They show gradual head expansion with suture diastasis but no other signs of intracranial hypertension. CT shows these findings: (1) no significant ventricular enlargement, (2) enlarged basal cisterns including sylvian cistern and (3) dilated supratentorial cortical sulci including interhemispheric fissure. It has been postulated that these enlarged CSF-filled spaces represent the initial stage of communicating hydrocephalus (Fig. 18–2). Several studies have reported that some patients subsequently develop ventricular enlargement that requires shunting,[7] whereas other studies have shown that this represents benign subarachnoid space enlargement.[8, 9] In shunted patients with external hydrocephalus there may be slowing of head size growth but questionable evidence that the neurological condition is benefited by shunting.

Cerebral atrophy resulting from impaired brain development or brain injury does not usually occur in a macrocephalic child unless there is concomitant CSF circulatory obstruction. In certain children CT shows mild CSF space enlargement caused by sepsis, dehydration, starvation and protein depletion. This may be reversible if the underlying condition is corrected.

Subdural Lesions

In children with macrocrania, CT may show enlarged extracerebral spaces. These may be caused by subdural effusion, subdural hygroma, and subdural hematoma. These may appear as crescent-shaped hypodense lesions overlying the cerebral convexities. Subdural effusions may develop in children with systemic illnesses such as sepsis, meningitis, gastroenteritis and dehydration. The hypodense lesion is usually associated with subarachnoid

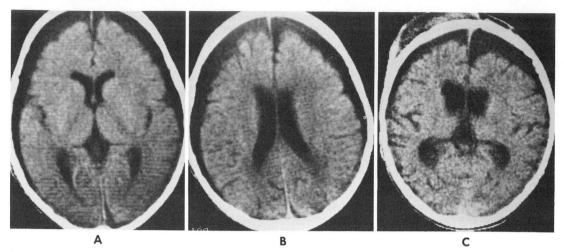

Figure 18–2. A 14-month-old child with delayed neurological development had increased head size. *CT findings:* bilateral semilunar-shaped hypodense extracerebral lesions with irregular medial interdigitations (*A*). The ventricles are enlarged (*B*). Following surgical drainage of subdural fluid with normal protein content, the head size progressively increased. *CT findings:* hypodense extracerebral lesions with further increase in ventricular size (*C*). This case of "external hydrocephalus" subsequently required diversionary shunt.

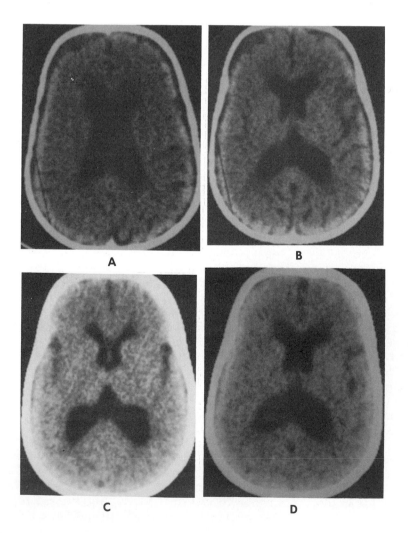

Figure 18–3. An 18-month-old girl had bacterial meningitis. Following treatment with antibiotics, the CSF formula became normal. *CT findings:* bilateral semilunar hypodense extracerebral lesions with medial hyperdense rim (*A*). The ventricles and subarachnoid spaces are enlarged (*B*). Several months later, CT shows resolution of the subdural effusions (*C*) with decrease in ventricular size and no evidence of enlarged subarachnoid spaces (*D*).

space and ventricular enlargement (Fig. 18–3). There is no enhancement in the medial membrane, although there may be diffuse cortical gyral enhancement underlying the effusion. On the basis of CT findings it is not always possible to differentiate subdural effusion from subdural empyema; however, in patients with meningitis, clinical features of rapid deterioration with significant neurological deficit (seizure, hemiparesis and papilledema) suggest subdural empyema.

Subdural hygromas usually result from trauma.[10] These extracerebral hypodense crescent-shaped lesions have density values consistent with CSF. There is no medial membrane enhancement. The ventricles may appear compressed and small or they may be enlarged because of associated communicating hydrocephalus (Fig. 18–4).

Chronic subdural hematomas appear hypodense but may have interspersed or layered hyperdense portions (solid clot). Mass effect is present and cortical sulcal spaces are effaced ipsilateral to the lesion. Enhancement may be seen in the medial border. Because CT findings do not always permit definitive diagnosis, subdural tap with fluid content analysis may be required in some cases. In addition, CT may not always define if extracerebral fluid-filled spaces are subdural, subarachnoid or combination of both.[11]

Hydrocephalus

If the macrocephalic child has CT evidence of moderate or severe ventricular enlarge-

ment, the location of CSF obstruction (intraventricular or extraventricular) and the cause of hydrocephalus must be determined. Hydrocephalus represents a pathophysiological condition characterized by imbalance of CSF production compared with reabsorptive capacity; this results in ventricular enlargement that is not caused by brain atrophy (Table 18–2). In infants, common causes of hydrocephalus include myelomeningocele (40 percent), extraventricular obstructive (communicating) process (30 percent) and intraventricular obstructive (noncommunicating) process (30 percent).

The most common locations for intraventricular obstruction are the aqueduct of sylvius, the intraventricular foramina and the outlet foramina of the fourth ventricle. Extraventricular obstructive hydrocephalus results from impaired CSF resorption at these locations: the basal cisterns, tentorial incisura, midconvexity cisterns and parasagittal region.

CT demonstrates ventricular dilatation in patients with hydrocephalus. In moderate to severe cases diagnosis of hydrocephalus is established on a single scan; however, in mild cases, serial scans are necessary to show progressive ventricular enlargement. In obstructive hydrocephalus, three features are characteristic: first, rounded enlargement of the superior-lateral portion of the frontal horns, second, temporal horn dilatation and third, periventricular hypodensities. CT is helpful in delineating the point of obstruction. This is represented by the transition from enlarged to nonenlarged (e.g., normal-sized) or nonvisualized CSF spaces (e.g., ventricles, cisterns). Enlarged lateral ventricles only indicate obstruction of the intraventricular foramina of Monro. If there is triventricular enlargement with nonvisualization of basal cisterns, this is consistent with obstruction at the fourth ventricular outlet foramina. Triventricular dilatation and basal cisternal enlargement indicates extraventricular incisural obstruction. Triventricular dilatation with enlargement of basal and sylvian cisterns and low-convexity cortical sulci indicates extraventricular obstruction at the midconvexity region. This anatomical localization of the site of CSF obstruction by these CT patterns is theoretically accurate; however, it is not always reliable. Some patients with extraventricular obstruction show enlarged lateral and third ventricles *without* CT evidence of dilated fourth ventricle. In addition, some patients with extraventricular obstructive hydrocepha-

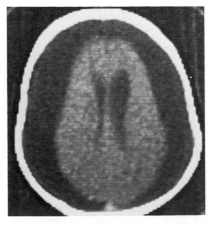

Figure 18–4. Following removal of choroid plexus papilloma, she remained obtunded. *CT findings:* bilateral semilunar shaped hypodense extracerebral lesions compressing the lateral ventricles. *Operative findings:* subdural hygromas.

TABLE 18–2. Classification of Hydrocephalus

Obstructive
A. Congenital lesions
    1. Aqueductal stenosis (true narrowing, septum, forking)
    2. Dandy-Walker syndrome (atresia of the foramina of Luschka and Magendie)
    3. Masses (cysts, neoplasms, vascular malformations)
    4. Arnold-Chiari malformation
B. Acquired lesions
    1. Aqueductal stenosis (gliosis)
    2. Ventricular inflammatory disorders (ventriculitis)
    3. Masses (cysts, neoplasms)
Communicating
A. Congenital lesions
    1. Arnold-Chiari malformation
    2. Encephalocele
    3. Leptomeningeal inflammation
    4. Congenital absence of arachnoid granulation
B. Acquired lesions
    1. Leptomeningeal inflammation
    2. Hemorrhage
    3. Masses such as cysts, neoplasms (especially causing leptomeningeal involvement)
    4. Platybasia

lus have secondary intraventricular sites of obstruction. In these cases, metrizamide CT ventriculogram may be necessary to determine appropriate shunt strategy.

Etiologies of Hydrocephalus

Aqueductal Stenosis. These patients show rapid head size growth and usually signs of intracranial hypertension. This diagnosis is most probable if CT shows lateral and third ventricular enlargement with a small fourth ventricle and nonvisualized basal cisterns (Fig. 18–5). The dilated proximal portion of the aqueduct is rarely seen on CT because of its small size and scanning angulation. The occipital horns appear larger than the frontal horns. There is a periventricular hypodense halo confined to white matter. This is most prominent surrounding the anterior pole; it is believed to represent transependymal CSF reabsorption. Marked lateral and third ventricular dilatation may cause low insertion of the tentorium and small posterior fossa. Since CT does not directly visualize the aqueduct, it is not possible to define the precise cause of aqueductal stenosis unless a gross pathological lesion such as a neoplasm is present. CT findings of congenital stenosis with forking of the aqueductal region and acquired lesions in which ependymal and subependymal layers of the aqueduct are replaced by gliotic tissue following hemorrhage or infection are identical.

The CT findings of aqueductal stenosis may be confused with fourth ventricular outlet obstruction if the fourth ventricle is not well visualized in the latter condition. Demonstration of the site of obstruction may require metrizamide cisternography. It is necessary to perform both noncontrast and intravenous medium–enhanced scans to exclude the presence of an occult mass that may be obstructing the aqueduct. In those cases of aqueductal obstruction caused by mass lesion in which the diagnosis of occult lesion was established by the enhanced scan or subsequent diagnostic studies such as metrizamide or air ventriculogram, the posterior third ventricle appeared abnormal on initial nonenhanced scan. In one study, Naidich et al. reported 15 percent of patients with "benign hydrocephalus" treated for six months to three years before CT showed an underlying neoplasm.[12] In aqueductal stenosis the third ventricle appears as an enlarged tubular structure; the dilated posterior portion has a convex shape directed posteriorly. If there is a mass causing obstruction at the level of the proximal aqueduct, the posterior third ventricle may be elevated with an indentation of the convex shape.

In severe hydrocephalus, suprapineal recess dilatation—with extension posteriorly into the quadrigeminal cistern and superior vermis—and medial atrial wall diverticula may be visualized by CT (Fig. 18–6). These probably represent the effect of prolonged increased intracranial pressure. These usually decrease in size after shunting. It is important not to confuse these hydrocephalus-related findings with primary arachnoid or ependymal cysts.

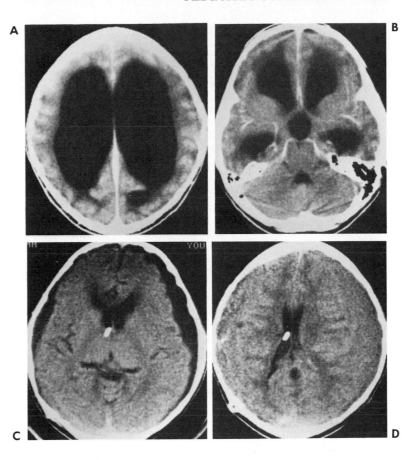

Figure 18–5. A 6-year-old developed headache and vomiting. He had papilledema and abducens nerve paresis. *CT findings:* marked lateral and third ventricular dilatation (*A*) with disproportionately smaller fourth ventricle (*B*). Immediately following shunt insertion he was asymptomatic; however, headache recurred two weeks later. *CT findings:* bilateral hypodense extracerebral lesions with ventricular compression (*C*). Three weeks following surgical drainage, he became lethargic. *CT findings:* bilateral isodense subdural hematoma with medial displacement of the white matter and lateral ventricular compression (*D*).

The CT findings of medial atrial wall diverticula include: (1) unilateral or bilateral atrial dilation, (2) ipsilateral shortening of the tentorial bands visualized on axial-enhanced scan, (3) focal defect of the ipsilateral tentorial band on coronal-enhanced scan, (4) extension of the atrial wall over the free margin of the tentorium to simulate posterior fossa cyst, (5) lateral displacement of the ipsilateral choroid plexus and (6) contralateral displacement of the internal cerebral veins.[12, 13]

Dandy-Walker Cyst.[14] In this condition there is cystic dilation of the fourth ventricle. There is accompanying hypoplasia of the cerebellar hemispheres and vermis. Other associated developmental anomalies occur in two thirds of patients. These include agenesis of the corpus callosum, aqueductal stenosis or

Figure 18–6. A child with aqueductal stenosis had shunt placement on multiple occasions. *CT findings:* dilatation of lateral and third ventricle with a hypodense lesion directly posterior to the third ventricle, representing dilated suprapineal recess (*A*). A child with severe hydrocephalus had shunt failure. *CT findings:* left atrial diverticulum causing lateral displacement of the choroid plexus and contralateral displacement of the internal cerebral veins (*B*).

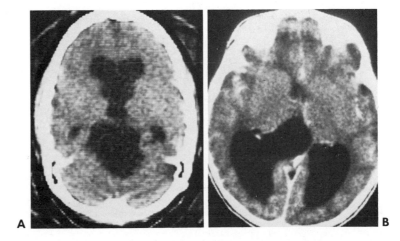

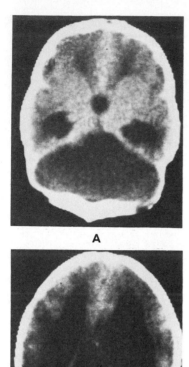

Figure 18–7. A 6-month-old child developed increasing head size with prominence of the posterior region. *CT* findings: large posterior fossa hypodense lesion pointing anteriorly (*A*). There is anterior displacement of the interpeduncular cistern. The fourth ventricle is not seen. The tentorium is elevated and there is biventricular enlargement (*B*).

leptomeningeal cysts. The occiput of the head appears prominent. Macrocephaly is caused by hydrocephalus. The characteristic CT finding is posterior fossa midline hypodense nonenhancing cyst. This represents encysted fourth ventricle. The fourth ventricle never appears normal in size or location. The vermis and cerebellar hemispheres are hypoplastic; they are replaced by cyst. There is usually marked elevation of the torcular; the cyst may extend above the tentorium. The lateral and third ventricles are enlarged (Fig. 18–7). If the cerebellar hypoplasia is limited to the inferior vermis (Dandy-Walker variant), CT shows a large posterior fossa cyst; this appears to be in continuity with the abnormal dilated fourth ventricle through the vallecula (Fig. 18–8). Other conditions may simulate CT findings of the Dandy-Walker syndrome, including mega cisterna magna,[15] extra-axial subarachnoid cyst,[16] and cystic neoplasms. Differentiation may require metrizamide cisternography and vertebral angiography (Table 18–3).

Arnold-Chiari Malformation Type II.[17, 18] This disorder is characterized by hydrocephalus and hindbrain anomalies. There is frequently associated spina bifida cystica. In the Arnold-Chiari malformation the cerebellar tonsils are displaced through the foramen magnum, and ventral displacement and caudal kinking of the lower pons and medulla develop. The fourth ventricle is elongated and angulated; posterior fossa basal cisterns are obliterated. Hydrocephalus may result from obstruction of the outlet foramina of the fourth ventricle or aqueductal stenosis. Characteristic CT findings of the Arnold-Chiari malfor-

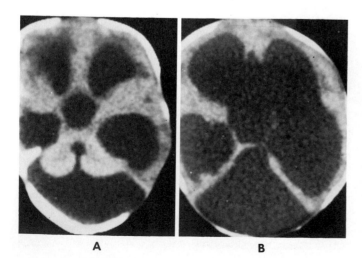

Figure 18–8. A 1-month-old developed rapid increase in head size with occipital protuberance. *CT findings:* large posterior cyst with connection to the fourth ventricle through the vallecula (*A*). The tentorium is elevated and there is biventricular enlargement (*B*).

TABLE 18–3. Diagnostic Features of Posterior Fossa Cysts

CT Findings	Mega Cisterna Magna	Dandy-Walker Syndrome	Dandy-Walker Variant	Extra-axial Posterior Fossa Cyst (Noncommunicating)	Extra-axial Retrocerebellar Cyst (Communicating)	Cystic Neoplasms Astrocytoma Hemangioblastoma
1. Cyst	Round or triangular–midline	Round or triangular–midline Points anteriorly	Round or triangular–midline Points anteriorly	Irregular shape; asymmetrical or unilateral	Irregular shape; asymmetrical, unilateral Points anteriorly	Round, unilateral or midline
2. IV ventricle size	Normal	Excysted	Enlarged—displaced	Displaced	Displaced	Displaced
3. Hydrocephalus	No	Yes	Yes	Yes	Yes	Yes
4. Cerebellar hypoplasia						
hemispheric	No	Yes	No	No	No	No
vermian	No	Yes	Yes	No	No	No
5. Cisterns						
cisterna magna	Enlarged	Not visualized	No	Not visualized	Not visualized	Not visualized
brain stem	Normal	Displaced	No	Displaced	Displaced	Displaced
vallecula	Not seen	Not seen	Visualized	Displaced	Displaced	Not visualized
6. Tentorium — position	Normal	Elevated	Elevated	Not elevated	Not elevated	Normal
7. Enhancement	No	No	No	No	No	Yes — nodular or ring
Metrizamide CT						
1. Cyst fills	Yes	Yes	Yes	No	Yes	No
2. IV ventricle fills	Yes	No	No	Yes	Yes	No
3. Cyst and IV ventricle separate	Yes	No	No	Yes	Yes	Yes
Vertebral angiography	Normal	Stretching of hypoplastic vessels surrounding cyst	Same as Dandy-Walker syndrome	Displacement of cerebellar vessels away from skull	Same as noncommunicating cyst	Consistent with cerebellar mass

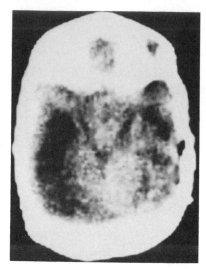

Figure 18–9. A 3-year-old child had Arnold-Chiari type II malformation. *CT findings:* the midbrain appears beaked, with elongation caudally and loss of indentations, which should represent superior collicular plates. (Courtesy of Dr. T. P. Naidich.)

mation in children include: (1) the falx is incompletely formed (hypoplasia, fenestrations); (2) the tentorial leaves are poorly developed, with the incisura being widened and elongated; (3) the posterior fossa is small and the foramen magnum is enlarged; (4) the midbrain is beaked and elongated caudally with loss of indentations that usually represent superior collicular plates (Fig. 18–9) and (5) the cerebellum bulges upward through wide incisura to extend above the tentorium. The cerebellar component is located contiguous with and slightly superior to the tentorium.

This appears bullet-shaped and extends above the incisura. These hindbrain and cerebellar abnormalities are sometimes better visualized by CT after shunt insertion (Fig. 18–10). Cervical cord cavities (hydromyelia and syringomyelia) may result from mechanical effects of fourth ventricular foramina obstruction and enhanced central cord canal pulsations. Spinal CT or myelography may be required to visualize these complicating conditions.

Masses. These include congenital midline tumors such as teratomas and gliomas, choroid plexus papilloma, and vein of Galen malformation. Cystic lesions such as porencephalic, subarachnoid and leptomeningeal are other causes of hydrocephalus. These mass lesions may present with progressive head enlargement without localizing neurological signs.

Arachnoid Cyst. These are extracerebral fluid-containing mass lesions that form within arachnoid membranes.[19, 20] Most common locations include the middle fossa, cerebral convexities, posterior fossa, suprasellar region, and collicular plate. In children under age 2, rapid increase in head size is the predominant clinical sign. Older patients present with clinical disturbances resulting from cyst location, as when chiasmal compression results from suprasellar mass or ataxia is caused by posterior fossa cyst. CT characteristics of arachnoid cysts include: (1) homogeneous hypodense (consistent with CSF) appearance, (2) sharp margination, (3) thinning of overlying contiguous bone and (4) no enhancement. Middle fossa cysts may cause sphenoid or temporal bone erosion; these are sometimes associated with middle fossa enlargement (Fig. 18–11).

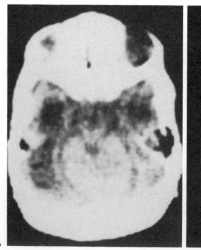
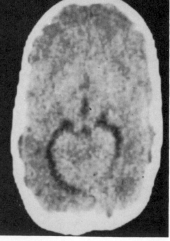

A   B

Figure 18–10. A 3-year-old had meningomyelocele and Arnold-Chiari type II malformation. Following placement of shunt, CT shows a midline bullet midline mass (A) that is surrounded by CSF and compresses the midbrain (B). This represents dysgenetic cerebellum growing upward through the incisura into the supratentorial region. (Courtesy of Dr. T. P. Naidich.)

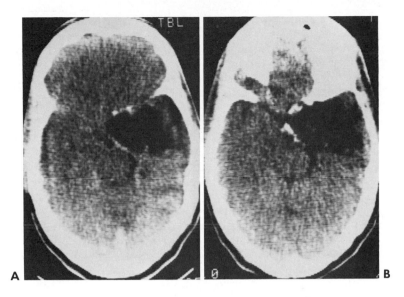

Figure 18–11. A 10-year-old child had left hemifacial spasm. EEG showed right temporal slow and spike focus. *CT findings:* right midline fossa hypodense sharply marginated lesion extending into the suprasellar region (A) with bone erosion (B). *Operative finding:* subarachnoid cyst.

The temporal lobe may be hypoplastic; this is reflected by a characteristic flat posterior margin of the cyst. Convexity cysts are elongated or globular in shape; their surface interphases with normal brain. They cause inner skull table erosion. Posterior fossa arachnoid cysts occur most commonly behind the cerebellum. They envelop the cerebellar hemispheres posterolaterally and extend anterosuperiorly over the vermis toward the quadrigeminal cistern. CT shows a unilateral hypodense nonenhancing sharply marginated retrocerebellar lesion that displaces the fourth ventricle and causes hydrocephalus. These may have a similar appearance to other posterior fossa lesions (see Table 18–2).

Communicating Hydrocephalus. CSF flow is obstructed external to the ventricles. These children have progressive head enlargement and show delay in development. The diagnosis of communicating hydrocephalus is usually established by CT; this shows symmetrical triventricular enlargement, usually with visualization of the posterior fossa cisterns (Fig. 18–12). The fourth ventricle is enlarged and midline in location. The basal cisterns, including the retrocerebellar ones, may be enlarged and this must be differentiated from posterior fossa cysts (see Table 18–3). Communicating hydrocephalus may result from thickened adhesions that obliterate the arachnoid villi reabsorptive space. Etiologies include infection, trauma, surgery, hemorrhage, or neoplastic cells obstructing the leptomeningeal spaces. In some patients with the Arnold-Chiari malformation, the hydrocephalus is

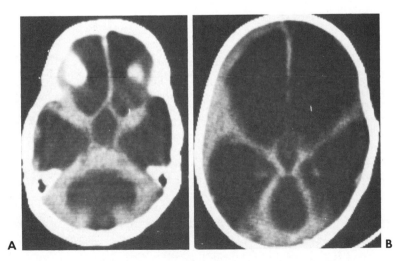

Figure 18–12. A 3-year-old child developed headache and vomiting. *CT findings:* triventricular enlargement (A) with minimal cortical mantle (B).

communicating (extraventricular). Diffuse meningeal neoplasm such as leukemia, lymphoma or medulloblastoma is a possible cause; this diagnosis is established by CSF cytology.

Progressive ventricular enlargement may also occur in children with normal CSF pressure (normal pressure hydrocephalus). Causes include intraventricular hemorrhage and posterior fossa surgery with obliterative arachnoiditis involving the posterior fossa cisterns.[21] There is a pressure gradient between ventricles and brain parenchyma; this results in slow ventricular expansion and white matter damage. Signs of increased intracranial pressure are not present. Progressive ventriculomegaly may cause developmental delay and impaired intellectual function. CT findings are consistent with communicating hydrocephalus. Arrested (compensated) hydrocephalus is a result of surgical or spontaneous termination of hydrocephalus such that the pressure gradient between the ventricles and brain parenchyma is no longer present. Therefore, further ventricular expansion ceases with reduction in pressure exerted upon white matter and brain parenchyma. In compensated hydrocephalus, CT shows ventricular dilatation with or without subarachnoid space enlargement. The finding of periventricular edema along the superior-lateral border of frontal horns is usually associated with transependymal CSF resorption and significant ventricular pressure gradients. This suggests active rather than arrested process. This is a *clinical condition* and its diagnosis is *not* established by CT findings; however, serial CT scans provide a useful means for following these patients.

Cerebral edema is discussed in Chapter 9.

Symptomatic Megalencephaly

As contrasted with benign familial megalencephaly, these patients with enlarged head size have clinical evidence of developmental delay, mental retardation, neurological disturbances and seizures. Head shape may be normal or they may have craniofacial disproportion with frontal bossing. The large brain may be caused by multiple conditions: (1) metabolic with accumulation of storage products as in leukodystrophy, mucopolysaccharidoses and gangliosodosis, (2) neurocutaneous syndromes such as tuberous sclerosis and neurofibromatosis, (3) dwarf-like states such as achondroplasia, (4) gigantism and (5) neoplasms with diffuse cellular infiltration. Assessment of these patients includes complete metabolic investigation and careful observation for cutaneous lesions. CT findings will depend upon the underlying condition.

Neurocutaneous Disorders

Tuberous Sclerosis.[22] Some children develop megalencephaly. The classic triad includes mental retardation, infantile spasms and hypopigmented macules. The absence of facial adenoma sebacum can obscure the diagnosis. Intracranial calcifications are demonstrated by radiography in 40 percent. They appear as round radiopaque areas located along the lateral ventricular surface and in the superficial cortex. Before the advent of CT, if the diagnosis of tuberous sclerosis was suspected and radiography was negative, air studies would sometimes outline nodular masses projecting into the ventricles. CT shows single or multiple hyperdense calcified nonenhancing ependymal masses (Fig. 18–13), and CT is more sensitive than skull radiography. The incidence of astrocytomas—frequently with giant cells—is increased in patients with tuberous sclerosis. These subependymal giant cell astrocytomas may obstruct the intraventricular foramina. They show the characteristic CT pattern of multilobulated hyperdense enhancing intraventricular mass with associated subependymal calcifications (Fig. 18–14).

Neurofibromatosis.[23] Megalencephaly is a common feature of this condition. Because of the increased incidence of neoplasms in patients with neurofibromatosis, the finding of an enlarged head should lead to CT to inves-

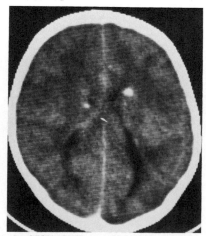

Figure 18–13. A 4-year-old boy had facial adenoma sebacum and seizure disorder. Skull x-ray showed no calcifications. *CT findings:* multiple periventricular nonenhancing calcified lesions.

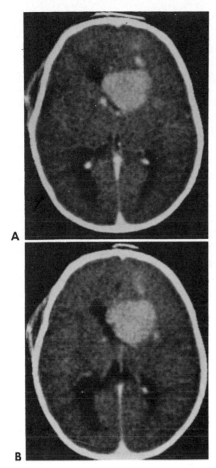

Figure 18–14. A 4-year-old child with tuberous sclerosis developed headache and vomiting. *CT findings:* periventricular calcified tubers (*A*) with hyperdense lesion that subsequently enhances (*B*) located at the intraventricular foramina. *Operative finding:* subependymal giant cell astrocytoma.

tigate the possibility of intracranial neoplasm or hydrocephalus. Megalencephaly may result from migratory phase congenital anomalies such as gray matter heterotopias. There is no correlation of head size with intellectual function or seizures.

Metabolic CNS Diseases[24]

The presence of storage product accumulation may lead to head enlargement, but this may be counterbalanced by cerebral atrophy. These disorders are diagnosed by specific laboratory techniques; however, CT abnormalities may reflect structural brain changes. CT findings are bilateral and usually symmetrical. These include ventricular enlargement, basal cisternal and cortical sulcal space dilatation, cerebral hemispheric white matter hypodensities and basal ganglionic hypodensities. The hypodensities may represent (1) increased water content; (2) defective myelination as in phenylketonuria or maple syrup urine disease; (3) abnormal myelin formation with active myelin destruction as in adrenoleukodystrophy,[25, 26] Alexander's disease and metachromatic leukodystrophy;[27] (4) spongioform degeneration as in Canavan's disease; (5) storage of abnormal metabolites as in gangliosidosis and (6) necrosis involving the basal ganglia as in Leigh's disease.[28]

Leukodystrophies

ADRENOLEUKODYSTROPHY. Initial CT findings are symmetrical parietal occipital hypodensities. There is diffuse enhancement at the anterior border of hypodense regions. Hypodense regions later extend into the temporal and frontal regions. In more advanced stages, there are extensive symmetrical hypodense nonenhancing regions.

ALEXANDER'S DISEASE.[28] CT shows prominent hypodensities in the frontal white matter and lenticular nucleus, and ventricular enlargement. Periventricular enhancement may be seen in the active stage; later stages show ventricular and subarachnoid space enlargement.

METACHROMATIC LEUKODYSTROPHY. CT shows symmetrical hypodensities in deep white matter of both hemispheres (centrum ovale). These hypodense regions show scalloped lateral edges. The ventricles are enlarged; there is no enhancement (Fig. 18–15). The hypodensities are believed to represent myelin loss and not lipid breakdown products.

CANAVAN'S SPONGIOFORM ENCEPHALOPATHY. CT shows extensive symmetrical hypodensities involving cerebral hemispheric white matter. Superficial cortical gray matter and deep gray matter (basal ganglion and thalamus) may be initially spared. They may be involved in more severely advanced cases.

KRABBE'S DISEASE. CT may show symmetrical deep cerebral hemispheric hypodensities. These are initially contiguous with the trigone of the lateral ventricles. This rapidly progresses to the atrophic stage, with ventricular and subarachnoid space dilatation.

AMINOACIDOPATHIES. These are conditions such as phenylketonuria and maple syrup urine disease. CT may show symmetrical bilateral hypodensities. These are initially located at the anterior and posterior portions of the

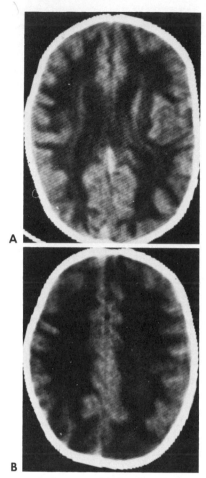

Figure 18–15. A 2-year-old developed spasticity and optic atrophy. He was diagnosed as having metachromatic leukodystrophy. *CT findings:* ventricular and subarachnoid space dilatation (A) with white matter hypodensities (B).

lateral ventricles. If there is defective myelination, white matter volume is reduced; CT shows dilatation of ventricles and subarachnoid spaces.

LEIGH'S DISEASE (SUBACUTE NECROTIZING ENCEPHALOMYELOPATHY). There may be symmetrical necrotic lesions in specific locations such as brain stem, basal ganglia and spinal cord. CT may show symmetrical sharply marginated hypodense nonenhancing ganglionic lesions; brain stem lesions are not seen.

GRAY MATTER METABOLIC DISORDERS. The gangliosidoses primarily involve gray matter. CT may show ventricular and subarachnoid space dilatation; white matter hypodensities are less consistently seen than with disorders primarily involving white matter. Macrocephaly is frequently seen in patients with mucopolysaccharidoses and Tay-Sachs disease. This

may be caused by accumulation of brain metabolites or communicating hydrocephalus resulting from meningeal involvement.

Microcephaly

This is defined as head circumference more than two standard deviations below mean for age, sex, race and gestation. The small head size reflects failure of normal brain growth. Microcephalic patients have mental retardation and seizures. Microcephaly may be primary; in this case it results from abnormal brain development during the first or second trimester. There may be other associated neurological developmental defects such as lissencephaly (smooth brain without normal gyral pattern), microgyria and agenesis of the corpus callosum. Secondary microcephaly may be of traumatic, vascular or infectious etiology, as in herpes simplex, cytomegalic inclusion body disease, rubella and toxoplasmosis. These develop in the third trimester or perinatal period. Pathological findings in secondary microcephaly include brain necrosis, multilocular cysts, encephalomalacia and porencephaly. The presence of dystrophic calcification is consistent with an infectious cause.

Hydrocephalus of an obstructive type may also be present in the microcephalic child. CT findings in microcephaly reflect an underlying pathological processes. This may help in genetic counseling of the parents. The presence of specific CT abnormalities suggests that microcephaly is either acquired or secondary, whereas the CT finding of small head with no abnormalities or congenital malformations suggests that microcephaly is either primary or familial.

Congenital Anomalies

These children present with delayed neurological development, neurological deficit, mental retardation or seizures. It is these clinical findings that suggest the need for CT.

Porencephalic Cysts.[30] These represent fluid-filled cavities usually located in the cerebral hemispheres. These develop most commonly in the third trimester or perinatal period. Causes may be varied, including intracranial hemorrhage, infarction, encephalitis and trauma; clinical abnormalities result from a causal lesion or from the cyst's mechanical properties, e.g., mass effect and ventricular enlargement. Clinical manifestations include head size enlargement and intracranial hypertension, seizures, developmental delay and neurological deficit. CT shows a hypodense homogeneous sharply marginated nonenhancing lesion. These appear round or wedge-shaped with the apex pointing toward the ventricular surface. There may be mass effect with midline shift toward the contralateral hemisphere. Communication of cysts with ventricles may not be well visualized with CT, and this may be visualized only with metrizamide cisternography. Large cysts may compress contiguous ventricles such that ventricular communication is not appreciated; therefore, lack of demonstration of this communication does not exclude the diagnosis of porencephalic cysts (Fig. 18–16).

Agenesis of Corpus Callosum.[31] This is frequently associated with absence of cingulate gyrus and septum pellucidum. Clinical symptoms are caused by other associated abnormalities such as micropolygyria, lissencephaly, gray matter heterotopia, hydrocephalus, lipomas and Dandy-Walker syndrome (Fig. 18–17). The severity or completeness of the callosal defect depends upon the embryonic stage at which malformation began to develop. CT findings of agenesis of corpus callosum include enlargement and elevation of the third ventricle, lateral displacement of frontal horns, and interhemispheric cysts (Fig. 18–18).

Hydranencephaly. This condition involves absence of the cerebrum. There is an intact cranial vault, meninges (falx, tentorium) and posterior fossa. This is believed to result from occlusion or agenesis of the supraclinoid internal carotid arteries. The cranium is normal sized or enlarged, and it is fluid filled. CT

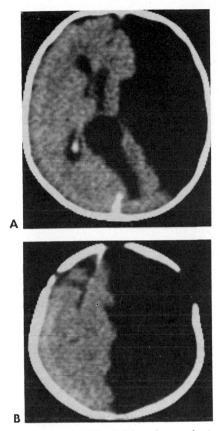

Figure 18–16. A child had delayed neurological development and increasing head size. *CT findings:* sharply marginated hypodense right hemispheric lesion (A) with contralateral ventricular displacement (B). Following injection of metrizamide into the cyst, there is no evidence of communication with the ventricles (not shown). *Operative finding:* porencephalic cyst.

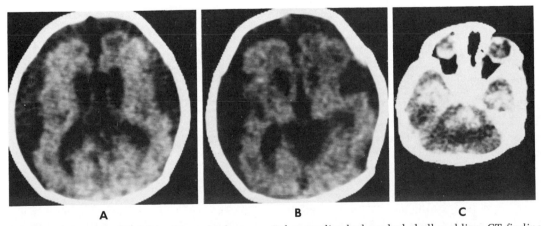

Figure 18–17. A 6-day-old child with multiple congenital anomalies had marked skull molding. *CT findings:* elevated anterior third ventricle (A) extending to the interhemispheric fissure with hypodense extracerebral lesions (B) and hypodense lesions throughout the cerebellum (C). *Necropsy findings:* agenesis of corpus callosum, lissencephaly and cerebellar hypoplasia.

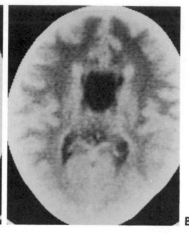

Figure 18–18. A 30-month-old child developed seizure disorder. *CT findings:* high-riding elevated anterior portion of the third ventricle with separation and lateral displacement of the lateral ventricles by a midline cyst (*A*). There are cerebral hemispheric white matter hypodensities (*B*). *Necropsy finding:* agenesis of the corpus callosum.

findings include: (1) the entire cerebrum is consistent with CSF density and normal ventricular structures are not visualized; (2) there are intact posterior fossa, thalamus and basal ganglia (brain stem model); (3) the falx and tentorium are intact and well-delineated on enhanced scan and (4) normal brain parenchymal enhancement is not seen (Fig. 18–19). CT findings of hydranencephaly may simulate other conditions (Table 18–4). Isotope scan may show absence of flow through the internal carotid arteries; this diagnosis may be confirmed by angiography if CT findings are equivocal.

Holoprosencephaly.[32, 33] This represents malformations whose common morphologic feature is a single monolocular ventricle. The defect is failure of the primary cerebral vesicle to cleave and expand bilaterally. It is usually associated with midline facial defects such as hypotelorism, median cleft lip and cyclopia. Skull roentgenograms show abnormalities of orbital, maxillary and ethnoid bones. CT findings include: (1) midline monolocular hypodense cavity, (2) nonvisualization of falx and tentorium and (3) normal posterior fossa and thalamus. In some cases frontal and occipital regions appear normal. There are two forms: *alobar,* which has a large monocular chamber without evidence of normally cleaved cortex, and *lobar,* in which the cerebrum is incompletely formed, with an intact interhemispheric fissure (Fig. 18–20). Associated abnormalities at the level of the aqueduct may cause obstructive hydrocephalus. We have identified certain similar severe developmental defects by tomograms that show no normal cerebrum; however, these lack pathological confirmations as of this writing (Fig. 18–21).

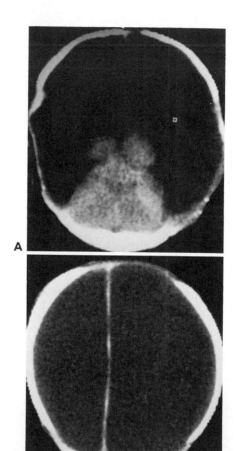

Figure 18–19. A 2-week-old infant developed prolonged seizures. The head was markedly enlarged and it transilluminated diffusely. *CT findings:* bilateral cerebral hemispheric hypodensities (*A*). The falx and tentorium are intact. The lateral and third ventricles are not visualized; the fourth ventricle is normal. The basal ganglion, thalamus and brain stem appear of normal density. There is no enhancement following contrast infusion (*B*). Angiography confirmed the diagnosis of hydranencephaly.

TABLE 18–4. Differential Diagnostic Entities in Hydranencephaly

	Hydranencephaly	Alobar Holoprosencephaly	Bilateral Porencephaly	Hydrocephalus	Subdural Hygroma	Hypoxic-Ischemia Brain Damage
Plain skull x-ray	Normal	Hypotelorism anterior-basal bone defects	Normal	Split sutures	Split sutures	May show overlapping sutures due to microcephaly
Isotope scan	Decreased flow	Normal	Decreased flow	Normal	Normal	Normal
Angiogram	Agenesis of supra-clinoid carotid arteries	Poorly formed intracranial vessels	Focal arterial obstruction	Vessels compressed against inner skull table	Inward compression of vessels	Normal
CT findings Hypodense lesion shape	Symmetrical bilateral hemispheric	Crosses midline	Wedge-shaped in vascular distribution	Dilated ventricles	Extracerebral semilunar-shaped hypodensities	Bilateral diffuse cystic hypodensities
Ventricles	Not formed	Single ventricular cavity	Enlarged	Enlarged	Compressed	Enlarged
Subarachnoid spaces	Not visualized	Not visualized	Enlarged	Not visualized	Not visualized	Enlarged
Meninges present	Intact	Not visualized	Intact	Normal	Intact	Intact
Normal parenchyma	Not visualized	May persist in frontal or occipital region	Normal in noninvolved region	Thin rim of overlying cortex	Inward displace-ment of gray-white matter inter-phase	Diffuse hypodensities throughout both hemispheres

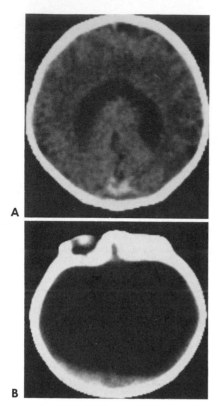

Figure 18–20. *A*, lobar holoprosencephaly with no evidence of the lateral ventricles. *B*, alobar holoprosencephaly with a single hypodense lesion with no evidence of ventricular system, brain parenchyma or meninges (falx, tentorium).

Perinatal Disorders. This may be caused by hypoxic ischemic damage or intracranial hemorrhage. Premature infants are more likely to develop germinal matrix intraventricular hemorrhages or leukomalacia. In full-term infants perinatal asphyxia (defined by an Apgar score of less than six at five minutes or apnea requiring assisted ventilation for more than several minutes) may cause cystic degeneration of superficial cortex, basal ganglia, and thalamus[34] or traumatic hemorrhages, e.g., subdural hematoma and subarachnoid hemorrhage. Clinical manifestations of ischemic or hemorrhagic perinatal disorders include developmental delay, mental retardation, motor dysfunction (hemiplegia, quadriplegia), epilepsy and microcephaly.

CT findings of perinatal ischemia include hypodensities in the cerebral hemispheres and periventricular regions. There may be ventricular compression; contrast enhancement does not usually occur. Ischemic damage is maximal in the parietal-occipital and basal ganglionic regions and less marked in the temporal and frontal cortex. Because of higher water content of brain tissue in normal premature infants, the diagnosis of ischemic damage may be overestimated. The higher protein content of neonatal CSF may obscure the ventricular–brain parenchyma interface; this makes delineation of ventricular compression difficult. Subcortical and periventricular encephalomalacia usually develops in three regions: the anterior frontal horn, the corona radiata, and the external and internal sagittal strata of the temporal and occipital horns. These represent arterial border zones that are frequently compromised in perinatal period. CT shows multiple bilateral hypodense regions in the cerebral white matter.[35] Certain infants with hypoxic-ischemic brain damage have poor neurological outcome but show no CT abnormalities.

Intraventricular hemorrhage is demonstrated by CT in 40 per cent of premature infants who do not survive; this correlates with necropsy findings.[36, 37] The germinal matrix is

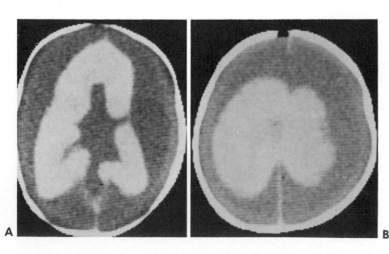

Figure 18–21. A 6-month-old had delayed neurological development. His head showed prominent transillumination. *CT findings:* prominent hyperdense tubular structure (*A*) with no normal intracranial structures suggestive of primitive neural tube (*B*).

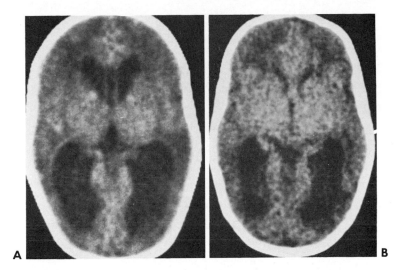

Figure 18–22. An 8-day-old premature child became increasingly tremulous and fed poorly. CSF was clear. *CT findings:* bilateral germinal matrix hemorrhages without ventricular dilatation (*A*). One month later he was neurologically normal. CT shows resolution of the hematoma with decrease in ventricular size (*B*).

the bleeding source. This is highly vascular subependymal tissue adjacent to the lateral ventricle at the caudate-thalamic groove. Germinal matrix–intraventricular hemorrhage occurs on the second to fourth day; it is not a complication of delivery. Clinical features of hemorrhages are varied in severity. Patients abruptly deteriorate or have a saltatory course; commonly, hemorrhage develops in a sick neonate on a respirator and its development may not be clinically apparent. In one study, ventricular hemorrhage in premature infants was clinically predicted in only 54 percent. Factors that indicated risk of hemorrhage included: fall of hematocrit, bulging fontanelles, decreased motor activity, hypotonia, and seizures.[31] These are classified: Grade I, subependymal hemorrhage without intraventricular extension (Fig. 18–22); Grade II, subependymal and intraventricular hemorrhage; Grade III, subependymal intraventricular hemorrhage with ventricular dilatation (Fig. 18–23); Grade IV, subependymal intraventricular hemorrhage with extension into the subcortical white matter and thalamus. False-negative findings may relate to the following factors: (1) hemorrhage is very small; (2) hemorrhage occurred *after* the initial scan; (3) scan is delayed and blood has resolved. Serial scans are necessary to follow these patients for development of hydrocephalus.

Ventricular hemorrhage may originate from the choroid plexus veins in full-term infants. The course is usually benign. Certain patients are neurologically asymptomatic; however, some patients subsequently develop hydrocephalus. Convexity or posterior fossa subdural and epidural hematomas may result from difficult delivery of full-term infants. Posterior fossa lesions are caused by tentorial tears. These may rapidly progress to cause brain stem compression. Subarachnoid hemorrhage may also result from physical injury during delivery.

Acute Infantile Hemiplegia. This includes hemiplegia of rapid onset that develops in children usually younger than six years old. The clinical history is a previously well child who suddenly becomes hemiplegic. Seizures (generalized or partial) develop in two thirds of cases. These may be prolonged and frequent. Sequelae include flaccid hemiplegia and recurrent seizures. Causes include: (1) trauma; (2) infection; (3) congenital cardiac disorders; (4) hemoglobinopathies, e.g., sickle cell; (5) cerebral angioma; (6) collagen vascular disorders and (7) occlusive vascular disease.[38]

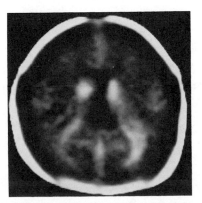

Figure 18–23. A premature male child developed increased jitteriness and poor feeding at 96 hours after delivery. CSF was bloody. *CT findings:* bilateral germinal matrix hemorrhages with intraventricular and subarachnoid blood.

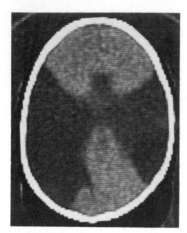

Figure 18–24. A child with infantile-onset right hemiplegia developed seizures at age 5. *CT findings:* bilateral wedge-shaped hypodense lesions in the territory of the MCA consistent with prior infarction.

CT scan should be the initial diagnostic procedure. It helps to define the nature of this lesion—whether it is an infarct (Fig. 18–24), hematoma, angioma, neoplasm, trauma-related cyst, hemispheric hypoplasia or cerebral atrophy. If CT shows findings of a neoplasm or angioma, angiography is necessary. Angiographic findings of occlusive vascular disease include stenosis or occlusion of one or both internal carotid arteries at the basal proximal supraclinoid origin or the proximal portion of the middle or anterior cerebral arteries. In certain cases abundant collaterals are visualized as a prominent telangiectatic network (moyamoya). This vascular pattern is transient and disappears within several weeks or months. If patients with this angiographic pattern have enhanced CT scan within the initial three weeks, a prominent gray matter enhancement pattern is seen (Fig. 18–25). In one report of patients who had angiographic findings of severe carotid stenosis with dense telangiectatic pattern, CT showed infrequent enhancement. There was cortical atrophy that was most marked in the frontal region and accompanied by single or multiple irregular hypodense lesions in the cortical, periventricular and ganglionic regions; however, these patients were studied at least 3 months later.[39] In children who have onset of hemiplegia before age 3, calvarial and brain atrophic changes may develop (Dyke-Davidoff-Masson syndrome). Skull roentgenogram may show skull thickening with dilatation and overdevelopment of nasal sinuses on the involved site. CT demonstrates ipsilateral ventricular dilatation.

Unexplained Coma. In one series of 75 children who were comatose but had not suffered head injury, intracranial infection (meningitis, encephalitis) represented 34.7 percent of cases.[40] Other etiologies included hypoxic-ischemic disorders (24 percent); epilepsy (14.7 percent); metabolic encephalopathy (14.7 percent) of hepatic, renal, toxic or septic (4 percent) origin; cerebrovascular lesions (4 percent) and nonaccidental injury (2.6 percent). Clinical history indicates hypoxic-ischemic injury or epilepsy. Laboratory studies are nec-

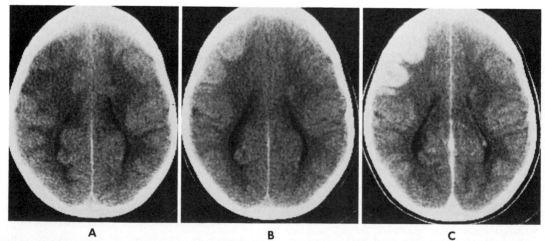

A   **B**   **C**

Figure 18–25. A 6-year-old child had a generalized seizure. Findings were flaccid right hemiparesis and hemianesthesia. Initial CT (24 hours later) showed no abnormality (*A*). Repeat CT (8 days later) showed a vague hyperdense left frontal-parietal lesion (*B*) with gray matter enhancement (*C*). Angiogram showed severe left supraclinoid carotid stenosis with basal telangiectatic blush (moyamoya).

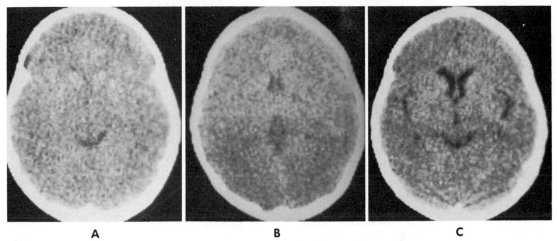

Figure 18–26. A 5-year-old child developed fever and vomiting. She became lethargic with decerebrate posturing. Laboratory studies were consistent with Reye's syndrome. CT findings: marked ventricular compression (A) with no abnormal density (B). Following symptomatic treatment, repeat CT shows increased in size of ventricles (C) and quadrigeminal cisterns. (Courtesy of Dr. T. P. Naidich.)

essary to exclude CNS infection by (lumbar puncture) and metabolic etiology.

For those children whose conditions are not diagnosed by history or metabolic studies, CT should be performed. These conditions cause unexplained coma, and CT may show Reye's syndrome, hypoxic-ischemic injury, acute onset of hydrocephalus, encephalitis, or the effects of child abuse. Reye's syndrome is an encephalopathy associated with fatty liver infiltration.[41] Clinical features include impaired consciousness and intracranial hypertension. CT may show small-sized ventricles with diffuse cortical enhancement. These findings reflect increased cerebral blood volume caused by vasodilatation or cerebral edema. Following supportive treatment and control of intracranial hypertension, clinical improvement may occur and CT normalizes. In other cases, rapid clinical deterioration is accompanied by the development of cerebral atrophy (Fig. 18–26). CT may show periventricular hypodensities caused by loss of myelin. In acute hydrocephalus, CT shows ventricular enlargement with periventricular edema. With high intraventricular pressure, consciousness is most likely to be disturbed and CT shows periventricular edema. In children who have suffered abuse, external stigmata such as bruises may not be apparent. Intracranial injuries include hematoma, and contusion; edema may cause coma. Convexity and interhemispheric subdural hematoma may develop. This latter lesion may be difficult to detect. CT shows eccentric thickening of the posterior falx with inferior extension to the tentorial region.[42] These are usually associated with such parenchymal injuries as edema and contusion.

REFERENCES

1. Milhorat TH, Hammock MK: Cranial computed tomography in infancy and childhood. Williams and Wilkins, Baltimore, 1981, pp 13–28
2. Quencer RM: Maturation of normal primate white matter: computed tomographic correlation. Am J Neuroradiol 3:365, 1982
3. Takao T, Dkuno T, Ito M: Normal CT in children. Comput Radiol 6:63, 1982
4. Naidich TR, Epstein F, Lin JP: Evaluation of pediatric hydrocephalus by computed tomography. Radiology 119:337, 1976
5. DeMeyer W: Megalencephaly in children. Neurology 22:634, 1972
6. Day RE, Schutt WH: Normal children with large heads—benign familial megalencephaly. Arch Dis Childh 54:512, 1979
7. Robertson WC, Gomez MR: External hydrocephalus. Arch Neurology 35:541, 1978
8. Ment LR, Duncan CC, Geehr R: Benign enlargement of the subarachnoid spaces in the infant. J Neurosurg 54:504, 1981
9. Kendall B, Holland I: Benign communicating hydrocephalus in children. Neuroradiology 21:93, 1981
10. Jackel K, Allen JH: Subdural hygromas: diagnosis with computed tomography. J Comput Assist Tomogr 3:201, 1979
11. Modic MT, Kaufman B, Bonstelle CT: Megalocephaly and hypodense extracerebral fluid collections. Radiology 141:93, 1981
12. Naidich TP, Schott LH, Baron RL: Computed tomography in evaluation of hydrocephalus. Radiol Clin North Am 20:143, 1982
13. Naidich TP, McLone DG, Hahn YS: Atrial diverticula

in severe hydrocephalus. Neuroradiology 3:257, 1982

14. Sawaya R, McLaurin RL: Dandy-Walker syndrome: clinical analysis of 23 cases. J Neurosurg 55:89, 1981

15. Archer CR, Darwish H, Smith K: Enlarged cisterna magna and posterior fossa cysts stimulating Dandy-Walker syndrome on computed tomography. Radiology 127:681, 1978

16. Drayer BP, Rosenbaum AE, Maroon JC: Posterior fossa extraaxial cyst: diagnosis with metrizamide CT cisternography. Am J Roentgenol 128:431, 1977

17. Naidich TP, Pudlowski RM, Naidich JB: Computed tomographic signs of the Chiari malformation. I. Skull and dural partitions. Radiology 134:65, 1980

18. Naidich TP, Pudlowski RM, Naidich JB: Computed tomographic signs of Chiari II malformation. II. Midbrain and cerebellum. Radiology 134:391, 1980

19. Leo JS, Pinto RS, Hulvat GF: Computed tomography of arachnoid cysts. Radiology 130:675, 1979

20. Banna M: Arachnoid cysts on computed tomography. Am J Roentgenol 127:979, 1976

21. Hill A, Volpe JJ: Normal pressure hydrocephalus in the newborn. Pediatrics 68:623, 1981

22. Barry JF, Harwood DC, Fitz CR: Unrecognized tuberous sclerosis diagnosed with CT. Neuroradiology 13:177, 1982

23. Riccardi VM: Von Recklinghausen neurofibromatosis. N Engl J Med 305:1, 617, 1981

24. Kendall BE: Cranial CT scans in metabolic diseases involving the CNS of children. Resident Staff Phys 32:33, 1982

25. Heinz ER, Drayer BP, Haenggeli CA: Computed tomography in white matter disease. Radiology 130:371, 1979

26. Eiben RM, Dichiro G: Computer-assisted tomography in adrenoleukodystrophy. J Comput Assist Tomogr 1:308, 1977

27. Buonanno FS, Ball MR, Laster DW: Computed tomography in late infantile metachromatic dystrophy. Ann Neurol 4:43, 1978

28. Hall K, Gardner-Medwin D: CT scan appearances in Leigh's disease. Neuroradiology 16:48, 1978

29. Holland I, Kendal BE: CT in Alexander's disease. Neuroradiology 20:103, 1980

30. Ramsey RG, Huckman MS: Computed tomography of porencephaly and other cerebrospinal fluid-containing lesions. Radiology 123:73, 1977

31. Guidert-Tanier F, Piton J, Billery J: Agenesis of the corpus callosum. J. Neuroradiol 9:135, 1982

32. Hayashi T, Yoshida M, Kuramento S et al: Radiological features of holoprosencephaly. Surg Neurol 12:261, 1979

33. Dublin AB, French BN: Diagnostic image evaluation of hydranencephaly and pictorially similar entities with emphasis on computed tomography. Radiology 137:81, 1980

34. Flodmark D, Becker LE, Harwood-Nash DC: Correlation between computed tomography and autopsy in premature and full-term neonates that have suffered perinatal asphysia. Radiology 137:93, 1980.

35. Taboada D, Alonso A, Olague R: Radiological diagnosis of periventricular and subcortical leukomalacia. Neuroradiology 20:33, 1980

36. Lazzara A, Ahmann P, Dykes F: Clinical predictability of intraventricular hemorrhage in preterm infants. Pediatrics 65:30, 1980

37. Volpe JJ: Neonatal intraventricular hemorrhage. N Engl J Med 304:886, 1981

38. Solomon GE, Hilal SK, Gold AP: Natural history of acute hemiplegia of childhood. Brain 93:107, 1970

39. Handa J, Nadano Y, Okuno T: CT in moyamoya syndrome. Surg Neurol 7:315, 1977

40. Seshia SS, Seshia MMK, Sachdeva RK: Coma in childhood. Dev Med Child Neurol 19:614, 1977

41. Giannotta SL, Hopkins J, Kindt GW: CT in Reye syndrome. Neurosurgery 2:201, 1982

42. Zimmerman RA, Bilaniuk LT, Generalli T: Cranial CT of craniocerebral injury in the abused child. Radiology 30:687, 1979

Chapter 19

VISUAL DISORDERS AND ORBITAL CT SCANNING

Orbital CT has been able to provide more detailed and accurate images because of thin tissue sections and coronal and sagittal plane scanning, which are possible with new-generation scanners. This has improved the diagnostic quality of orbital images. Optimal technique for orbital examination is dependent upon the specific types of scanner utilized; however, certain general guidelines are applicable.

For axial sections, patients are positioned in either supine or prone position. Although the majority of patients are scanned supine, the prone position is safer because incident x-ray beam is directed through the back of the skull. If this method is utilized, the radiation dose to the lens and cornea is one sixth that received if the patient is supine. The patient's head is adjusted relative to Reid's orbitomeatal baseline. This extends from the inferior orbital rim to the middle of the external auditory meatus. Scanning angulation is usually parallel (zero degree) or 10 to 20 degrees from the orbitomeatal line.

For coronal scans, two positions may be used: first, prone with chin elevated; incident x-ray is directed to back of skull and second, supine with head angulated downward (hanging head) at 90 degrees. In the latter position, the x-ray beam is directed toward the lens. Technique and angulation for coronal views may require modification because of metallic dental materials. These create artifacts that degrade image quality.

Because of the small size of the orbit, thin tissue sections are necessary for optimal diagnostic imaging. If scan sections are 1.5 to 2 millimeters, the optic nerve and extraocular muscles may not be seen completely in one section. This may falsely magnify the size of these structures. Thin sections are necessary

to obtain high-quality reformated coronal and sagittal images. Complete orbital scan with 2-mm tissue sections requires 20 to 30 images. Images that are made up of very small and numerous pixels, such as 320 × 320 and 512 × 512, provide excellent detail. Ability to improve spatial resolution is limited by two factors: first, the lens is so radiosensitive that increased radiation does may cause damage, and second, thin sections cause greater statistical fluctuation in photon counts, e.g., noise level. This produces a mottled (grainier) image that may obscure anatomical detail. Because the orbit is a high-contrast region (high density of bone and very low density of retro-orbital fat), contents are best viewed with wide window width, e.g., +200 to +500 HU, and window level of +60 to +200 HU. To visualize detail of the orbital bone, it may be necessary to utilize even wider window settings.

NORMAL ANATOMICAL STRUCTURES[1]

Axial Sections (Fig. 19–1)

Orbital Walls. The medial and lateral walls of the orbit meet at the posterior orbit (apex) to form a triangular space with a globe at the anterior junction. The lateral wall separates the orbit from the temporal and middle fossa. This wall is made up of the orbital surface of the greater sphenoid bone (posteriorly) and the orbital zygomatic bone (anteriorly). The medial orbital wall consists of four bones (frontal process of the maxilla, lacrimal bone, orbital plate of the ethmoid bone, and body of the sphenoid). Ethmoid and sphenoid sinuses are contiguous with the thin medial orbital wall.

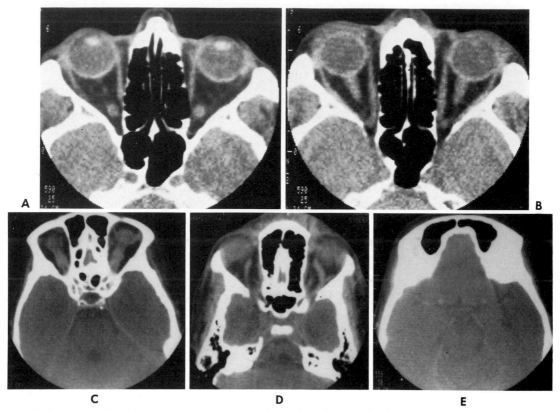

Figure 19–1. *Normal axial orbital sections. A,* Inferior region shows globe, lens, scleral ring, apex of inferior rectus, sphenoid bone, orbital fat, middle fossa, nasal cavity, nasal sinus. *B,* Midorbital region shows lateral rectus, medial rectus, optic nerve, superior orbital fissure, medial orbital bone. *C* and *D,* Superior region shows superior rectus, lacrimal gland, superior ophthalmic vein, sella turcica, cavernous sinus. *E,* Orbital roof region shows frontal sinus, anterior fossa.

Paranasal Sinuses. These include: (1) maxillary sinus, located ventral to orbit; (2) ethmoid sinus, located contiguous to the medial orbital wall; (3) sphenoid sinus, located in the body of the sphenoid bone and inferior to the sella turcica and (4) frontal sinus, located within the frontal bone at the dorsal level.

Extraocular Muscles. The medial rectus is separated from the medial orbital wall by a thin rim of fat. It is the thickest muscle. Because of its size and orientation, that is, parallel to the scanning angulation, it is the most consistently visualized muscle on axial CT. The lateral rectus is located parallel to the lateral orbital wall. It is better seen anteriorly because in the posterior portion it may blend with the sphenoid bone. The muscle apex is a wedge-shaped mass. This corresponds to the origin of the inferior rectus. The superior rectus appears medially on dorsal sections. It is sometimes confused with the optic nerve; however, the superior rectus is thicker and located more dorsally. The supe-

rior rectus may blend with the levator palpebrae muscle. The superior rectus is seen on both axial and coronal sections; the inferior rectus is rarely seen on axial but usually seen on coronal sections. The extraocular muscles attach to the globe and extend posteriorly to the orbital apex. This conforms to the conical shape. The globe is the base and the muscles converge toward the apex. Orbital tumors are classified as intraconal or extraconal.

Optic Nerve. This originates from the posterior globe; it passes posteromedially and upward to the optic foramina. It is 4 to 6 mm in thickness. It has a uniform hyperdense appearance; however, shifts in patient gaze cause movement artifact that may alter the shape or density of the optic nerve. In its course from the apex to the posterior globe, it may have an undulating course. At certain positions it may no longer be parallel to the x-ray beam; therefore, it may appear heterogeneous in shape and size. To compare the size of both optic nerves in an individual patient requires that the patient be positioned perfectly straight in the scanner.

Retro-orbital Fat. This is of uniform low density. It provides effective contrast for the interspersed soft tissues and thin bones of the orbit. No abnormalities of this structure have been delineated with CT.

Eyeball. The globe is spherical in shape. It appears hypodense because of fluid-containing media, e.g., aqueous and vitreous. It is surrounded by a hyperdense scleral rim. The lens is biconvex in shape and appears hyperdense anterior to the globe. The anterior-posterior dimension of the globe is 50 to 55 percent of the size of the entire orbit.

Lacrimal Gland. This is an oval or wedge-shaped structure. It is located on the medial portion of the zygomatic process in the dorsal orbit. It appears hyperdense and sometimes shows normal enhancement.

Superior Orbital Vein. This originates at the medial orbital canthus and is derived from the nasofrontal vein. It is seen on postcontrast scan and appears as a curvilinear structure in the dorsal orbit. It crosses over the optic nerve to extend to the medial orbit.[2]

Coronal Sections (Fig. 19–2)

Orbital Walls and Paranasal Sinuses. The orbital roof is formed by the orbital plate of the frontal bone and lesser sphenoid wing. It comprises the floor of the anterior cranial fossa. The orbital floor is formed by the orbital plate of the maxilla and the orbital surface of the zygomatic bone. This defines the roof of the maxillary sinus. The relationships of the orbital roof, frontal sinus and anterior intracranial fossa are well delineated.

Extraocular Muscles. The superior rectus-levator palpebrae complex is seen in the superior (dorsal) orbit. The inferior rectus is seen inferior to the globe. The superior oblique may be seen medial to this structure. The medial and lateral recti are well delineated; however, the inferior oblique is not visualized by CT.

The optic nerve is well visualized as a homogeneous hyperdense mass in the central orbital region.

PATHOLOGICAL CONDITIONS

Alterations of Normal Structures

Proptosis. The globe comprises 50 to 55 percent of the anterior-posterior (AP) orbital contents. If the patient's head is tilted and asymmetrically aligned in the scanner, a false impression of forward protrusion of the globe in the eye, which is closer to x-ray beam, may be created. In patients with proptosis, AP dimension of the orbit (the globe plus the

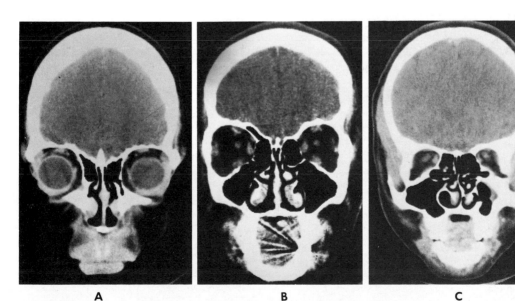

A	**B**	**C**

Figure 19–2. *Normal coronal orbital sections. A,* Anterior orbit shows frontal bone forming orbital roof, maxillary bone forming orbital floor, medial walls, formed by frontal, lacrimal and maxillary bone, globe, orbital fat. *B,* Midorbit section shows maxillary sinus, medial rectus, lateral rectus, lateral wall formed by greater sphenoid wing, levator palpebrae superior rectus muscle, inferior rectus, optic nerve. *C,* Posterior orbital apical section.

retroglobal region) increases and the proportion occupied by globe decreases. Hilal and Trokel utilize the measurement from the anterior cornea to a line drawn on the zygomatic process; this should not exceed 21 mm in normal persons.[4] It should be remembered that proptosis and exophthalmus are readily and reliably determined by clinical examination utilizing an inexpensive hand-held exophthalmometer.

Globe Size. MICROPHTHALMUS. A small eyeball, with diameter of less than 10 mm, is usually caused by ocular disorders such as trauma, congenital cataracts and retrolental fibroplasia. Less common causes include toxoplasmosis, rubella and genetic disorders, or the condition may be sporadic without identifiable etiology.

BUPHTHALMOS. Congenital or secondary glaucoma developing early causes enlarged globe (Fig. 19–3). An enlarged globe may also be seen in some patients with axial myopia.

Eyelid and Soft-Tissue Swelling. This has been reported in palpebral cellulitis, plexiform neurofibromatosis, orbital pseudotumor, and orbital trauma. The orbital septum is dense; therefore, it is an effective barrier to soft-tissue swelling. CT is reliable in defining if swelling is anterior (preseptal) or orbital (postseptal). This distinction may not always be reliably defined by clinical examination.

Scleral Thickening. This has been seen in orbital inflammatory disease, including pseudotumor. Thickened sclera may enhance following contrast injection.

Lacrimal Gland Enlargement. This structure is sometimes visualized as a lateral dorsal mass in normal persons. This may be falsely diagnosed as orbital tumor. Abnormal lacrimal gland enlargement is seen in several disorders: granulomatous conditions such as sarcoidosis and Wegener's granulomatosis, orbital pseudotumor, and neoplasm.

Superior Ophthalmic Vein Prominence. This is a characteristic finding in carotid-cavernous fistula; however, it may be seen in other conditions, such as endocrine ophthalmopathy and orbital pseudotumor. In these conditions, this is believed to represent orbital venous congestion.

Cavernous Sinus Enhancement. Utilizing high-accuracy fourth-generation technology, cavernous sinus is routinely visualized. It is seen directly lateral to the sella turcica on postcontrast scan. The normal enhancement of cavernous sinus appears as symmetrical vertically oriented enhancing linear bands. If this enhancement is more intense or extensive on one side, it suggests parasellar mass. This finding has been reported in extrasellar extension of pituitary adenoma, parasellar meningioma, carotid-cavernous fistula and carotid aneurysm. The cranial nerves located within the cavernous sinus may appear as round hypodense regions. An extensive asymmetrical hypodense nonenhancing region within the cavernous sinus may represent cavernous sinus thrombosis.

Optic Nerve Enlargement. The optic nerve is 4 to 6 mm in diameter. It is best visualized in midorbital sections, that are performed at zero-degree angulation. Four- to 6-mm sec-

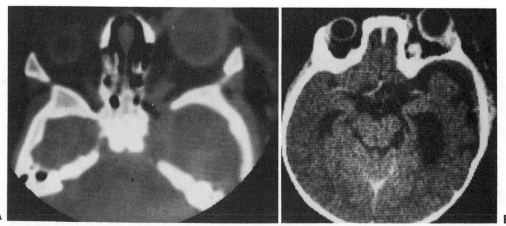

Figure 19–3. A child with neurofibromatosis developed amaurosis in the right eye caused by glaucoma. CT *findings:* enlarged globe that is proptotic (A) with poorly formed sphenoid bone and two retroglobal soft-tissue masses (B). The temporal lobe appears hypoplastic with markedly enlarged temporal horn and extracerebral spaces.

tions provide good assessment of optic nerve size. If thinner sections (2 mm) are utilized, optic nerves may appear enlarged. This may be artifactual resulting from partial volume effect because the nerve is never seen in its entirety in one section. If the scan is straight and symmetrical, there should be minimal difference in optic nerve size on two sides. Optic nerve enlargement may be caused by infiltration of the optic nerve or surrounding sheath by neoplasm or granuloma, such as glioma, meningioma, neurofibroma, metastases and sarcoid. This enlargement may result from distention of the subarachnoid sheath surrounding the optic nerve, as with papilledema, optic neuritis or endocrine ophthalmopathy. Unilateral optic nerve enlargement is most consistent with tumor or optic neuritis. Bilateral enlargement is more consistent with papilledema or systemic disorder, such as endocrine ophthalmopathy, but certain tumors may be bilateral (glioma, neurofibroma).

Extraocular Muscle Enlargement. This may be unilateral or bilateral. It may involve single or multiple muscle groups. Bilateral muscle enlargement is most common with endocrine ophthalmopathy. It is less common in orbital pseudotumor. The finding of a round or wedge-shaped hyperdense thick mass at the orbital apex represents the origin of the inferior rectus; this is characteristic of endocrine ophthalmopathy. Bilateral orbital apical masses are characteristic of endocrine ophthalmopathy; however, if unilateral, differentiation from orbital tumors may not be possible. Other causes of unilateral muscle enlargement include orbital pseudotumor, granuloma, orbital cellulitis, carotid-cavernous fistula, and plexiform neuroma. In rare cases, single-muscle thickening is caused by tumor (Fig. 19–4). Examples are carcinoma of the ethmoid or maxillary sinus (medial rectus), sphenoid or orbital meningioma (lateral rectus) and intracranial glioma or metastases (superior rectus).

Optic Canal and Superior Orbital Fissure. Marked enlargement of this region may be seen with CT; however, conventional tomograms are more sensitive. Enlargement of the optic canal may sometimes be better visualized with reversed image mode—bone appears black rather than white.

Pathological Findings

Bone Changes. With CT, it is sometimes possible to delineate bone erosion, fractures and bone thickening (hyperostosis). In certain benign tumors (dermoid, hemangioma, meningioma), the entire orbit may be enlarged.

Calcification. This may occur in the globe or retroglobal region. The anterior pattern is usually dystrophic, in which case it is commonly caused by local ocular conditions such as glaucoma, infection and trauma. Posterior calcification may be caused by retinal (Fig. 19–5) or choroidal tumors as well as hypercalcemic states. Bilateral global calcification in a child with no previous history of eye disease is highly suggestive of retinoblastoma. Retroglobal calcification most commonly occurs in meningiomas or vascular lesions such as orbital varices and arteriovenous malformations. In rare instances, optic gliomas calcify.

Orbital Mass Lesions. Utilizing axial and coronal sections, it is possible to define the presence and location of the mass, its relationship to the muscle cone, and any unilateral or bilateral abnormalities. Analysis of these characteristics of orbital mass should be made: (1) location (ventral, dorsal, anterior, posterior, medial, lateral), (2) morphology (shape, margination), (3) attenuation values (homogene-

Figure 19–4. A woman developed diplopia and had left abducens nerve palsy. Skull x-ray and isotope scans were negative. *CT findings:* left medial sphenoid wing erosion with soft-tissue mass. The left lateral rectus muscle is enlarged (*A*). There is a parietal osteolytic lesion and epidural mass (*B*).

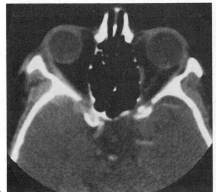
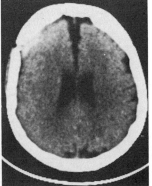

A   B

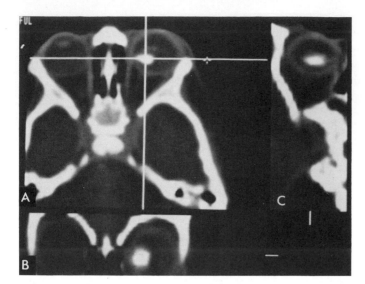

Figure 19–5. A 2-year-old child became blind in the right eye. *CT finding:* a dense calcified global mass seen on axial (*A*), coronal (*B*) and sagittal (*C*) views. This represents retinoblastoma.

ous, heterogeneous), (4) enhancement patterns, (5) effect on normal orbital structures, (6) bone changes and (7) evidence of paranasal sinus or intracranial extension (parasellar, middle fossa, frontal lobe). CT is less accurate in predicting the histological features of lesions. Supplemental diagnostic studies such as ultrasound, conventional tomography, carotid angiography, orbital venography and ultimately surgical biopsy are usually necessary.

Orbital Foreign Bodies. Metallic foreign bodies in the globe and retro-orbital region of very small size may be accurately delineated by CT (Fig. 19–6). Less dense substances such as wood and glass are less reliably detected. It may be difficult to differentiate these objects from granulomatous response to the foreign body.

SPECIFIC PATHOLOGICAL CONDITIONS

Endocrine Ophthalmopathy.[6-8] This is the most common cause of unilateral or bilateral exophthalmos. Clinical findings include proptosis, limitation of ocular motility, visual loss and corneal ulceration. The superior and medial recti muscles are initially involved. Most patients have clinical or laboratory evidence of abnormal thyroid function. Some patients are euthyroid; however, they have antithyroid antibodies, elevated titer for long-acting thyroid stimulator (LATS), and abnormal response to tri-iodothyroxine suppression test.

Ultrasonography is quite sensitive for detecting enlarged muscles. Both ultrasound and CT show abnormalities even if patients have

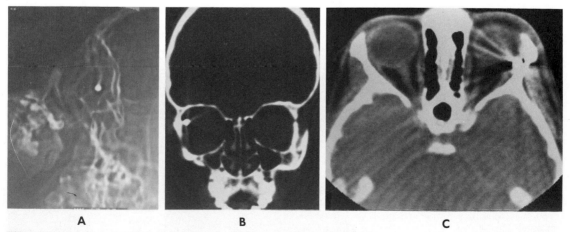

Figure 19–6. A boy was shot in the left eye. Skull x-ray shows a bullet fragment in the orbit (*A*). *CT findings:* bullet is well seen in the superior-lateral orbit on coronal view (*B*) but not well seen on axial section (reader's right) because of artifact (*C*).

minimal or no ophthalmoparesis. They may also show bilateral abnormalities even if clinical findings are unilateral. In 7 to 15 percent of cases, CT and ultrasound orbital abnormalities are unilateral in endocrine ophthalmopathy. If there is a unilateral apical mass, orbital venography may be necessary to exclude neoplasm (Fig. 19–7). Orbital neoplasms cause compression and displacement of the superior ophthalmic vein; this is not seen in ophthalmopathy despite swelling of the apical muscle cone.

CT findings in endocrine ophthalmopathy are quite characteristic (Fig. 19–8). Superior rectus enlargement is well appreciated on dorsal axial sections and coronal projections. Swelling or orbital apex represents the origin of the inferior rectus, but the individual course of this muscle is not usually seen. Enlargement of the medial rectus is best visualized in midorbital sections. The lateral rectus is less frequently enlarged; this is never seen as an isolated finding. There is usually a correlation between grades of muscle enlargement and clinical findings. In patients with visual loss caused by endocrine ophthalmopathy, CT may show thickening of the optic nerve. CT has not demonstrated abnormalities of retrobulbar fat to correspond with erosion of fat, which is seen with ultrasound.

Orbital Inflammatory Disease (Pseudotumor). Orbital pseudotumor includes a heter-

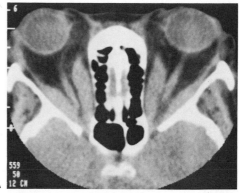
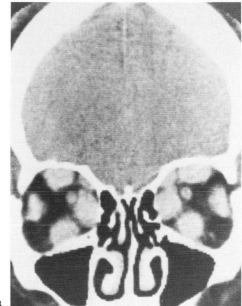

A

B

Figure 19–8. A woman with Graves' disease developed double vision and left eye prominence. CT findings: marked enlargement of all extraocular muscles (A), which is well visualized on coronal projection (B).

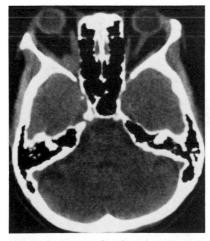

Figure 19–7. A woman developed vertical diplopia. She had exophthalmos with restricted movement of the left inferior rectus. *CT findings:* left-sided proptosis with marked apical enlargement. The lateral and medial recti are also enlarged. The patient was subsequently found by laboratory studies to have hyperthyroid activity.

ogeneous group of inflammatory disorders. This may affect one, several or all the structures of the orbit—extraocular muscles, lacrimal gland, globe, ligaments, blood vessels and optic nerve.[9, 10] It may represent several diverse conditions: (1) localized orbital inflammatory process of unknown etiology, (2) response of orbital tissue to foreign body or (3) orbital manifestation of systemic disease such as sarcoidosis, Wegener's granuloma and periarteritis nodosum. Clinically these patients may present with proptosis, impaired ocular motility, visual loss, and orbital pain. If clinical findings are unilateral, orbital pseudotumor may simulate neoplasm or endocrine ophthalmopathy; if bilateral, it must be differentiated from endocrine ophthalmopathy. In pseudo-tumor, ultrasound may detect generalized or focal areas of widely dispersed echoes. Skull x-ray and conventional tomography are negative. Orbital biopsy shows edema, granuloma formation with lymphocytic infiltration, fibrosis and normal retrobulbar fat. Dramatic response of clinical symptoms to systemic corticosteroids is quite characteristic.

CT findings depend upon the structures involved. In myositic pseudotumor, there is diffuse and symmetrical thickening of extraocular muscles (Fig. 19–9). In some cases dense muscle enhancement is seen. In nonmyositic form, these abnormalities have been reported: (1) hyperdense ovoid or wedge-shaped sharply marginated multilobulated retro-orbital mass that may extend and appear contiguous with the posterior portion of the globe (Fig. 19–10); (2) scleral thickening and

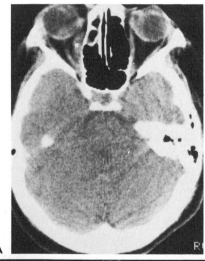

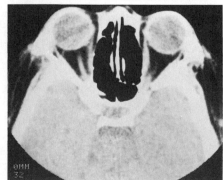

Figure 19–9. A girl developed bulging left eye and diplopia and had medial rectus paresis. *CT findings:* left-sided proptosis and medial rectus enlargement (*A*). Following treatment with corticosteroids, there was a decrease in the size of the medial rectus (*B*).

enhancement; (3) enlargement of the optic nerve, which appears more prominent at the posterior edge of the globe; (4) enlargement of the lacrimal gland and (5) obliteration of hypodense retro-orbital fat. Following treatment with corticosteroids, there is usually a marked decrease in these CT abnormalities.

Orbital Tumors. The clinical features of these neoplasms are quite similar. These include proptosis, visual loss, ophthalmoparesis and orbital pain. Conventional radiography—including tomography—with special views to visualize optic canal and superior orbital fissure should be the initial studies. The finding of an optic canal diameter that is larger than 6.5 mm or asymmetry of more than 1 mm is suggestive of optic glioma or meningioma. Paranasal sinuses and nasopharynx are assessed for evidence of tumor (bone erosion and abnormal densities). The sphenoid bone and sella turcica should be carefully studied for intracranial extension.

Ultrasound is a highly sensitive procedure to detect global and retroglobal masses. It should be utilized as a complementary procedure. Orbital tumors distort the retro-orbital fat pattern and produce echo patterns based upon their characteristic acoustical transmission properties. These lesions are classified as solid if they have poor acoustical transmission properties, whereas good acoustic transmission qualities characterize cystic or vascular tumors because of their fluid content. Cystic tumors have round regular borders and vascular tumors have irregular borders. Of solid tumors, malignant neoplasms have irregular borders and neurogenic tumors (gliomas, meningiomas) have regular round borders reflecting their benign nature.

In evaluation of patients with suspected orbital tumors, carotid angiography is utilized to detect intracranial tumor components or to define vascular nature, as in carotid-cavernous fistula or orbital arteriovenous malformation. Angiography is not sensitive in detecting orbital mass effect. It may be negative in certain vascular lesions such as hemangioma, even if magnification and subtraction angiographic techniques are used. This is because the orbital venous system is more likely to show abnormal vessels. Orbital venography is more sensitive than angiography in detecting mass effect by tumor as manifested by displacement of the superior orbital vein and for defining the presence of abnormal vessels such as hemangioma and orbital varices.

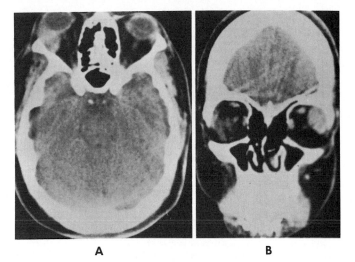

Figure 19–10. A woman developed left-sided proptosis and severe retro-orbital pain. *CT findings:* left lateral extraconal mass seen on axial (*A*) and coronal (*B*) views (reader's right).

A   **B**

CT is complementary to orbital radiography, hypocycloidal tomography and ultrasound. Angiography and venography are necessary, especially if a vascular lesion is suspected. CT is superior to ultrasound in detecting posterior orbit and small optic nerve sheath tumors. The accuracy of ultrasound and CT is approximately 99 percent in detecting orbital tumors. False-negative orbital CT and ultrasound results may occur rarely in patients with small optic nerve sheath tumors.

Hemangioma. Characteristic clinical features include pulsatile proptosis and dilated vessels of the eyelid and conjunctivae. Other common findings are proptosis, visual loss and ophthalmoparesis. Roentgenogram may show optic canal erosion and enlargement, abnormal soft-tissue densities or orbital calcification. Ultrasound shows an irregularly shaped mass with excellent acoustical transmission properties that are caused by blood-filled spaces. Orbital venography most reliably defines abnormal vessels. CT shows a retroglobal sharply marginated mass. It may be oval, round or elliptical in shape (Fig. 19–11). It is frequently located laterally and superiorly in the retroglobal region. It causes medial and downward deviation of the globe. The mass appears hyperdense. With thin sections interspersed, low-density cystic spaces that represent vascular sinuses may be appreciated; this creates a honeycombed appearance. Seventy percent show homogeneous enhancement and 30 percent do not enhance. Ultrasound pattern is sometimes more specific than CT; however, CT better outlines posterior extension of the hemangioma.

Orbital Meningioma. Primary orbital meningiomas may be of two types: first, lesions originating from the optic nerve sheath or optic foramina within the optic canal (Fig. 19–12) and second, extradural lesions occurring within or outside the muscle cone (Fig. 19–13). Secondary lesions may extend into the orbit from the sphenoid ridge, olfactory groove, parasellar or basofrontal region.[11] Patients with orbital meningiomas may develop slowly progressive visual impairment; the diagnosis of "chronic optic neuritis" may initially be incorrectly considered. The problem of diagnosis is further exacerbated because visual symptoms caused by meningioma may transiently respond to corticosteroids. In extradural meningiomas, skull x-rays may show enlargement of the optic foramen, hyperosto-

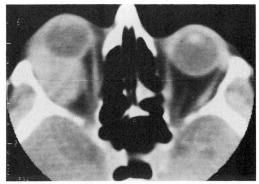

Figure 19–11. A man developed left-eye bulging and the eye was displaced downward. *CT findings:* a hyperdense homogeneous nonenhancing intraconal mass displacing the globe and optic nerve medially. *Operative finding:* hemangioma.

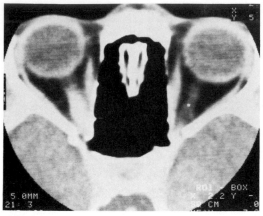

Figure 19–12. A woman developed progressive visual acuity impairment and was found to have optic atrophy and pupillary afferent defect. *CT findings:* markedly enlarged and hyperdense left optic nerve. *Operative finding:* optic nerve sheath meningioma.

sis or calcification; however, in small intraorbital meningiomas x-rays are frequently negative. Ultrasound is quite sensitive in detecting small tumors of the optic nerve sheath, but differentiation from other neurogenic tumors such as gliomas, and neurofibromas is not usually possible. CT may show enlargement of the optic nerve and a retroglobal mass that may or may not appear contiguous with the optic nerve. The mass is hyperdense and it may contain calcified portions. It is ovoid, sharply marginated and regularly shaped; there may be visible attachment to bone. Dense homogeneous enhancement is seen in 90 percent, whereas 10 percent do not enhance. Intracranial CT scan sections, including those of the parasellar region, middle fossa and frontal region, are necessary.[12]

Optic Glioma. These tumors most commonly occur in young patients. They cause visual impairment and a lesser degree of proptosis than seen with meningiomas. These gliomas originate near the optic foramen and extend anteriorly or posteriorly into the optic chiasm along visual pathways. They are usually unilateral but they may be bilateral, including in patients with von Recklinghausen's disease. Skull roentgenogram and tomograms show enlargement or asymmetry of optic canals, and if there is intracranial extension, a J-shaped deformity of the sella turcica may be seen. Ultrasound is highly reliable in defining localized widening of the optic nerve by a mass that has sharply defined borders and poor acoustic transmission properties.

CT findings in optic glioma include: (1) fusiform enlargement of the optic nerve, (2) homogeneous hyperdense sharply marginated mass, (3) enlargement of the optic foramina and (4) diffuse enhancement seen in 60 percent and no enhancement seen in 40 percent. Size and shape of the optic nerve should be evaluated in both axial and coronal sections. Intracranial extension must be evaluated by postcontrast scan that includes the sella region.[13]

Neurofibroma. Plexiform neurofibroma may involve eyelids, soft tissues (anterior to the globe) or optic nerves in patients with von Recklinghausen's disease. The CT appearance of neurofibroma is that of a hyperdense noncalcified sharply marginated mass. This is located laterally in the superior and posterior retroglobal region. The mass does not show evidence of enhancement. There may be associated bone anomalies such as dysplasia of the sphenoid bone and agenesis of the tem-

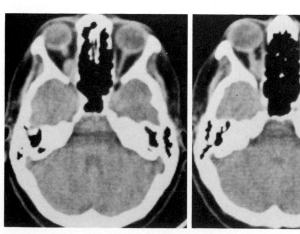

A B

Figure 19–13. A woman developed decreased vision in her left eye and was found to have central scotoma and decreased pupillary reactivity. *CT findings:* posterior apical mass (A) and enlarged optic nerve (B). *Operative finding:* orbital meningioma.

poral lobe. On the basis of CT characteristics, it is not possible to differentiate neurofibromas from optic nerve gliomas or meningiomas.

Malignant Neoplasms. Certain tumors extend directly into the orbit from contiguous structures such as paranasal sinus, lacrimal gland and nasopharynx, whereas other tumors reach the orbit by hematogeneous dissemination (lymphoma, neuroblastoma, bronchogenic or breast carcinoma).[14] In metastatic orbital lesions, CT shows a homogeneous speckled hyperdense sharply marginated lesion. This is round or ovoid in shape; it usually shows dense enhancement (Fig. 19–14). There is usually orbital bone erosion; this is best

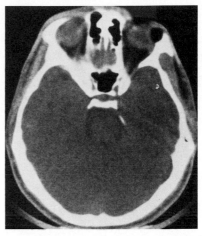

Figure 19–15. A man developed pain and swelling of upper lid region. Skull x-ray showed a radiolucent area in the superior orbit. *CT findings:* homogeneous hypodense sharply marginated superior-lateral orbital mass. *Operative finding:* dermoid cyst.

visualized at wide window width. Lymphomas occur in the anterior and inferior orbits. They have associated soft-tissue swelling and palpable skin nodules. CT shows a sharply marginated ovoid nonenhancing orbital mass, usually with no evidence of bone erosion. Neuroblastoma is the most common tumor that occurs in children and metastasizes to the orbit. CT findings include: (1) involvement of orbital soft tissues located anterior to the globe, (2) bone erosion, (3) homogeneous round multilobulated sharply marginated hyperdense mass, (4) dense enhancement of the mass and (5) enlargement of medial rectus muscles.

Dermoid Cyst. This is the most common type of congenital orbital lesion. These masses are located in the superior and lateral orbital region. Since they are slow-growing benign lesions, they may enlarge the orbit. Because these cysts contain dermal elements such as fat and calcium, they have CT density values that reflect the presence of these contents— fat causes very hypodense lesion and calcium results in hyperdense lesion. They are sharply marginated and show no evidence of enhancement (Fig. 19–15).

Vascular Lesions

Orbital Arteriovenous (AVM). These are the most common vascular lesions. Characteristic clinical findings are pulsatile proptosis, orbital bruit, prominent lid and conjunctival vessels. Diagnosis is established by carotid angiography and orbital venography. Feeding vessels originate from the internal and external

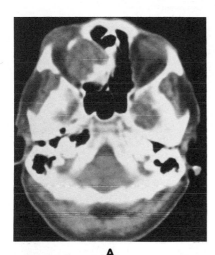

A

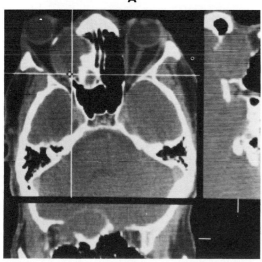

B

Figure 19–14. A man with maxillary sinus carcinoma developed proptosis and diplopia. *CT findings:* hyperdense nonenhancing maxillary sinus mass causing marked bone erosion (*A*). This extends into the orbit and anterior fossa (*B*).

carotid system. These angiomas are located in the dorsal orbit. CT shows a hyperdense lesion with interspersed calcification. It is irregular in shape and margination. Postcontrast enhancement pattern may suggest the presence of abnormal vessels. Orbital varices characteristically show calcified regions (phleboliths) on CT and skull roentgenograms (Fig. 19–16).

Carotid-Cavernous Fistula. These usually result from trauma or a vascular cause. The characteristic clinical pattern is that patients develop sudden onset of proptosis, orbital pain and diplopia. Findings include ophthalmoparesis and orbital bruit. CT findings are: (1) enlargement of the superior ophthalmic vein, (2) proptosis, (3) diffuse muscle thickening and (4) dense parasellar enhancement (Fig. 19–17). In cases of traumatic origin, associated findings include orbital foreign bodies, air or hematoma formation. Diagnosis is suggested by CT findings but must be confirmed by carotid angiography.

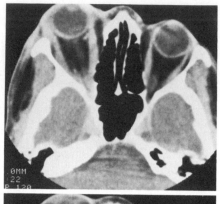

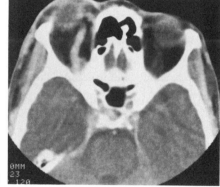

Figure 19–17. A man had severe head and facial trauma two years previously. He developed pulsatile proptosis and had bruit over the left eye. *CT findings:* left-sided proptosis with enlargement of the extraocular muscles (A). The cavernous sinus is enlarged (B) and the superior orbital vein is dilated. Angiogram shows carotid-cavernous fistula.

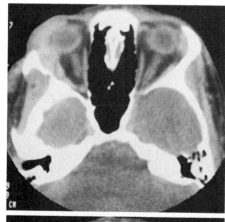

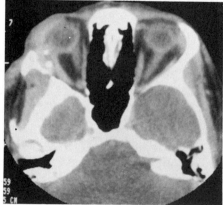

Figure 19–16. A child developed proptosis and diplopia. Findings were conjunctival vein injection and orbital bruit. *CT findings:* lateral orbit soft-tissue nonenhancing mass (A) with interspersed calcification (B). Angiogram showed orbital varix.

Orbital Trauma

This may result from a direct blow to the face or penetrating missile injuries. Soft-tissue facial injury and bone fractures usually accompany orbital injury. In patients with suspected orbital trauma, CT scan should include sections inferior to the orbitomeatal line to assess injury to the paranasal sinus. Coronal sections are also necessary to determine the integrity of the floor and roof of the orbits.[15] CT may identify the following abnormalities: (1) soft-tissue swelling, (2) orbital hematoma, (3) orbital air, (4) bone fracture and displacement, (5) entrapment of extraocular muscle in bone fracture, (6) foreign bodies, (7) absence of globe or lens and (8) clouding and fluid level in paranasal sinuses. Coronal CT is necessary to exclude the presence of blowout fracture of the orbital floor. Because of the thinness of the orbital bones, orbital fracture may not be identified with skull roentgenogram or conventional tomography. In orbital trauma, CT

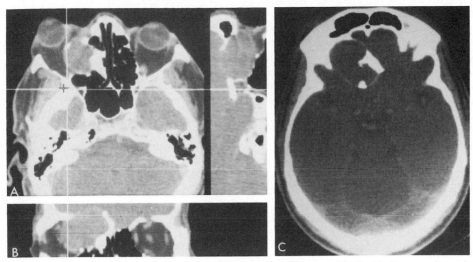

Figure 19–18. A man had multiple episodes of sinusitis and developed proptosis. Skull x-ray showed clouding of the maxillary sinus. *CT findings:* soft-tissue mass in sinus extending into orbit (*A,B*) and intracranially (*C*). *Operative finding:* mucocele.

is complementary to orbital roentgenogram because roentgenogram better defines bone fractures and CT shows accompanying soft-tissue abnormalities and delineates the full extent of injury.[16]

Orbital Infectious-Inflammatory Disorders

Postseptal Cellulitis. CT is the definitive diagnostic procedure to determine if an infectious process has entered the posterior orbit.[17] If this has occurred, surgical drainage is required because vision is threatened and intra-cranial extension is a potential complication. If cellulitis has not passed the orbital septum, conservative antibiotic therapy without drainage is indicated.

Orbital Abscesses. This may result from postseptal cellulitis or more commonly develops because of the presence of an orbital foreign body. CT shows a hyperdense orbital mass that has no characteristic morphology and does not usually enhance. This nonspecific pattern is quite different from CT findings in intracranial abscesses in which there is relatively specific ring-enhancing CT pattern.

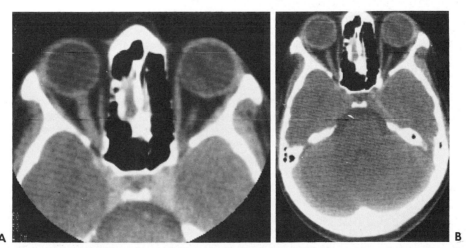

Figure 19–19. A woman developed visual blurring in the left eye. Findings were optic pallor, centrocecal scotoma and afferent pupillary defect. *CT findings:* markedly dilated optic nerve sheath (*A*). Following one week of corticosteroid treatment, visual acuity improved. *CT findings:* decrease in size of left optic nerve (*B*). *Clinical diagnosis:* optic neuritis.

Mucocele. The presence of mucoid material or pus within the paranasal sinus may lead to formation of pyomucocele. This may enlarge to cause orbital and sinus bone erosion. Skull roentgenogram shows clouding of sinuses usually accompanied by bone erosion. CT shows a hyperdense mass within the sinus. This may extend into the retroglobal region (Fig. 19–18). Coronal sections demonstrate the ventral-dorsal extent and assist in defining the presence of intracranial extension.[18]

Optic Neuritis. In most cases, CT shows no abnormalities; however, in rare instances optic nerve may appear enlarged (unilateral or bilateral). The enlargement is fusiform and uniform throughout its length (Fig. 19–19). Following treatment or during spontaneous remission, there may be reduction in nerve size.[19, 20]

REFERENCES

1. Jacobs L, Weisberg LA, Kinkel WR: Computed Tomography of the Orbit and Sella Turcica. Raven Press, New York, 1980, pp 27–67
2. Weinstein MA, Modic MT, Risius B: Visualization of the arteries, veins and nerves of the orbit by sector computed tomography. Radiology 138:83–87, 1981
3. Tadmor R, New PFJ: Computed tomography of the orbit with special emphasis on coronal sections. J Comput Assist Tomogr 2:24–44, 1978
4. Hilal SK, Trokel SL: CT of the orbit using thin sections. Semin Roentgenol 12:137, 1977
5. Brismar J, Davis KR, Dallow RL: Unilateral endocrine exophthalmos. Neuroradiology 12:21, 1976
6. Enzmann D, Marshall WH: CT in Graves' ophthalmopathy. Radiology 118:615, 1976
7. Enzmann DR, Donaldson SS, Kriss JP: Appearance of Graves' disease on orbital computed tomography. J Comput Assist Tomogr 3:815–819, 1979
8. Smigiel MR, McCarty CS: Exophthalmos. Mayo Clin Proceed 50:345, 1975
9. Jellinek EH: The orbital pseudotumor syndrome and its differentiation from endocrine exophthalmos. Brain 92:35, 1969
10. Nugent RA, Rootman J, Robertson WD: Acute orbital pseudotumors. Classification and CT features. Am. J Neuroradiol 2:431–436, 1981
11. Macpherson P: The radiology of orbital meningioma. Clin Radiol 30:105–110, 1979
12. Lloyd GAS: Primary orbital meningioma: a review of 41 patients investigated radiologically. Clin Radiol 33:181, 1982
13. Byrd SE, Harwood-Nash DC, Fitz CR: Computed tomography of intraorbital optic nerve gliomas in children. Radiology 129:73–78, 1978
14. Hesselink JR, Davis KR, Weber AL: Radiological evaluation of orbital metastases with emphasis on computed tomography. Radiology 137:363–366, 1980
15. Grove AS: Orbital trauma evaluation by computed tomography. Comput Tomogr 3:267–278, 1979
16. Zilkha A: Computed tomography of blow-out fracture of the medial orbital wall. Am J Neuroradiol 2:427–429, 1981
17. Zimmerman RA, Bilaniuk LT: CT of orbital infection and its cerebral complications. Am J Roentgenol 134:45–50, 1980
18. Hesselink JR, Weber AL, New PFJ: Evaluation of mucoceles of the paranasal sinuses with computed tomography. Radiology 133:397–400, 1979
19. Salvolini U, Cabanis AE, Rodallec A et al: Computed tomography of the optic nerve. J Comput Assist Tomogr 2:141–155, 1979
20. Forbes G: Computed tomography of the orbit. Radiol Clin North Am 20:37, 1982

Chapter 20

EVALUATION OF TREATMENT MODALITIES

CT is the most reliable diagnostic study to evaluate the results of therapy in many neurological disorders in which there are gross pathological changes of the brain structure. It is possible to assess the completeness of resolution of those pathological conditions that may not require specific treatment, such as cerebral infarct, intracerebral hematoma and multiple sclerosis; in these cases CT may obviate the need for such invasive diagnostic investigations as angiography and surgical biopsy. Other noninvasive diagnostic studies (EEG, isotope scan) may not accurately reflect improvement or worsening of the pathological processes and may not correlate with the clinical condition. For example, the size of EEG slow wave focal discharge may decrease as neoplasms increase in size, whereas slow wave focus caused by cerebral infarction may increase in size instead of decreasing several months later. Development of EEG spike discharge after surgery or radiotherapy may represent the effect of cortical gliotic scar or tumor recurrence. EEG findings may reflect summated and not individual pathological effects such as hemorrhage, edema, necrosis, neoplastic tissue, calcification and gliosis.

Isotope scan findings may be difficult to interpret in the early postoperative period or following head trauma. Superficial isotope uptake may result from craniotomy site, bone fracture or scalp lacerations; this uptake may persist for several months and may simulate subdural lesion.[1] Isotope scan may remain abnormal for 8 to 16 weeks following radiotherapy despite marked tumor shrinkage.[2] Because of these discrepancies in clinical and pathological features, angiography is sometimes required to assess adequacy of treatment, especially if clinical deterioration occurs. However, angiography may be less sensitive in the postoperative period. Angiographic findings usually define the presence of hydrocephalus, mass effect and vascular changes such as vasospasm. It is less reliable in defining the mechanism of mass effect, as in hematoma, edema and neoplasm.

Clinical condition is usually the most reliable indicator of adequacy of therapeutic modalities. If clinical improvement does not occur or deterioration develops following treatment, several possible mechanisms should be considered: (1) recurrence or progression of the initial pathological process, (2) complication of therapy (infection, hematoma), (3) occurrence of an unrelated neurological disorder and (4) systemic complication such as sepsis, dehydration and hypoxia. Before CT came into use, delineation of the underlying pathological process sometimes required angiography, air studies or surgical exploration.[3]

CORTICOSTEROIDS

Vasogenic edema is most prominent in white matter. It occurs with neoplasms, trauma, infectious-inflammatory disorders, intracranial hemorrhage and, less commonly, cerebral infarction. CT shows a hypodense lesion with irregular margination, frond-like projections and mass effect. Enhancement may occur in a linear or gyral pattern at the periphery of the lesion. This is the result of impairment of the blood-brain barrier caused by the effect of edema. Following treatment with corticosteroids, there may be marked decrease in edema and mass effect.[3, 4] There may also be a decrease in contrast enhancement caused by stabilization or repair of the lipid component of the endothelial cell membrane. In patients with cerebritis and abscess

339

treated with corticosteroids and antibiotics, CT following successful treatment shows an isodense region. In patients treated with antibiotics but without steroids, the lesions appeared hypodense following therapy. The significance of this difference in CT patterns—hypodense or isodense lesions resulting from the two treatment modalities—is unclear.

Corticosteroids decrease the thin peripheral enhancing rim that develops within the initial 14 days of intracerebral hematoma; however, the enhancing rim that develops in the third to fifth week is not modified by corticosteroids. In gliomas, the response of edema to corticosteroids is variable. Reduction in edema is most marked in glioblastoma multiforme and least in low-grade gliomas. In meningiomas there is usually minimal clinical improvement and minimal effect on edema volume following treatment with corticosteroids. Edema due to cerebral metastases is markedly decreased by

corticosteroids.[3] Following long-term and high-dosage corticosteroid treatment, CT may show the development of ventricular and subarachnoid space enlargement (Fig. 20–1). This CT evidence of cerebral atrophy may be reversible after reduction in dosage or discontinuation of medication. Two possible mechanisms for steroid-induced cerebral atrophy include: protein catabolism and decreased brain volume caused by cerebral dehydration.[5] This CT finding is most common in patients with neuropsychiatric manifestations of systemic lupus erythematosus (lupus cerebritis); however, it also occurs in patients without clinically apparent CNS disease who are treated with corticosteroids. There are usually neurobehavioral changes in patients who develop this cerebral atrophy caused by corticosteroids; however, some patients with these CT findings show no neurobehavioral abnormalities.

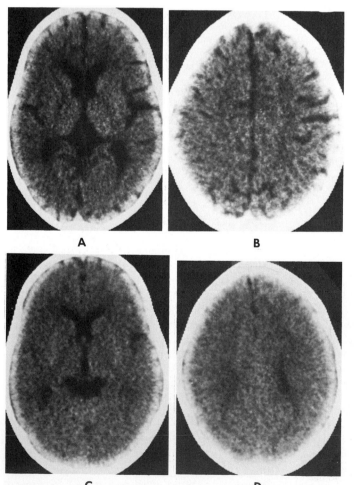

A　　　**B**

C　　　**D**

Figure 20–1. A child with rhabdomyosarcoma of the jaw received irradiation and chemotherapy including high-dose corticosteroids. *CT findings:* Ventricular (*A*) and subarachnoid space enlargement (*B*). Six months later she was receiving no medication. *CT findings:* decrease in ventricular (*C*) and subarachnoid space size (*D*).

SURGICAL CHANGES

Early Postoperative Period[6-8]

CT may be performed immediately post-operatively to determine baseline condition; however, this is rarely indicated unless the clinical condition warrants. This baseline study may be helpful in determining the mechanism of subsequent clinical deterioration that may result from hydrocephalus or mass effect. Mass effect is usually present in the early postoperative phase even if patients show good recovery. This mass effect may result from multiple factors such as edema, tissue necrosis, infarction and hematoma. Postoperative edema may persist for several weeks, and its presence does not necessarily correlate with clinical state. However, severe edema with mass effect and herniation is seen only in patients with poor clinical condition. Acute postsurgical extracerebral hematomas appear as hyperdense lenticular or semilunar lesions. Small residual amounts of blood seen under bone flap may have a similar density with little mass effect. This may be seen in the first seven days after surgery. The CT finding of a thin hyperdense epidural layer is not usually associated with marked mass effect. This blood resolves usually within 7 to 14 days.

Following surgery, air may be seen intracranially. This may be widely dispersed and usually spontaneously resolves (Fig. 20–2). Pneumocephalus is a common finding following surgery; however, a large focal collection may form and be under pressure. This tension pneumocephalus is most commonly seen in

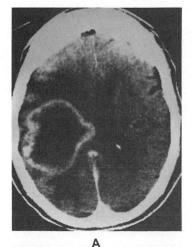

A

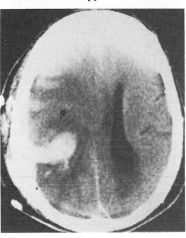

B

Figure 20–3. A 51-year-old man had right hemiparesis. *CT findings:* left temporal-parietal hypodense lesion with variable thickness ring enhancement (*A*). Following surgical removal of glioblastoma, he remained lethargic. *CT findings:* left hypodense neoplastic mass with intracerebral hematoma (*B*).

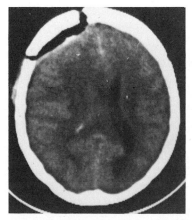

Figure 20–2. Following removal of convexity meningioma, this patient remained lethargic. *CT findings:* air is seen under the bone flap with ventricular distortion and displacement.

the frontal subdural spaces (Fig. 20–3). If clinical condition does not improve and CT shows subdural air with mass effect, surgical relief may be necessary.[9] Resolution of benign pneumocephalus (air not under pressure) may not be complete for four to five weeks.

Intracerebral blood is frequently seen in the immediate postoperative period (Fig. 20–4). This appears as a hyperdense region with surrounding edema. Blood may also be seen in cortical sulcal spaces. Certain surgical hemostatic materials such as Gelfoam, Surgicel and microfibrillar collagen may appear slightly hyperdense to simulate the presence of intracerebral blood; however, they are rarely applied in sufficient volume to result in mass

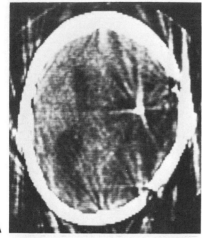

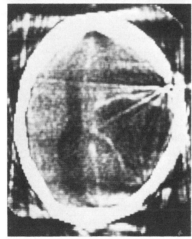

Figure 20–4. Following surgical resection on AVM, this woman remained obtunded with worsening of left hemiparesis. *CT findings:* right hemispheric hypodense lesion (*A*) with peripheral enhancing rim (*B*).

effect to appear as localized clot on CT. Surgicel consists of oxidized cellulose. It is applied as a thin open mesh to help form thin clot. Gelfoam is bovine collagen that has been soaked in thrombin. It is used to line craniotomy sites. It is resorbed within several weeks. Immediately following surgery, the CT finding of a slightly hyperdense component without mass effect at the surgical site may represent surgical material rather than intracerebral hematoma. However, in many cases these materials have been utilized and the postoperative site does not appear hyperdense; therefore, the finding of a hyperdense lesion at the operative site most probably represents hematoma. Hematoma resolution may be observed by serial CT.

Necrotic tissue at the postoperative site may appear hypodense, with a thin peripheral enhancing rim. Enhancement may result from surrounding vascular granulation tissue (Fig. 20–5). If this hypodense central region and peripheral enhancing rim develops within the initial postoperative week, it may not represent hematoma, abscess or residual tumor. This most probably represents necrotic tissue with impaired blood-brain barrier. Superficial dural enhancement underneath the craniotomy site may simulate subdural empyema or hematoma. There is no associated mass effect and there is normal position of the gray-white interface (Fig. 20–6). Residual neoplasm usually has an identical CT appearance to that seen on preoperative scan. Scan quality may be degraded by surgical hardware such as shunt tubes and metallic clips.

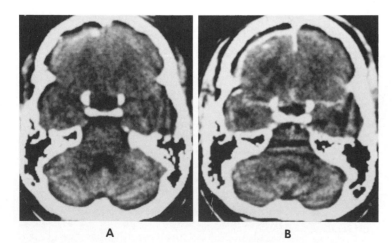

Figure 20–5. After surgical excision of suprasellar pituitary adenoma, this man developed fever, headache and skin pallor. He was hypotensive but had no new focal neurological deficit. CSF was normal. *CT findings:* left frontal air under frontal craniotomy site with hyperdense dura (*A*) that densely enhances (*B*). There is no mass effect. He clinically responded to increased dosage of corticosteroids.

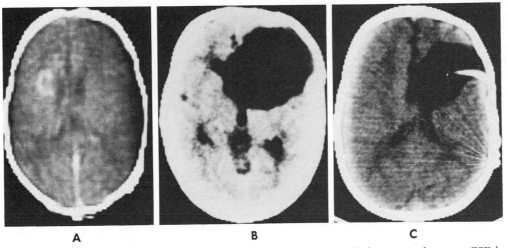

Figure 20–6. A 3-month-old child had neonatal meningitis and had multiple ventricular taps. CSF became normal; however, he developed right hemiparesis. CT showed left isodense periventricular ring-enhancing lesion (*A*). Following surgical excision of brain abscess, right hemiparesis worsened. *CT finding:* hypodense left (reader's right) hemispheric lesion (*B*). Porencephalic cyst was shunted. Six months later, hemiparesis worsened. CT showed hypodense cyst with shunt in cyst (*C*).

Following tumor resection, there is usually good correlation between the clinical condition of the patient and CT findings; however, there is poor correlation in 10 to 15 per cent of cases.[10, 11] In patients with improved clinical condition, CT usually shows decreased lesion size, mass effect and intensity of contrast enhancement, although the latter is not a consistent finding.[12] There may sometimes be an increase in edema caused by breakdown of the blood-barrier barrier. Following surgical treatment of brain abscess, CT may determine the completeness of surgical excision. CT may show a small superficial ring-enhancing lesion contiguous with the surgical site. This may represent the effect of luxury perfusion or granulation tissue rather than recurrent abscess.

Following surgical evacuation of epidural hematomas, CT usually appears normal if in these cases patients show good clinical recovery; however, substantial hemisphere edema may be seen, even in those with good clinical outcome. Immediately following surgical removal of subdural hematoma, mass effect may persist for several weeks, although extracerebral lesion is no longer present and clinical improvement occurs. In some patients with subdural hematoma, clinical improvement may not occur. This may be the result of underlying parenchymal lesions such as contusions and cerebral infarction; these are usually well visualized on postoperative CT studies.

Later Postoperative Period

Within two to three weeks following surgery, CT findings that represent edema, mass effect, air, necrosis and blood should have decreased but may not have resolved completely. At this time, the CT finding of a hypodense region with a peripheral enhancing rim may be difficult to interpret. The presence or absence of mass effect is an important associated finding. If the ring-enhancing lesion has minimal mass effect, possible mechanisms are vascular granulation tissue, reactive gliosis, resolving hematoma or infarction, and granuloma formation caused by surgical material. Ring enhancement due to these conditions usually resolves within six months.[13] After this time, the CT finding of a hypodense lesion with ring enhancement supports the diagnosis of a complicating procedure such as recurrent tumor or abscess (Fig. 20–7). Jeffries et al. have reported that the persistence of ring enhancement beyond six months is not caused by normal or spontaneously reversible postoperative changes.[8] However, CT findings resulting from reactive gliosis and granuloma formation may persist beyond that time. These may be followed by serial CT if patients are neurologically stable.[14, 15]

The CT findings that are believed to represent reactive gliosis may persist or spontaneously resolve;[16, 17] however, there is probably no resolution of the underlying pathological condition. This may appear as a

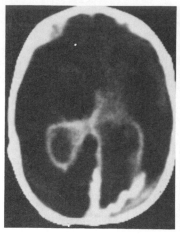 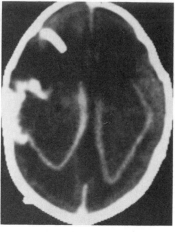

A   B

Figure 20–7. A child with meningomyelocele and hydrocephalus had ventriculoperitoneal shunts and developed CSF infection. CSF was purulent and culture grew gram-negative organisms. *CT findings:* marked ventricular dilation (*A*) with ependymal enhancement (*B*) with shunt tube in the left frontal horn.

ring enhancing lesion or it may show other patterns—hypodense nonenhancing or isodense nodular enhancing. We have seen CT patterns of gliosis that simulated neoplastic recurrence in patients who had had surgical and irradiation therapy as long as two decades previously. In patients who are clinically asymptomatic but in whom CT shows abnormal density and enhancing lesions, the possibility of reactive gliosis must be considered. A second course of irradiation should not be undertaken without surgical biopsy.

Following surgical removal of a parenchymal lesion, the operative site may appear hypodense. This may represent loss of brain mass and may be accompanied by ventricular and subarachnoid space enlargement. Porencephalic cysts appear as hypodense lesions that may subsequently increase in size. Communication of cysts with ventricles is best assessed by metrizamide, which may be injected directly into the cyst. Hydrocephalus that develops postoperatively is more likely caused by an underlying pathological process rather than surgical effect.

Shunting Procedures

Shunting for hydrocephalus may utilize silver-impregnated polyethylene tubing. The catheter is radiopaque and may be visualized with skull roentgenogram or CT. The catheter causes only slight surrounding tissue reaction. Following insertion of an intraventricular shunt catheter through a frontal or parietal-occipital burr hole, there is usually a rapid decrease in ventricular size. Reduction in ventricular size is frequently asymmetrical; it is more marked in the ventricle containing the

shunt catheter. Frontal horns may be decreased to a greater extent than are atrial and occipital regions. As ventricles decrease in size, cisterns and sulcal spaces may increase in size. If extracerebral CSF-filled cerebral convexity spaces are enlarged after shunting, this implies loss of normal brain parenchyma. Shunt catheters in the frontal horn may extend to the contralateral side if the septum pellucidum is abnormal—perforated, absent or fenestrated.[18]

Complications of shunt insertion include hemorrhage along the shunt tract. Intraventricular blood accumulation may result from damage to the highly vascularized choroid plexus by the shunt catheter. Blood is frequently seen in the dependent portion of the occipital horns; this usually resolves within several days. Less commonly, intracerebral hematoma develop—this is probably because of perforation of brain parenchyma by the catheter. Catheters may perforate the septum pellucidum and extend into the contralateral frontal horn. Catheter tips may become extraventricular if ventricles collapse rapidly to slit-like dimensions. The proximal portion of the shunt catheter may be obstructed by choroid plexus or brain parenchyma, especially if ventricles are slit-like or if the catheter is improperly positioned. Subdural hematoma may develop following shunting for the following reasons: (1) ventricular decompression is too rapid, (2) ventricular decompression is too complete and (3) decompression is associated with reduced cortical mantle.

Infection may complicate shunt systems. There may be cerebral abscess contiguous with shunt catheter. If CSF becomes infected, ependymitis and ventriculitis may develop

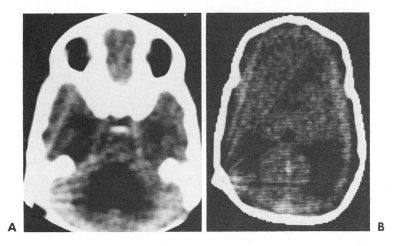

Figure 20–8. A child with congenital hydrocephalus had multiple shunt procedures. She was lethargic with headache and vomiting. *CT findings:* marked dilatation of the fourth ventricle (*A*) with relatively small size (*B*) of the lateral and third ventricle. *Diagnosis:* entrapped fourth ventricle.

(Fig. 20–8). CT shows the abnormalities of dense ependymal enhancement, marked asymmetrical ventricular enlargement, multiple hypodense intraventricular and periventricular cysts, and separation or entrapment of the fourth ventricle (Fig. 20–9) or temporal horns caused by adhesions along CSF pathways. Because portions of the ventricles may be separated or isolated from the remainder of CSF pathways, multiple shunt catheters may be required to obtain ventricular decompression.[19]

If a shunt malfunctions, symptoms of hydrocephalus recur. In pediatric patients, clinical

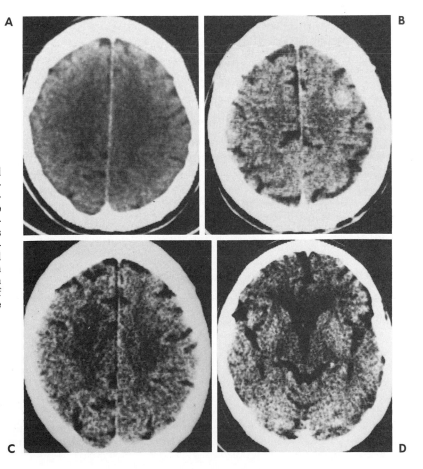

Figure 20–9. This 50-year-old man with bronchogenic carcinoma had dizziness and headache. EEG and isotope scan were negative. *CT findings:* no abnormality is seen (*A*). Four weeks later he had left focal motor seizure. *CT findings:* right parietal hyperdense enhancing lesion (*B*). Following head irradiation there is complete resolution of the lesion (*C*) with CSF space enlargement (*D*).

features include vomiting, headache, lethargy, altered consciousness, suture separation, and bulging fontanelles. With shunt failure, CT may show ventricular dilatation with bulbous contour of frontal horns, temporal horn enlargement and periventricular hypodensities. In other patients who develop symptoms of shunt failure, CT shows small-sized ventricles and nonvisualization of cisternal and cortical subarachnoid spaces (slit ventricle syndrome). This may result from ependymal fibrosis with intraventricular gliosis. This causes ventricles to appear small; however, intraventricular pressure is high. Because ventricles may appear equally small in size whether or not the child is symptomatic, CT does not provide evidence of shunt malfunction unless metrizamide or radionuclide ventriculography is performed through the shunt system to determine CSF flow.[20] Shunt malfunction caused by slit ventricles may be intermittent and produce intermittent symptoms. Therefore, these shunt studies may not be of value in determining shunt patency.

Stereotactic Surgery

CT-guided stereotactic surgery may be used to provide accurate target coordinates. Because the usual stereotactic frame contains hardware that creates unacceptable artifact in CT, it has been modified and constructed with low atomic number materials. The patient and frame are imaged together by the CT system and the target is identified. The CT system must have a computer software program that converts CT scan coordinates to stereotactic frame coordinates. The frame is adjusted and the probe is then advanced. CT may be repeated to confirm the appropriate position of the probe prior to biopsy or aspirations of the lesion. The actual operation may be done in the CT scan suite. This technique is suited for tumor biopsy, cyst aspiration and abscess drainage. This technique is especially suited for deep-seated lesions (ganglionic, thalamic, pineal). Following the surgical procedure, CT may be repeated to assess results and potential complications.[21]

Radiation Therapy (RT)

METASTASES

Neoplastic cells reach the brain by hematogenous dissemination or direct contiguous extension. The smallest tumor nodules de-

tected by high resolution CT are 3 to 6 mm in size; however, some larger lesions are not always detected (Fig. 20–10). Small metastases usually appear as isodense homogeneously enhancing lesions. There is no mass effect or surrounding edema. These smallest lesions contain approximately 10^6 to 10^7 tumor cells. Cell kinetic studies indicate that the initial tumor nidus grows to this just-detectable size in two months. As metastatic neoplasm exceeds 1 cm, surrounding vasogenic edema and central necrotic component are commonly seen.[22] Following irradiation, radioresponsive tumors show a decrease in size and enhancement, and this is usually maximal by the time of completion of RT. Some studies have reported that resolution of lesion size was incomplete, that is, there was one half shrinkage, by completion of RT; however, there was continued resolution as long as four months later as delineated by serial CT studies. Differences in temporal sequence of tumor disappearance may be related to variables of RT technique such as dosages, build-up phase and time interval. Those patients with metastatic intracranial tumors who showed complete resolution of the lesion(s) had better clinical response and longer time interval before recurrent than those in whom CT showed less striking changes. In one study, no patient who had complete disappearance of neoplasm as manifested by CT findings subsequently died of recurrent CNS metastatic disease.[23] In patients who have undergone surgery or irradiation for metastatic neoplasm, CT should be performed when the patient has been taken off corticosteroids because this drug reduces enhancement pattern and edema to mask the presence of a residual neoplasm.[23]

PRIMARY BRAIN NEOPLASMS

RT is chiefly employed for gliomas and pituitary adenomas; however, it has been utilized for other tumors including medulloblastoma, neuroblastoma, germ cell tumors, neuroectodermal tumors and even some recurrent meningiomas. Prior to initiation of RT, it is usually mandatory to have biopsy confirmation of the diagnosis of malignant glioma except if biopsy represents a potential risk to the patient (brain stem neoplasm). Biopsy confirmation is crucial because CT and angiographic features for neoplasms are not always specific. There is conflicting evidence concerning correlation of CT features with radioresponsive-

Figure 20–10. A 60-year-old man with bronchogenic carcinoma had nonspecific headache and dizziness. CT was normal (*A*). Eight months after he received prophylactic brain irradiation, he developed confusional episodes. *CT findings:* marked ventricular and subarachnoid space enlargement with symmetrical white matter hypodensities (*B*).

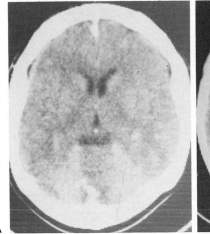

A

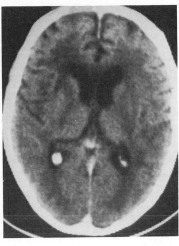

B

ness. Gliomas with these findings decrease in size most dramatically following RT: (1) isodense nodular enhancing lesion and (2) hypodense lesion with complex ring enhancement. If the lesion showed hypodense nonenhancing lesion or dense calcification, CT showed less change following RT. Recurrence was not correlated with specific CT pattern.

Irradiation Effects

Occurrence of untoward effects of brain irradiation may be according to three patterns. These are: (1) acute reactions occurring during initial RT phase, (2) early delayed reactions occurring several months after RT is completed and (3) late delayed reactions developing several months to many years later.[24] Following initiation of RT, there may be increased edema and necrosis; this may result in intracranial hypertension causing progressive mass effect and clinical deterioration. CT shows increased edema and mass effect, and in some cases there is CT evidence of cerebral herniation. This complication may be treated by corticosteroids. In patients with brain metastases who receive high-dosage corticosteroids prior to irradiation, CT does not subsequently show an increase in peritumoral edema unless a complicating pathological process such as hemorrhage develops. Enlargement of pituitary adenomas may develop during the initial stage of RT. Surgical intervention may be necessary if visual function significantly worsens and does not respond to corticosteroids.

Early delayed irradiation reactions most commonly involve the spinal cord but may involve the brain. Symptoms include tingling, paresthesias and electrical shock radiating down the back, especially when precipitated by neck flexion (Lhermitte's sign). This radiation myelopathy is usually transient and rapidly clears. It is caused by demyelination. There is also a cerebral syndrome that is caused by similar mechanism. It is characterized by transient worsening of neurological symptoms. This occurs 6 to 20 weeks after RT. Symptoms resolve in four to six weeks. If clinical worsening was caused by tumor growth, it would be expected that progressive deterioration would occur rather than spontaneous clinical improvement. The natural history of this radiation-induced disorder may be complicated by neoplastic recurrence.

Corticosteroids may be associated with good clinical response, although early delayed reaction usually spontaneously resolves. Because of the self-limited nature of the condition, pathological studies are limited. This early delayed reaction is believed due to radiation-induced demyelination. CT may show hypodense regions scattered throughout the cerebral hemispheric white matter (Fig. 20–11). This is sometimes associated with diffuse enhancement and mass effect. These findings are widespread and usually reversible within several months. This pattern is distinct from rapid tumor recurrence (focal lesion, vasogenic edema, dense enhancement).

Late delayed reactions to irradiation may be parenchymal tissue necrosis or vasculopathy involving small and medium-sized blood vessels. Radiation necrosis may follow irradiation therapy to the extracranial head region (skin, nasopharynx) or to the brain for intracranial tumor, but it is quite unusual to develop in

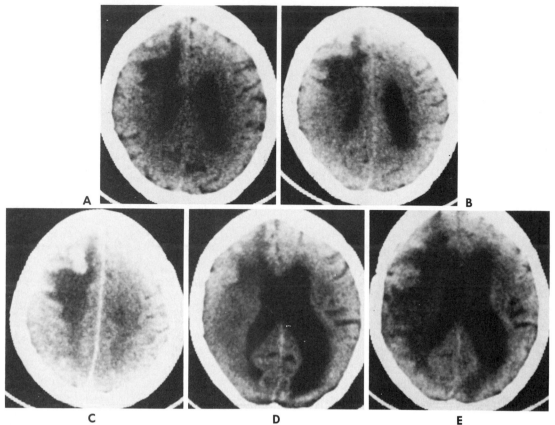

Figure 20–11. A 52-year-old woman had radical mastectomy and one year later suddenly developed right hemiparesis. EEG and isotope scan were negative. *CT findings:* left frontal white matter hypodense nonenhancing lesion with slight mass effect (*A*). She received irradiation for presumed metastasis without surgical biopsy. Three months later, she developed hemiplegia. *CT findings:* left frontal irregularly marginated hypodense lesion (*B*) with dense nodular enhancement (*C*). Angiogram showed avascular mass. Following surgical excision of necrotic lesion, CT showed a hypodense lesion with slight increase in mass effect (*D*). Two months later, she was demented and bedridden. *CT findings:* enlarged hypodense lesion with mass effect (*E*).

patients without intracranial disease. Clinical and neurodiagnostic evidence of radiation necrosis may develop as early as four months or as late as four years following RT.[24, 25] Clinical features of radiation necrosis may simulate tumor recurrence. Isotope scan may show abnormal uptake; however, this may be caused by other lesions (postsurgical changes, recurrent tumor, reactive gliosis, abscess or granuloma formation, diffuse white matter damage). Angiography shows radionecrotic masses as avascular masses. Angiographic evidence of tumor stain or neovascularity is consistent with tumor recurrence. The pathological findings in radiation necrosis are more prominent in white than gray matter (Fig. 20–12). White matter is edematous with necrotic, cystic and multifocal demyelinated components.

Mikhael correlated CT findings with total and fractional doses and duration of treatment in patients with radiation necrosis. Patients who have received a total dose of 5000 to 5500 rads in 180- to 200-rad fractional doses over 36 to 42 days may develop RT-related complications. CT may show the following abnormalities: (1) diffuse hypodense white matter irregularly marginated lesions, (2) minimal mass effect and (3) lack of enhancement (Fig. 20–13). Areas of the brain that show evidence of radiation necrosis have received at least 4500 rads. In patients who have received a total dose of 6000 to 7000 rads in 30 to 35 fractions administered over 46 to 72 days, CT findings of radiation necrosis were more varied. These findings included: (1) hypodense irregularly marginated lesion with mass effect, some of these showing enhancement (Fig. 20–14), (2) diffuse (bilateral white matter lesion (hypodense, isodense or hypodense) with mass effect and (3) varied pattern of contrast en-

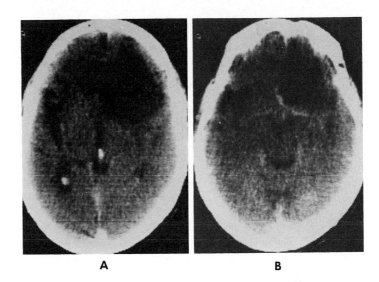

Figure 20–12. Two years following surgical excision and irradiation of craniopharyngioma, this patient developed dementia and urinary incontinence. *CT findings:* hypodense right frontal (A) and anterior suprasellar (B) nonenhancing lesion with mass effect. *Necropsy finding:* radionecrosis of frontal lobe.

hancement. These lesions occur in brain regions that have received at least 6000 rads. CT findings of radiation necrosis cannot always be differentiated from recurrent tumor, although these findings should be correlated with radiation doses. In many cases, however, surgical biopsy may be required.[25, 26]

Radiation-induced vasculopathy may involve small and medium-sized intracranial blood vessels. This results in ischemia and infarction. Blood vessel lumen is narrowed because of fibrinoid necrosis and endothelial hyperplasia. Angiography shows irregular narrowing of intracranial vessels. This is consistent with vasculitis. Isotope scan may show localized uptake. CT findings may be consistent with infarction. These vascular changes are not believed to be a mechanism for delayed radiation necrosis.

Pneumographic studies have demonstrated cerebral atrophy following RT. Wilson and colleagues have reported symmetrical lateral ventricular enlargement that developed within three to five months in one half of patients who received 3000 to 6000 rads of cranial irradiation.[27] Robertson demonstrated posterior fossa atrophy in patients who had RT for brain stem gliomas.[28] These effects are believed caused by oligodendrocyte damage with white matter demyelination. Brain neoplasm

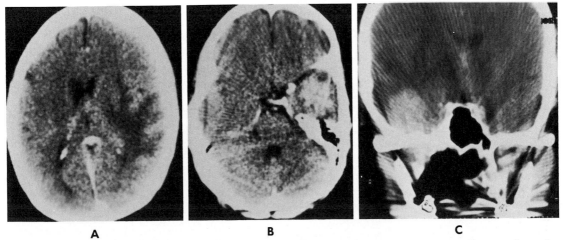

Figure 20–13. A 57-year-old man had head and face irradiation for basal cell carcinoma. One year later, he developed seizures. EEG showed right temporal delta focus; angiogram showed right temporal avascular mass. *CT findings:* irregularly marginated hypodense right temporal lesion (A) with dense nodular enhancement (B) seen on coronal (reader's left) projections (C). *Operative finding:* radionecrosis.

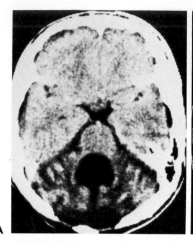
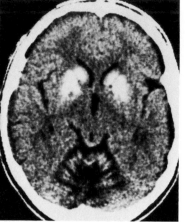

Figure 20–14. Ten years following surgical biopsy and irradiation of brain stem glioma, clinical condition of this patient was stable. *CT findings:* posterior fossa surgical defect with enlarged fourth ventricle and basal cisterns (*A*) with bilateral basal ganglionic calcification (*B*).

shrinkage may contribute to decreased brain mass, but this should not contribute to symmetrical ventriculomegaly. Intracranial calcification has been detected following RT. In some cases, tumor calcification is denser and more extensive after RT. Calcification that develops in patients who receive methotrexate and low-dose RT is believed caused by multiplicative synergistic toxicity.

ANTINEOPLASTIC DRUG THERAPY

Methotrexate

Children who have survived acute leukemia have received intrathecal methotrexate and cranial RT. Neurological disorders have developed in long-term survivors; however, it is not known if these are caused by the leukemia or therapy. These are impaired intellectual function, necrotizing leukoencephalopathy and microangiopathy with dystrophic calcification. Necrotizing leukoencephalopathy develops several months following treatment. Symptoms include mental deterioration that may progress to coma, seizures and motor weakness. CSF shows elevated protein and pleocytosis but negative cultures. EEG shows marked symmetrical slowing. CT shows symmetrical periventricular white matter hypodense lesions without mass effect or enhancement. These lesions may subsequently calcify. Cerebral cortex and basal ganglia are spared. This disorder is most common in patients who have received both cranial RT and methotrexate.

Mineralizing microangiopathy with dystrophic calcification involves gray matter (cerebral cortex, putamen, cerebellar hemispheres). Pathological studies have shown mineralized calcified material occluding small intracranial blood vessels. Intracranial calcification occurs in necrotic gray matter after methotrexate and cranial RT in 25 to 30 percent of patients. These patients may be neurologically normal.[29, 30]

Bromocriptine

Shrinkage of prolactin-secreting pituitary tumors with bromocriptine has been documented with serial CT. Reduction in size may occur immediately (within one month) or be delayed (two to six months). This occurs in both macroadenoma and microadenoma. Medical treatment should be continued for six months before resorting to surgery if the clinical condition, as indicated by visual function and pituitary function, remains stable. Decrease in tumor size correlates with reduction in serum prolactin level. It is clear that CT changes and reduced prolactin levels are not permanent after bromocriptine is discontinued.[31, 32] It is important to be aware that as these pituitary neoplasms are treated with bromocriptine, degenerative change in the form of hemorrhage and necrosis may develop. This may lead to increased tumor size and clinical deterioration.

REFERENCES

1. Waxman AD, Siemsen JK, Wolfstein RS: Evaluation of postcraniotomy patients by radionuclide scan. J Neurosurg 43:471, 1975
2. Handel SF, Malcolm MR, Wilson CB: Scintophoto-

graphic evaluation of response of brain neoplasms to systemic chemotherapy. J Nucl Med 12:292, 1971

3. Hatam A, Yu ZY, Bergstrom M: Effects of dexamethasone on peritumoral brain edema: evaluation by CT. J Comput Assist Tomogr 6:586, 1982

4. Laster DW, Moody DM, Ball MR: Resolving intracerebral hematoma; alteration of the ring sign with steroids. Am J Roentgenol 130:935, 1978

5. Bentson J, Reza M, Winter J: Steroids and apparent cerebral atrophy on computed tomography scans. J Comput Assist Tomogr 2:16, 1978

6. Krishna Rao CV, Kishore PRS, Bartlett J: Computed tomography in the postoperative patient. Neuroradiology 19:257, 1980

7. Lin JP, Pay N, Naidich TP: CT in the postoperative care of neurosurgical patients. Neuroradiology 12:185, 1977

8. Jeffries BF, Kishore PRS, Singh KS: Postoperative computed tomographic changes in the brain. Radiology 135:751, 1980

9. Monajati A, Cotanch WW: Subdural tension pneumocephalus following surgery. J Comput Assist Tomogr 6:902, 1982

10. Marks JE, Gado M: Serial CT of primary brain tumors following surgery, irradiation and chemotherapy. Radiology 121:85, 1977

11. Norman D, Enzmann DR, Levin V: CT in the evaluation of malignant glioma before and after therapy. Radiology 121:85, 1977

12. Pay NT, Carella RJ, Lin JR: The usefulness of CT during and after radiation therapy in patients with brain tumors. Radiology 121:79, 1976

13. Grand W, Kinkel WR, Glasauer FE: Ring formation on computerized tomography in the postoperative patient. Neurosurgery 2:107, 1978

14. Epstein AJ, Russell EJ, Berlin L: Suture granuloma: an unusual cause of an enhancing ring lesion in the postoperative brain. J Comput Assist Tomogr 6:815, 1982

15. Feely MP, Dempsey PJ: Assessment of postoperative course of excised brain abscess by CT. Neurosurgery 5:49, 1979

16. Weisberg LA: CT findings in intracranial gliosis. Neuroradiology 21:253, 1981

17. Weisberg LA: Non-neoplastic gliotic cerebellar cyst. Neuroradiology 24:53, 1982

18. Naidich TP, Schott LH, Baron RL: CT in evaluation of hydrocephalus. Radiol Clin North Am 20:143, 1982

19. Zimmerman RA, Bilaniuk LT, Gallo E: CT of the trapped fourth ventricle. Am J Roentgenol 130:503, 1978

20. Faria MA, O'Brien MS, Tindall CT: Technique for evaluation of ventricular shunts using Amipaque and computerized tomography. J Neurosurg 53:92, 1980

21. Lundsford LD, Rosebaum AE, Perry J: Stereotactic surgery using the therapeutic CT scanner. Surg Neurol 18:116, 1982

22. Takakura K, Sano K, Hojo S: Metastatic tumors of the central nervous system. Igaku-Shoin, Tokyo, 1981, p 1939

23. Brown SD, Zawadzki J, Eifel P: CT of irradiated solid tumor metastases to the brain. Neuroradiology 23:127, 1982

24. Deck MDF: Imaging techniques in the diagnosis of radiation damage to the central nervous system. In Radiation Damage to the Nervous System. HA Gilbert, AR Kagan (eds). Raven Press, New York, 1980, pp 107–127

25. Mikhael MA: Radiation necrosis of the brain: correlation between CT, pathology and dose distribution. J Comput Assist Tomogr 2:71, 1978

26. Mikhael MA: Radiation necrosis of the brain: correlation between patterns on computed tomography and doses of radiation. J Comput Assist Tomogr 3:241, 1979

27. Wilson GH, Byfield J, Hanafee WN: Atrophy following radiation therapy for CNS neoplasms. Acta Radiol (Therap) 11:361, 1972

28. Robertson EG: Pneumoencephalography. Charles C Thomas, Springfield, 1967, p 377

29. Bjorgen JE, Gold LHA: CT appearance of methotrexate induced necrotizing leukoencephalopathy. Radiology 122:377, 1977

30. Bleyer WA, Griffin TW: White matter necrosis, mineralizing microangiopathy and intellectual abilities in survivors of childhood leukemia: associations with CNS irradiation and methotrexate therapy. In Radiation Damage to the Nervous System. HA Gilbert, AR Kagan (eds). Raven Press, New York, 1980, pp 155–174

31. Bonneville JF, Poulignot D, Cattin F: Computed tomographic demonstration of the effects of bromocriptine on pituitary microadenoma size. Radiology 143:451, 1982

32. Scotti G, Scialfa G, Pieralli S: Macroprolactinomas: CT evaluation of reduction of tumor size after medical treatment. Neuroradiology 23:123, 1982